DRUG FATE
AND METABOLISM

DRUG FATE AND METABOLISM
Methods and Techniques

VOLUME 2

Edited by

EDWARD R. GARRETT

*The Beehive, College of Pharmacy
University of Florida
Gainesville, Florida*

JEAN L. HIRTZ

*Ciba-Geigy Biopharmaceutical
Research Center
Rueil-Malmaison, France*

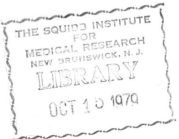
MARCEL DEKKER, INC.   New York and Basel

LIBRARY OF CONGRESS CATALOGING IN PUBLICATION DATA (Revised)

Main entry under title:

Drug fate and metabolism.

    Includes bibliographies and indexes.
    1. Drugs—Analysis. 2. Drug metabolism.
3. Pharmacokinetics. I. Garrett, Edward R. II. Hirtz,
Jean L. [DNLM: 1. Drugs—Metabolism. QV38 D792]
RS189. D78   615'. 7   76-28081
ISBN: 0-8247-6603-2

MARCEL DEKKER, INC.
270 Madison Avenue, New York, New York 10016

Current printing (last digit):
10 9 8 7 6 5 4 3 2 1

PRINTED IN THE UNITED STATES OF AMERICA

Historically, the major emphasis in drug development was on the isolation and synthesis of active principles and the evaluation of their safety and efficacy in animals and man. The fate of drugs in the body, which includes their absorption, distribution, metabolism, and elimination, was not emphasized. Systematic studies on the fate of drugs in the body have been conducted only within the last several decades.

Such studies were inhibited by the inadequacies of analytical techniques and methods to isolate, identify, and assay the drugs and their metabolites in the biological tissues and fluids of the organism. Drug metabolism studies were performed as long as a century ago on quinine (1869), salicylic acid (1877), and morphine (1883) with the simple techniques then available. However, such studies were infrequently done and in limited depth until B. B. Brodie elaborated a general method for the discriminatory extraction of drugs and metabolites from biological fluids during World War II in connection with the United States' antimalarial screening program. At about the same time, L. C. Craig developed countercurrent distribution procedures for separation and identification purposes. By modern standards, methods of quantification then available, which included colorimetry, fluorometry, and ultraviolet absorption spectroscopy, were insensitive and in the microgram per milliliter range.

Pharmacokinetics, the study of the time course of a drug's absorption, distribution, metabolism, and elimination, is another aspect in the fate of drugs and was of even later vintage. Its maturation also depended on the development of sensitive and reliable assays in biological fluids. Probably the first publication in this field of adequate sophistication was on ethanol in 1922. The basic principles of pharmacokinetics were elaborated by Torsten Teorell of Uppsala in 1937, and the first book on the subject was published by F. H. Dost of Berlin, later of Giessen, in 1953. However, this field did not truly flower until the 1960s, and its initial blossoming was observed at the first international conference on the subject in 1962 held under the initiative of Ekkehard Krueger-Thiemer at Borstel Forsch- ungsinstitut in Germany.

The burgeoning of these studies on drug fate in the organism was ferti- lized by the development of radiometric techniques when radiolabeled drugs became available. Gas-liquid chromatography, now the most widely used method, provided a simple and inexpensive technique to separate and quantify drugs and their metabolites. Sensitive detectors were developed to provide picogram monitoring of nonlabeled materials. Other analytical and separative methods of high sensitivity and precision became common- place in the laboratory. Instrumentation became available and less expensive for detection (NMR, spectrofluorimetry, infrared, gas and mass spectrometry, immunoassay) and for separation (thin-layer and high pressure liquid chromatography, etc.).

Today, it can be stated that the sensitivity of analytical detection no longer limits investigation into the fate of drugs. Separation and purification still is a rate-determining factor in assay development and demands a multidisciplined expert in biological, physical, organic, and analytical chemistry.

Similarly, the theoretical bases of pharmacokinetics and the technology of its applications have been expanded and refined within the last two decades. The generalized use of computers has permitted quantification of the models used to describe the totality of processes contributing to the time course of the drug in the body and to relate this time course to that of observed pharmacodynamics and pharmacological and toxicological action. The foundations of a modern pharmacology have been laid down, upon which structure personalized dosage regimens can be predicted for individualized optimum treatment with minimum toxicities; it is upon these premises that action and toxicities in one species can be predicted from studies performed on another.

The insights gained into the mechanisms of drug action provide clues to molecular modification that can best embody the active principal of action. Metabolic engineering can be construed as that practice which modifies the design of the molecule to take advantage of extant metabolic pathways to prolong or shorten the time of drug presence in the body. The clinical awareness that the rate and extent of drug release from a dosage form can perturb the availability and delivery of therapeutic agents has led to the necessity of establishing standards for bioequivalences of formulations. Pharmacokinetics now serves as a basis for these biopharmaceutical necessities.

It is therefore not suprising that the study of drug absorption, distribution, metabolism, and excretion constitutes a large part of the modern research for new and more efficient therapeutic agents. Governmental regulatory agencies in various countries now require precise data on the fate of new drugs and their formulations in animals and man and are increasingly insistent on stricter compliance.

Although there are several books dealing separately with drug metabolism, drug disposition, pharmacokinetics, and the like, a proper compendium has been lacking which encompasses the various fields and provides a delineation and appropriate critique of the useful methods and techniques that can be applied in them.

One of the editors (JLH) published (1968) a book on the analytical techniques (Les Méthodes Analytiques dans les Recherches sur le Métabolisme des Médicaments, Masson, Paris) which was later translated by editor ERG into English (Analytical Metabolic Chemistry of Drugs, Marcel Dekker, New York, 1971). The reception of this book was gratifying and prompted us to bring out the present more comprehensive and modernized series of volumes which includes other methods and techniques in the study of drug fate, not only analytical procedures. Since this ambitious goal exceeded the expertise of only one or a few authors, a multi-author series was projected. Experts were chosen who were highly respected in their fields. We reserved the right, and exercised it, to edit and revise to maintain a reasonable level of homogeneity in conformance with the objectives of the series. We hope we have succeeded.

The intent of these volumes is to review all the techniques, physical, chemical, biological, medical, and mathematical, which can be applied to the study of drug fate in the organism. It is addressed primarily to the research scientist and is devoted to methods, with only the minimal theory given for perspective, appreciation, and proper evaluation of results. The intent was not to compete with the many fine theoretical texts available, but to provide a broad spectrum of information that can be readily utilized by the research worker.

The practical use of these methods is explored fully. The limitations are explained. Necessary precautions and sources of error are delineated. Examples are given of applications in the study of the fate of drugs. When possible, each chapter includes tables that condense the appropriate literature on the particular topic. Each chapter has a selected, adequate, but not exhaustive, bibliography. For a more complete bibliographic survey, the reader is referred to the series edited by editor JLH (The Fate of Drugs in the Organism: A Bibliographic Survey, Marcel Dekker, New York: Vol. 1, 1974; Vol. 2, 1975; Vol. 3, 1976; Vol. 4, 1977).

It was deemed proper to include chapters on methods that would not be modern methods of choice but are of historical importance in evaluating the significance and limitations of the earlier studies in these fields. Whenever possible, a critique is provided, the future development is predicted, and the utility of a considered technique is evaluated.

It is our sincere hope that these endeavors of our dedicated authors will serve the desired purpose.

Edward R. Garrett   Jean L. Hirtz
Graduate Research Professor   Director, Ciba-Geigy
The Beehive, College of Pharmacy   Biopharmaceutical Research Center
Box J-4, University of Florida   B. P. 308
Gainesville, Florida 32610   92506 Rueil-Malmaison Cedex
U.S.A.   France

CONTENTS

MARVIN A. BROOKS
Department of Biochemistry and Drug Metabolism, Hoffmann-La Roche, Inc., Nutley, New Jersey

J. ARTHUR F. de SILVA
Department of Biochemistry and Drug Metabolism, Hoffmann-La Roche, Inc., Nutley, New Jersey

JOSEPH HAIMOVICH
Department of Chemical Immunology, The Weizmann Institute of Science, Rehovot, Israel

PETER JENNER
University Department of Neurology, The Institute of Psychiatry and King's College Hospital Medical School, London, England

DATTA V. NAIK
Department of Chemistry, Manhattanville College, Purchase, New York

STEPHEN G. SCHULMAN
Department of Pharmaceutical Chemistry, College of Pharmacy, University of Florida, Gainesville, Florida

MICHAEL SELA*
Department of Chemical Immunology, The Weizmann Institute of Science, Rehovot, Israel

---

*Established Investigator of The Chief Scientist's Bureau, Ministry of Health.

BERNARD TESTA
School of Pharmacy, University of Lausanne, Lausanne, Switzerland

JELKA TOMAŠIĆ*
Section on Carbohydrates, Laboratory of Chemistry, NIAMDD, National
Institutes of Health, Bethesda, Maryland

W. J. A. VANDENHEUVEL
Department of Animal Drug Metabolism and Radiochemistry, Merck Sharp
& Dohme Research Laboratories, Rahway, New Jersey

A. G. ZACCHEI
Department of Drug Metabolism, Merck Sharp & Dohme Research
Laboratories, West Point, Pennsylvania

---

*Present address: Tracer Laboratory, Rudjer Bošković Institute, Zagreb,
Yugoslavia.

CONTENTS OF VOLUME 1

(Other volumes in preparation)

DRUG FATE
AND METABOLISM

Chapter 1

VOLTAMMETRIC METHODS

J. Arthur F. de Silva and Marvin A. Brooks

Department of Biochemistry and Drug Metabolism
Hoffmann—La Roche, Inc.
Nutley, New Jersey

I. INTRODUCTION

The well-documented [1-7] electroanalytical methods for the assay of bulk chemicals, intermediates, and dosage forms are often methods of choice since their relative simplicity and rapidity facilitate the large number of analyses involved in quality assurance studies. The electroanalytical procedures of potentiometry, coulometry (constant current and potential), and voltammetry (polarography and amperometry) typically employed are applicable to the analysis of raw materials and finished products with usual required sensitivities of 2 to 5 $\mu g/ml$ (10^{-5} M).

The assays of drugs in biological fluids, however, require specific assays with sensitivities in the submicrogram range and are frequently performed with spectrophotometric or chromatographic methods and, more recently, by radioimmunoassay (RIA) rather than by electrochemical methods. Examples of early electrochemical methods used to measure drugs directly in biological fluids are the direct current polarographic assays of 2-ethyl-4-thioureidopyridine [8] and 1,4-benzodiazepines [9,10]. These assays were relatively insensitive (detection limits of >10 μg per ml biological fluid) and were inherently nonspecific in that compounds of similar structure such as metabolites and endogenous biological materials could interfere.

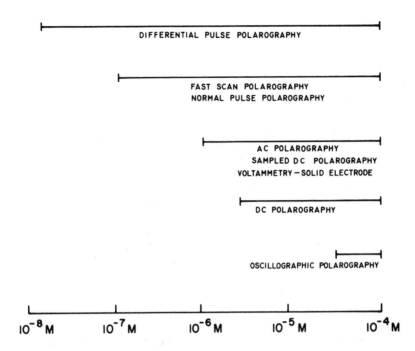

FIG. 1. Range of practical usefulness of voltammetric techniques.

However, recent advances in instrumentation have resulted in newer forms of polarography, capable of greater sensitivity (see Fig. 1) and specificity. Voltammetric methods can now routinely assay drugs with specificity in biological fluids at concentrations as low as 10 ng/ml [11]. The low electroactive background signal from the biological specimen relative to that of the species to be analyzed facilitates analyses on simple extracts, protein-free filtrates, diluted specimens (e.g., urine), or eluted thin-layer chromatography (TLC) separated extracts.

The purpose of this chapter is to review the basic theory involved in voltammetric methods, especially the newer polarographic methods used for drug analysis in biological samples. Specific attention will be given to the compounds and derivatives which can be assayed and the preparation of the sample for analysis. Section VI will review the literature of the voltammetric measurement of drugs in biological fluids. These examples will serve to demonstrate the utility of voltammetric methods in toxicological analysis, in bioavailability and pharmacokinetic studies on drugs, and in metabolite identification.

II. THEORY

A. Definitions

Voltammetry is an oxidative or reductive electrolysis at a microelectrode, completely controlled by the rate at which ions diffuse from the body of the solution to the electrode. The change in current at the microelectrode is proportional to the concentration of electroactive material and is monitored as a function of the applied potential. The forms of voltammetry differ in the application of the changing potential to the microelectrode. The studies are typically performed in cells of 1- to 50-ml capacity and employ a working and reference electrode with, if necessary, a counter of auxiliary electrode. The working electrode in the reductive processes for polarography is a dropping mercury electrode (DME) or a hanging mercury drop electrode (HMDE). Solid electrode voltammetry is typically employed for anodic (oxidation) processes and uses either rotating platinum or gold, wax-impregnated graphite, carbon paste, pyrolytic graphite, or glassy carbon for electrodes.

The widely-used technique of voltammetry permits both qualitative and quantitative analyses to be performed simultaneously on a wide variety of samples and yields information on different electroactive species in the same system. The technique is versatile, has a wide linear dynamic range, and yields accurate reproducible and easily interpretable results.

B. Direct Current Polarography

Jaroslav Heyrovsky developed direct current polarography as one of the first instrumental analytical techniques in 1922 and applied it to inorganic analysis [12] for which he was awarded the Nobel Prize in 1959. Shikata first demonstrated the usefulness of the technique in organic chemical analysis [13] in 1925 by the polarographic analysis of nitrobenzene. The advances of organic polarography are evidenced by texts [1, 14] and reviews [15, 16].

In its simplest form, DC polarography is a voltammetric process in which a linearly varying DC potential ramp is applied between two electrodes: one small and easily polarizable (the working electrode) and the other large and relatively resistant to polarization (the reference electrode). The components of a typical polarographic cell are shown in Figure 2. In addition to the DME (the working electrode) and the saturated calomel electrode (the reference electrode), a platinum wire serves as an electrode to monitor potential. The purpose of this "auxiliary electrode" is to com-

THE POLAROGRAPH

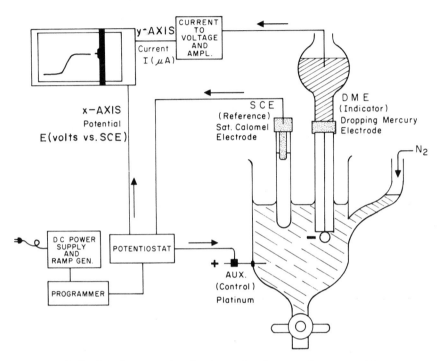

FIG. 2.   Components of a typical polarographic assembly.

pensate for the potential drop due to poor conductivity of the solution by
means of a potentiostat (Fig. 2) which compares the applied potential differences between the reference and auxiliary electrodes with that between
the working and reference electrodes.   This assures that the desired potential is applied to the working electrode.   This compensation circuit is now
a standard feature in modern voltammetric equipment.

   Increasing potential applied to the working electrode generates currents
due to the migration and diffusion of ions to the electrode.   The current
due to the migration of ions is suppressed by the use of electroinactive
salts as the supporting electrolyte, so that only the current due to the diffusion of ions which is proportional to the concentration is measured.   The
resulting current flow between the working and reference electrodes is

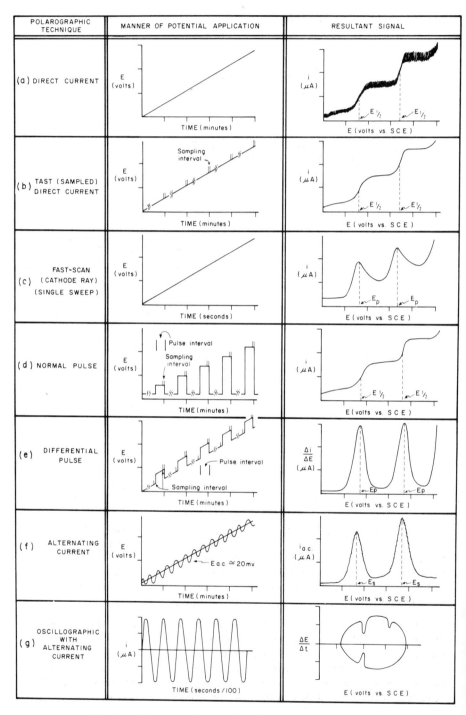

FIG. 3. The basic forms of voltammetric analysis.

recorded as a function of the applied potential, and a characteristic cur-
rent-potential relationship (i vs. E) curve or DC polarogram is obtained
as shown in Figure 3a. A characteristic feature of the DME is that the
surface area of the electrode (mercury drop) repeatedly grows to a maximum and then suddenly falls to zero as the drop detaches and a new one
begins to grow. Since the current flowing in the system is proportional to
the surface area of the electrode, it constantly fluctuates in the same fashion, producing a characteristic saw-toothed pattern superimposed upon the
step-like transitions of the DC polarogram.

Examination of the DC polarogram in Figure 3a shows that initially a
small increasing current (the residual current) flows as the potential increases until a large increase in current is produced by the reduction of an electroactive species. The current increases with increasing
potential until a plateau is reached (the limiting current), at which time
the current is proportional to the rate of diffusion. The same process can
occur with further increasing potential when a second, less readily reducible electroactive species is present. Finally, a large increase in potential
occurs for the electrodecomposition of the supporting electrolyte. The difference between the residual and limiting currents is defined as the diffusion
current (i_d) and is proportional to the concentration of the electroactive
species in solution. The fundamental equation was derived by Ilkovic [17].

$$i_d = 607 n D^{1/2} C_0 \times m^{2/3} t^{1/6} \qquad\qquad (1)$$

$$\underbrace{\phantom{607 n D^{1/2} C_0}}_{\substack{\text{Solution} \\ \text{factors}}} \quad \underbrace{\phantom{m^{2/3} t^{1/6}}}_{\substack{\text{Electrode} \\ \text{factors}}}$$

where i_d = diffusion current (μA)
    n = number of electrons involved in the redox reaction
    D = diffusion coefficient (cm^2/sec)
    m = mass of mercury flowing per sec (mg/sec)
    t = drop time of the mercury electrode (sec)
    C_0 = concentration of electroactive species (mM/liter)

The factors n, D, m, and t are constant since the chemical nature of the
solution analyzed and the electrochemical processes taking place at the
DME are kept constant over the period of analysis. Therefore, a linear
relationship of diffusion current (i_d) and the actual concentration of the
electroactive species in solution is obtained. The Ilkovic equation thus
reduces to: $i_d = k \times C_0$, where the diffusion current (i_d) is proportional
to the concentration (C_0) of the electroactive species, analogous to Beer's
Law in spectrophotometry.

The half-wave potential ($E_{1/2}$) is the value of the potential of the dropping
mercury electrode at the point on the current-voltage curve at which the
current is one-half of its limiting value. This is a characteristic of the
particular electroactive species in a particular supporting electrolyte that
causes the step-like transition and is independent of the concentration of
the substance and the electrode employed. The $E_{1/2}$ value is a qualitative

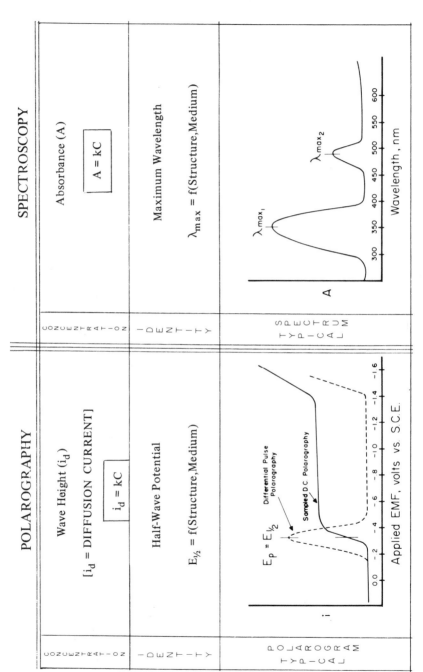

FIG. 4.　Analytically significant analogies between polarography and spectroscopy.

parameter employed in DC polarography and is analogous to λ_{max} in absorption spectroscopy (Fig. 4). The reader is referred to several excellent texts on the subject of DC polarography for further details of the theory of the technique [18-22].

C. Polarographic Methods for Trace-level Assay

The total diffusion current measured in the DC polarographic process results from the sum of two individual currents, the faradaic and capacitance currents. The faradaic current results from the transfer of electrons across the electrode-solution interface and is the component of the total current that is due to the reduction or oxidation of the electroactive species. The capacitance current results from the capacitive nature of the electrode-solution interface. Since the current required to charge this capacitor is additional to that required by the reacting species (faradaic current) more current is measured than is directly proportional to the concentration of the electroactive species present. New mercury surface is exposed to the solution as the drop grows, and thus current is always needed to charge the drop. This capacitance current in DC polarography is primarily due to the change in electrode area and is exhibited in the form of noise with a diminished signal/background ratio which limits the sensitivity to the order of 5×10^{-6} M.

The magnitude of the capacitive current in solutions less than 5×10^{-6} M can be greater than the faradaic current and can completely obscure the signal due to the reduction process. This is particularly important when increased sensitivity is required to measure drugs in biological fluids and demands higher amplification of the electrical signal for proper assay.

The newer polarographic techniques discriminate against capacitance currents and thus yield the higher signal-to-noise ratio necessary for higher sensitivity than conventional DC polarography. For the most part this is accomplished through the use of controlled drop timers and sampling circuits which measure faradaic currents when capacitance currents have decayed to a minimum value. This is usually accomplished by measuring currents just prior to drop dislodgment when the faradaic component is fairly high and the capacitance component is low.

1. Tast (Sampled DC) Polarography

This modification utilizes controlled drop time and a predetermined measuring interval just prior to drop dislodgment. The ratio between faradaic and capacitive current is high, and sensitivities approximately 1.5 times the conventional DC signal are obtained. Also, the sampling circuit employed minimizes or eliminates the characteristic drop-induced fluctuation patterns of DC polarography and yields well-defined curves (Fig. 3b) which can be easily interpreted for qualitative and quantitative analysis.

2. Fast Scan (Single Sweep or Cathode Ray) Polarography

In this technique the entire potential ramp is applied during a small fraction of the lifetime of a single drop. Since the total time of analysis is extremely short, the process can be monitored on a cathode ray oscilloscope. The scan sweep is synchronized with the dropping rate of the DME and is confined to the last few seconds of its drop life when the growth of the surface area of the drop is minimal. In a typical analysis the drop time is usually 7 to 10 sec, the sweep time is about 2 sec, and the initiation of the scan is delayed about 5 to 8 sec. The discriminatory current sampling time and the elimination of drop fluctuations due to growth and fall of successive drops yields a higher current signal-to-noise ratio for this method with sensitivities on the order of 10^{-7} M.

A typical polarogram (or polarotrace) is shown in Figure 3c. The residual current, as in DC polarography, is that current measured prior to the initiation of reduction of the material of interest. The limiting current is that current measured from the peak potential (E_p) of the polarogram until the initiation of the next reduction. Peaks result from the exhaustion of reducible material at the electrode surface with a consequent fall in current. The diffusion current, which is proportional to the concentration, is measured from an extension at the base-line or residual current to the peak potential and is proportional to the concentration. The peak potential closely resembles the $E_{1/2}$ of conventional DC polarography and is usually about 0.05 V more negative than this conventional half-wave potential. This method resolves mixtures better than with DC polarography; only a 30 to 35 mV separation is required to quantitate equal amounts of two reducible compounds.

Further increases in sensitivity have been reported employing differential cathode ray polarography where two dropping mercury electrodes with equal size drops are synchronized and used for the sample and reference cells respectively. The observed difference in the currents flowing through both cells give high sensitivities, even in the presence of extracts from biological fluids.

3. Pulse Polarographic Techniques

The parameters which affect the analytical utility of pulse polarography, a technique conceived by Barker and Gardner [23] approximately 15 years ago, have been evaluated [24-26]. These methods have higher sensitivity than DC polarography and are excellent for trace analysis. There are essentially two pulse polarographic techniques: pulse (normal or integral pulse), and differential pulse polarography which discriminates the faradaic current from the capacitative current with the use of controlled drop time interval and current sampling procedures.

a. Normal pulse polarography

This method employs potential pulses of successively increasing amplitude applied from a fixed initial potential to the working electrode (DME) at a fixed time during the drop life or timing period (see Fig. 3d). The pulses are usually applied for 50 to 60 msec prior to drop dislodgment, and the current is measured at some fixed time (usually 40 msec) after pulse application. Since the pulses are applied toward the end of the drop life, the change in area of the electrode with time is very small, and the electrode may be considered a stationary electrode. As a result the capacitive current is minimal and the signal represents only faradaic current. The polarogram obtained by this method has the same shape as the DC polarogram without the drop oscillation. The diffusion limited current for pulse polarography is approximated by the Cotrell equation which is applicable to diffusion to a stationary electrode [19].

$$i_d = nFA \left(\frac{D}{\pi t}\right)^{1/2} \times C_0 \qquad (2)$$

where n = number of electrons involved in the redox reaction
   F = faraday constant
   A = area of electrode
   D = diffusion coefficient
   t = time of current measurement after pulse application
   C_0 = concentration

The current ratio obtained [26] from the diffusion limited currents of the Ilkovic and Cotrell equations is:

$$\frac{i_d \text{ (pulse)}}{i_d \text{ (DC)}} = \left(\frac{3t_1}{7t_2}\right)^{1/2} \sim 5\text{-}10 \qquad (3)$$

where t_1 = drop time in the DC case
   t_2 = time of current measurement after pulse application

Theoretical considerations predict a sensitivity increase of approximately 5- to 10-fold using normal pulse polarography in comparison to DC polarography. In practice, however, pulse polarography is about two orders of magnitude (10^{-7} M as compared to 10^{-5} M) more sensitive than DC polarography. The increase in sensitivity comes through the ability to discriminate and electronically amplify the faradaic current from the capacitive currents.

b. Differential pulse polarography

In contrast to normal pulse polarography where large pulses of increasing height are used, differential pulse polarography (DPP) employs short duration, small amplitude pulses of constant height which are super-imposed on a slowly varying potential ramp (see Fig. 3e). These pulses occur toward the end of the drop life for a DME and last for about 51 msec (Princeton Applied Research instrumentation). Since the electrode area changes only slightly during pulse application, the electrode can be consid-ered a stationary electrode.

This technique involves two current sampling intervals during the life of each drop: one prior to pulse application and one toward the end of pulse application when the capacitive current has decayed (typically 40 msec after pulse application). The difference (hence "differential") current is displayed on the recorder in the shape of a first derivative signal (see Fig. 3e).

Parry and Osteryoung [26] have derived an equation for the fundamental processes involved in differential pulse polarography:

$$\Delta i_p = \frac{n^2 F^2}{4RT} \, AC\Delta E \, \frac{D}{\pi t} \tag{4}$$

where Δi_p = peak current (μA)

$\quad$ t $\quad$ = time of current measurement after pulse application

$\quad$ n $\quad$ = electron change involved in Redox reaction

$\quad$ F $\quad$ = faraday constant

$\quad$ R $\quad$ = gas constant

$\quad$ T $\quad$ = temperature

$\quad$ A $\quad$ = area of drop

$\quad$ C $\quad$ = concentration (mM/liter)

$\quad$ ΔE = pulse height (mV)

$\quad$ D $\quad$ = diffusion coefficient

The equation is applicable for pulse heights (ΔE) no greater than 40 to 50 mV. The peak current potential (E_p) for DPP is related to the $E_{1/2}$ of DC polarography:

$$E_p = E_{1/2} - \Delta E/2 \tag{5}$$

and demonstrates the dependence of E_p on pulse amplitude.

Although theory predicts that DPP is inherently less sensitive than pulse polarography, modern instrumentation shows the contrary. Although both techniques have eliminated capacitive current, the more sensitive DPP provides relatively noise-free Gaussian peaks which are more amenable to signal amplification than the step-like wave form of the normal pulse meth-od. Sensitivity limits for the method approach 10^{-8} M. A comparison of the sensitivity using DC polarography and DPP for the electroreduction of chlordiazepoxide is shown in Figure 5. The three peaks correspond to the reduction of the N_4-oxide, 4,5-azomethine, and 1,2-azomethine, respec-

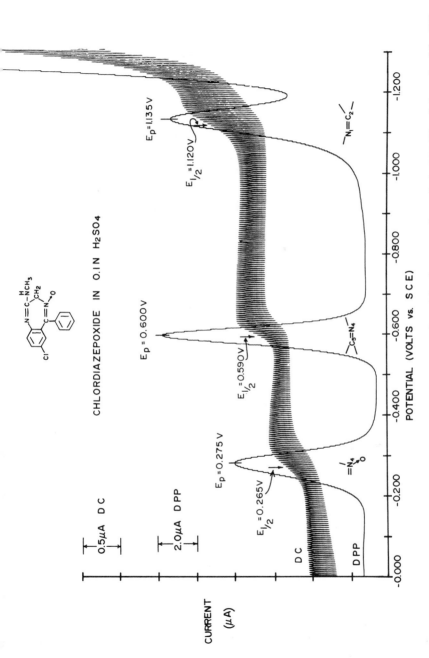

FIG. 5. Typical current vs. potential (i vs. E) curve for chlordiazepoxide in 0.1 N H₂SO₄ determined by DC and DPP polarography. (Reprinted from Ref. 58 by permission of the American Chemical Society.)

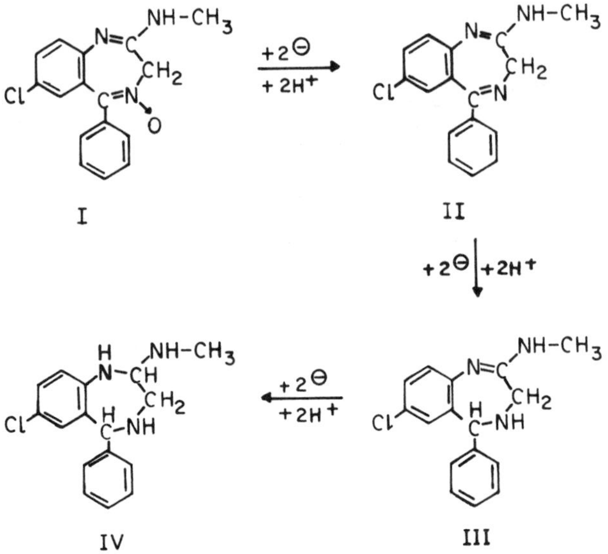

FIG. 6. Polarographic reduction mechanism of chlordiazepoxide in
acidic supporting electrolyte at the DME. (Reprinted from Ref. 27 by
courtesy of Verlag Chemie GmbH.)

tively. The polarographic mechanism for this compound is shown in
Figure 6 [27].

D. Alternating Current Polarographic Methods

Several alternating current polarographic methods have been employed for
the quantitation of pure materials and drugs in dosage forms at levels of
10^{-6} M or higher and to study the mechanism of polarographic reduction.
These methods are treated only superficially in this section since they cannot usually be applied to the analysis of drugs in biological fluids.

1. Alternating Current (AC) Polarography

In AC polarography [28, 29], a small constant amplitude (10-50 mV) alternating potential is superimposed upon a DC voltage ramp (see Fig. 3f). At
any point on the potential ramp where a redox reaction occurs, the super-
imposed AC voltage produces a periodic change in the concentration of the
oxidized and reduced forms at the electrode surface and thus produces an

AC current. Since the AC signal is not produced prior to the redox reaction and the material is being electrolyzed as fast as it approaches the electrode surface, the result is an AC peak (which approximates the $E_{1/2}$ of DC polarography) when both the oxidized and reduced forms are present at the electrode surface. Adsorption and desorption of surface-active substances at the electrode also yield characteristic peak currents in AC polarography (tensammetry). The height of the peak above baseline from the redox reaction can be used to quantitate with a sensitivity limit of 10^{-6} M.

Both AC polarography and tensammetry are typically limited to the measurement of inorganic ions which show the ability to exist periodically in the oxidized and reduced form (reversible reaction) and can only be used for a small number of organic substances which show a high degree of reversibility.

2. Oscillographic Polarography with Alternating Current

This "multisweep" method is cathode ray oscillopolarographic and was developed by Heyrovsky and Foreyt [30] (see Fig. 3g). The DME is polarized from 0 to 2.0 V in 0.01 sec and reversed to 0 V in the next 0.01 sec by an AC current of constant amplitude (0.05-5 mA) and frequency (in general, 50 cps). The frequency of the time sweep is synchronized with the applied alternating current-voltage to produce a stationary potential time figure on the oscilloscope. Any process resulting in a flow of current at the DME produces a horizontal inflection, proportional to concentration, on the potential-time curve. Reversible reactions are denoted by inflections in the curve in both polarization directions. The method is relatively insensitive (10^{-3} to 10^{-4} M).

E. Other Voltammetric Methods

Voltammetric methods which employ working electrodes other than the DME are typically not employed for the analysis of drugs in biological fluids due to their inherent lack of sensitivity (usually no greater than 10^{-5} to 10^{-6} M). Working electrodes such as the rotating platinum and gold electrodes and various carbon electrodes are typically used for oxidative processes since mercury oxidation occurs at potentials more positive than approximately +0.3 V vs. SCE. These electrodes have been employed for the analysis of bulk pharmaceuticals and drugs in dosage forms. They can be used in micropolarographic cells (10-20 μl) as detectors for liquid chromatography [31], capable of measuring drugs in the subnanogram range [32].

III. INSTRUMENTATION FOR VOLTAMMETRIC ANALYSIS

A. Electrodes

1. Working Electrodes

The DME is by far the most common electrode used in voltammetric analysis. The electrode consists of marine barometer tubing (usually about 6 in. long) with an i.d. of 0.05 to 0.08 mm attached to a reservoir of mercury. The electrode has the distinct advantage of presenting a clean, renewable surface of definable area with no memory effects to the solution. It can be used for DC, tast, pulse, and AC polarography. With proper timing circuits it can also be used for fast scan polarography. The hanging mercury drop electrode (HMDE), a stationary electrode, is often used in place of the DME for fast scan voltammetry. The electrode is particularly useful because a large electrode surface is obtained which yields increases in faradaic current and sensitivity of analysis. The electrode can be used in the differential pulse mode. The major drawback is that the commercial electrodes have only sufficient mercury reservoir to perform approximately ten assays.

The DME and HMDE electrodes are typically employed for reductive processes, whereas precious metal or carbon electrodes are used for oxidative processes. The mercury electrodes are restricted to reductive processes because of their oxidation to mercurous and mercuric ions. Platinum and gold electrodes, initially used in oxidative measurements, frequently do not yield reproducible responses due to changes in the electrodes surface or condition. They have been replaced by carbon electrodes which can be designed with renewable surfaces of constant area and which are inert to the chemical processes occurring at them. There are four basic carbon electrodes: the glassy carbon, pyrolytic graphite, carbon paste, and wax-impregnated graphite electrodes. The nature and construction of these carbon electrodes has been described elsewhere [33]. In general, these electrodes have a sensitivity limit of 10^{-6} M.

2. Reference Electrode

The mercury pool electrode was the first reference electrode employed, and was used in systems in which it was required to act as both reference and counter electrodes. In modern day instrumentation the saturated calomel electrode (SCE) or silver-silver chloride (Ag/AgCl) electrode is used either with or without a salt bridge. The salt bridge is used in those cases in which it is absolutely necessary to keep the salts out of the solution to be assayed.

The miniaturized Ag/AgCl electrode, which consists of anodically coated silver chloride on a silver wire, is especially useful in micro cells for trace-level assays.

3. Counter Electrode (Auxiliary)

This electrode is an inert conductive material, usually platinum or carbon, immersed directly in the solution to be assayed.

B. Electrochemical Cells

The glass cells employed for voltammetric analysis have been reduced in size over the years from the typical 25- to 50-ml "H cells" in which the working and reference electrodes were individual compartments separated by an agar plug, to cells of 2 to 4 ml (Fig. 7a) and 0.5 ml (Fig. 7b). The three electrodes are contained in one chamber and the SCE (a) and the Ag/AgCl, and DME (b) have been miniaturized. In addition, the cells incorporate stop-cocks to facilitate the removal of the sample for disposal after assay. Commercial cells of smaller volumes are also available. Princeton Applied Research (PAR) offers a cell assembly with a positioned electrode and a removable base for rapid sample interchangeability.

C. Instrumentation

Table 1 lists the commercially available voltammetric analyzers. The Chemtrix and Southern Analytical Laboratory instruments have been popular in fast scan polarography with DPP frequently performed on Melabs or PAR instruments. The PAR moderately priced Model 174 is often the unit of choice and has sophisticated electronics and versatility. With two minor auxiliary modules it can perform all the common modes of voltammetric analysis. The newly introduced PAR Model 374 with a built-in microprocessor and pressurized DME encompasses the state of the art in voltammetric analyzers. The microprocessor controls each stage of the actual analysis, examines experimental data for validity, and provides the status of the analysis through the display. The instrument has built-in capabilities for the storage of data, electronic background subtraction, and a higher limit of sensitivity than any other commercially available voltammetric instrument. In addition, PAR has introduced an autocell sequencer which can be used in conjunction with Models 174 and 374. The unit also employs the pressurized DME and can analyze as many as 36 samples completely unattended.

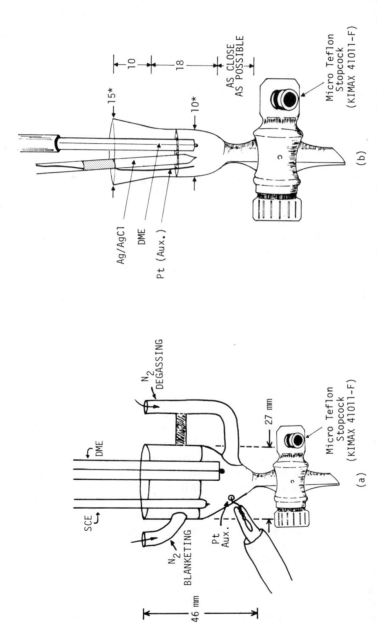

FIG. 7. Electrochemical cells for polarography. (a) Macrocell 2- to 4-ml capacity. (b) Semimicrocell of 0.5-ml capacity: *, i.d.'s; all dimensions in mm. (Reprinted from Refs. 58 and 11, respectively, by permission of the American Chemical Society.)

TABLE 1

Commercially Available Voltammetric Instrumentation and Their Operational Modes

Manufacturer	Model	Polarographic technique						
		DC	AC	Sampled DC	Normal pulse	Fast scan	Differential pulse	Oscillopolarography
Chemtrix Beaverton, Oregon	SSP-5					+		
Heath Richmond, Mich.	Digi-scan					+		
Laboratorni Pristroje Prague, Czechoslovakia	LP-7 LP 600 Polaroscope	+		+ 				+
McKee Pederson Danville, Calif.	MP-1000 2001	+ +	+	+ +	+	+	+ +	+
Melabs Palo Alto, Calif.	CPA-3	+		+	+	+	+	
Metrohm (Brinkman) Westbury, N.Y.	E 261-R E 506	+ +	+ (E393) +	+	+	+		
National Instrument Laboratories Rockville, Md.	Electrolab	+				+		
Princeton Applied Research Princeton, N.J.	170 174 374	+ + +	+ + (174/50) +	+ + +	+ +	+ + (174/51) +	+ + +	
Radiometer (London Company, Cleveland, Ohio) or Copenhagen, Denmark	PO4	+		+				
Sargent Chicago, Ill.	XVI	+						
Southern Analytical Camberly, England	A 1660 A 1300				+ +	+		
Taucussel (Ryaby Assoc.) Passaic, N.J.	PRG-34 PRG-3 PRG-4 PRG-5	+ + +	+ +	+ +	+ +	+	+ + +	

IV. ASSAY PARAMETERS FOR VOLTAMMETRIC ANALYSIS

The use of voltammetry in the analysis for drugs in biological fluids is based on the redox properties of organic molecules. The proper choice of the supporting electrolyte, the control of pH, and the choice of working electrode are all essential to the development of accurate, precise, and sensitive procedures.

A. Chemical Structure and Polarographic Activity

Whereas inorganic voltammetry involves simple cations (e.g., Fe^{2+}, Cu^{2+}, Mn^{2+}) and anions (e.g., cyanide) in the reversible electron transfer processes, organic voltammetry involves the participation of the whole electroactive species. Most organic reactions are irreversible and involve specific functional groups which are electroactive, e.g., nitro, nitroso, carbonyl, azomethine, ethylinic or acetylinic double bonds, N-oxide, diazo, sulfoxide, etc. The main portion of the molecule, which may be a hydrocarbon chain, a benzene nucleus, or heterocyclic system remains unaffected although it will influence the potential at which the functional group is reduced or oxidized by inductive or electrometric effects. Consequently, the $E_{1/2}$ values for specific functional groups lie within a narrow range of potential rather than at the fixed values of inorganic ions (Fig. 8). Examples of different types of functional groups assayed in a wide variety of pharmaceuticals are shown in Table 2 (Section VI).

B. pH Requirements

Hydrogen ions are involved in the redox reaction of most organic compounds. The solution pH can influence the course of the electrochemical reaction in organic polarography as well as the potential at which it occurs.

C. Choice of Supporting Electrolyte

Since hydrogen ions are involved in these voltammetric processes, it is essential that adequate buffering be provided in the supporting electrolyte to avoid changes in pH during analysis and resultant changes in the electrochemical system. Typical aqueous buffers which show no electroactivity per se are acetate, phosphate, and ammonia. If the compound is insoluble

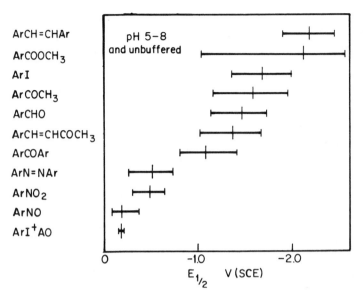

FIG. 8. The ranges of half-wave potentials in which the reduction of monosubstituted benzoid compounds at pH 5 to 8 and in unbuffered solution take place, provided that the reduction follows the same mechanism as that for parent compound. (Reprinted from Ref. 14.)

in aqueous media, organic cosolvents such as alcohols, dioxane, acetonitrile, dimethylsulfoxide, and dimethylformamide can be employed. Occasionally, completely nonaqueous solvents of high dielectric constant such as dimethylformamide, acetonitrile, dimethylsulfoxide, pyridine, or glacial acetic acid containing dissolved tetraalkyl salts as supporting electrolytes may be required to attain highly negative potentials (greater than -1.8 V vs. SCE) without decomposition of the supporting electrolyte. A review of nonaqueous solvents, reference electrodes and solvent potential ranges for electrolysis has been reported [34]. Generally nonaqueous polarography has not been successful at the microgram level because of irreproducibilities and impurities in the supporting electrolytes or solvents which tend to distort or mask the voltammetric peak.

D. Removal of Oxygen

Deaeration of a sample prior to reductive analyses is essential since dissolved oxygen (usually present at a concentration of 8 mg/liter or approx-

imately 0.001 N at room temperature) produces significant waves which
interfere in the analysis. Dissolved oxygen is reduced at the DME producing a double wave by a two-step reduction as follows:

$$O_2 \xrightarrow{2H^+} H_2O_2 \xrightarrow{2H^+} 2H_2O$$

The interference is further complicated in an unbuffered solution during
the reduction of oxygen since hydrogen ions are consumed and an excess
of hydroxyl ions occurs in the neighborhood of the electrode. These ions
can react with substances which diffuse from the bulk of the solution to the
electrode surface and consequently change their wave-form and wave-height.

The most common method for removing oxygen is by deaeration with a
polarographically inactive gas such as N_2 or CO_2. Nitrogen is usually
preferred for deaeration, but hydrogen, methane, inert gases, and in acid
solution even carbon dioxide can also be used. Deaeration is best effected
by bubbling in dry N_2 (Matheson, prepurified) into the solution for 5 min
through a coarse porosity micro filter stick (Scientific Glass Apparatus
Inc., Bloomfield, N.J., Model JM-5385) immediately prior to analysis.
The sample is then transferred into the cell and further blanketed with N_2
flowing over the surface of the solution during analysis.

E. Chemical Derivatization

When no intrinsic electrochemical activity is observed in either aqueous
or nonaqueous media, derivatization methods can convert the compound
into an electroactive species. The derivatization reactions most commonly used include nitration, nitrosation, condensation, addition, substitution,
oxidation, hydrolysis, and complex formation [14, 15].

1. Formation of Nitro Derivatives

The formation of nitro derivatives is the most common means of introducing polarographic activity. Benzenoid systems can be nitrated by reacting
the compound with a mixture of KNO_3 in concentrated H_2SO_4 or with mixtures of concentrated HNO_3 in concentrated H_2SO_4 ("mixed acid"). The
active nitrating agent in such a mixture is the nitronium ion ($-NO_2^+$)
formed according to the equation.

Nitration of phenyl rings

1) $HNO_3 + 2H_2SO_4 \rightleftharpoons NO_2^{\oplus} + 2HSO_4^- + H_3O^{\oplus}$.

2)

Phenyl   Nitronium
Compound   ion   Nitro-derivative

Unsubstituted phenyl compounds are nitrated in the para position while those containing a para substituent (e.g., $-CH_3$) are meta directing in the phenyl ring.

Nitration is most rapid in systems which are above 90% in sulfuric acid. The reaction mixture is diluted with water and the nitro derivatives formed can be extracted at acidic pH and analyzed with high sensitivity and specificity, usually in 0.1 N NaOH. Nitro derivatives may also be formed with primary aliphatic or aromatic amines and phenols using 2,4-dinitrofluorobenzene (DNFB) in a base catalyzed medium to yield intensely yellow colored dinitrophenyl (DAP) derivatives.

Dinitrophenyl (DNP) Derivatives

2,4-dinitrofluorobenzene   DNP derivative
(DNFB)

2. Dinitrophenyl-hydrazone Derivatives of
    Aldehydes and Ketones

Aliphatic and aromatic aldehydes and ketones react with 2,4-dinitrophenylhydrazine in aqueous ethanolic sulfuric acid to form hydrazones:

2,4-dinitrophenylhydrazone derivatives

The yellow-colored high melting derivatives have two functional groups: the $-NO_2$ (nitro) and $>C=N-$ (azomethine) which are very sensitive to electroreduction.

3. Diazotization of Primary Aromatic Amines

Diazotization of primary aromatic amines such as the sulfonamides with $NaNO_2$ in HCl to yield a diazonium salt which is then coupled to either α-naphthol or N-(1-naphthyl)ethylenediamine $\cdot$ 2HCl to form characteristic purple- or crimson-colored azo-dyes can be analyzed polarographically by the reduction of the diazo bond ($-N=N-$).

Diazotization and Coupling

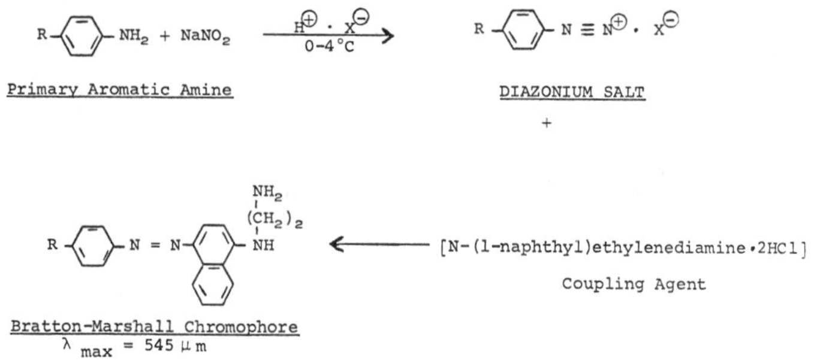

$$R\text{—}\langle \bigcirc \rangle\text{—}NH_2 + NaNO_2 \quad \xrightarrow[\text{0-4°C}]{H^{\oplus} \cdot X^{\ominus}} \quad R\text{—}\langle \bigcirc \rangle\text{—}N \equiv N^{\oplus} \cdot X^{\ominus}$$

Primary Aromatic Amine   DIAZONIUM SALT

+

$$R\text{—}\langle \bigcirc \rangle\text{—}N = N\text{—}\langle \bigcirc\bigcirc \rangle\text{—}\overset{\overset{\displaystyle NH_2}{\overset{|}{(CH_2)_2}}}{\underset{|}{NH}} \quad \longleftarrow \quad [N\text{-}(1\text{-naphthyl})ethylenediamine \cdot 2HCl]$$

Coupling Agent

Bratton-Marshall Chromophore
$\lambda_{max} = 545\ \mu m$

V. DETERMINATION OF DRUGS IN BIOLOGICAL FLUIDS

The availability of commercial instrumentation capable of measuring drug concentrations in the range of 10^{-6} to 10^{-8} M has facilitated the analysis of drugs in biological fluids by voltammetric methods. DPP and cathode ray polarography (CRP) are the only techniques capable of determining drugs routinely at concentrations of less than 5×10^{-5} M ($\sim 10\ \mu g/ml$) in biological fluids.

A. Analytical Utility

The determination of drugs in biological fluids is required for toxicological analysis, in determining bioavailability of generic dosage forms, in drug metabolism studies, and in clinical pharmacokinetic evaluation [35]. Although spectrophotometric, spectrofluorometric, chromatographic, and spectrometric methods have been the techniques predominantly used in drug analysis in biological fluids [36], electrochemical methods have recently taken their rightful place in these fields of analytical endeavor [6, 7, 33].

B. Development of a Voltammetric Assay

The following criteria have to be evaluated in determining whether a given compound can be assayed by voltammetric methods.

1. Supporting Electrolyte and Chemical Structure

Inspection of the chemical structure of a compound will permit the prediction of intrinsic polarographic activity and the proper choice of a supporting electrolyte. Compounds containing diazo ($-N=N-$), azomethine ($>C=N$), and carbonyl ($>C=O$) groups near a center of high electron density (aromatic or heterocyclic nucleus) usually show electrochemical activity in acidic supporting electrolytes, whereas compounds containing a nitro group usually show activity in basic supporting electrolytes. If intrinsic electrochemical activity cannot be deduced by inspection, the compound should be analyzed in acidic, neutral, and basic aqueous media, usually 0.1 to 1.0 M phosphate buffers ranging in pH from 2 to 13. The medium in which optimal electrochemical signal ($\mu A/\mu g/ml$) is obtained is then used for quantitation. In certain cases nonaqueous supporting electrolytes may have to be used [34]. If no intrinsic polarographic activity is noted, derivatization reactions such as nitration and nitrosation, condensation reactions to yield azomethines (e.g., semicarbazones and hydrazones), chemical hydrolysis or oxidation to yield benzophenones, and diazotization and coupling to yield azo-dyes will give chemical derivatives with polarographic activity.

2. Sensitivity

Sensitivity depends upon the actual signal obtained ($\mu A/\mu g/ml$) in the electrochemical process taking place at the DME. It can be affected adversely by the background signals derived from endogenous interferences in the biological samples. Interferences are manifested as high background signals or as spurious peaks in the reduction area of interest. These interferences can be removed by selective solvent extraction and/or a chromatographic separation step (usually thin-layer) for effecting suitable sample clean-up.

The dose of drug administered, the metabolic pathway, the tissue and body fluid distribution of the drug, and its rate of elimination can significantly influence the actual blood concentration measured as a function of time and therefore determine the sensitivity required of the assay. Drugs that are administered at doses ranging from 0.1 to 1.0 mg/kg of body weight can usually be quantitated by voltammetric methods. If the drug is rapidly metabolized and/or extensively distributed into the tissues, the resultant plasma concentrations are usually low and voltammetric analysis becomes difficult. However, many drugs are eliminated in the urine in sufficient amounts to make this medium quite suitable for voltammetric methods. Urine or the stomach contents can be frequently used for confirmatory analysis in cases of overdosages.

3. Specificity

A method is deemed to be specific when the parent drug can be determined
in the presence of its known metabolites, concomitantly administered drugs,
and endogenous biological materials. Specificity of an assay can be ensured by selective extraction of the parent drug alone or following chromatographic separation prior to quantitation. Thin-layer chromatographic
separation (TLC) is most useful since it provides a qualitative (visual)
evaluation of the sample extract in the identification of the parent drug,
its major metabolites, and any other drugs present. The components can
then be eluted separately and quantitated by a suitable method. Establishing
the specificity of the assay also ensures greater overall accuracy and
reproducibility of the analysis.

4. Analytical Parameters

The instrumental operational conditions must be optimized for each drug
or metabolite quantitated. Meticulous attention must be paid to all the
steps involved in the physical processing of the sample to minimize in-
determinate errors. Proper analytical procedures must be used throughout to ensure the accuracy, precision, and reproducibility of the analysis
[36]. The assay developed must also be fairly straightforward and amenable to routine analysis to be of clinical utility.

VI. APPLICATION OF VOLTAMMETRIC METHODS
     TO DRUG ANALYSIS

All the main forms of voltammetric analysis have been applied to the
analysis of drugs in biological fluids [1, 2, 6, 7, 14, 15, 37]. The examples
listed in Table 2 are selected for their diversity of chemical structures
and functional groups and for their specific application in toxicological
or therapeutic level determinations.

The measurement of blood levels using polarographic assays demands
high sensitivities. DPP is the only voltammetric method presently capable
of quantitating drugs at concentrations below 1.0 μg/ml of blood. The majority of the examples employ an extraction step prior to analysis whereas
only a few are analyzed directly in biological fluids. They are arranged
in alphabetical order by generic name. The references listed in Table 2
are numerically continuous with the general references in the text.

A. Analyses Using Intrinsic Electrochemical Activity

1. Direct Assays in Biological Material

Early assays used DC polarography for the analysis of drugs directly in
biological material or after dilution with an appropriate supporting elec-

trolyte. Kane [38] was the first to report on the analysis of the anti-
tubercular agent ethionamide directly in serum, urine, and cerebro-
spinal fluid using DC polarography. They also reported on the analysis of
the histamonostat, dimetridazole, and the trichomonicide, metronidazole
(two 5-nitroimidazole drugs) in serum and tissue by sampled DC polarography [39].

The facile reduction of the azomethine group in the 1,4-benzodiazepines
led to the development of a toxicological assay to determine diazepam
directly in whole blood with a lower limit of detection of 20 μg/ml [40].
In this analysis, 1 ml of whole blood was diluted with 9 ml of methanol-
Britton-Robinson buffer (pH 2.8); one drop of n-octanol and 3 drops of
0.5% gelatin were added as maxima suppressors, and DC polarography was
performed ($E_{1/2}$ = -0.82 V vs. SCE). Direct assays have also been reported for acenocoumarol [41], chlordiazepoxide [42], nitrazepam [43],
phenidione (2-phenylindan-1,3-dione) [44] in serum, isoniazid in cadaver
material [45], nitrofurantoin [46], and prothionamide [47] (see Table 2).

Two major shortcomings of these direct assays were that (1) they were
usually only sensitive enough to measure the drug after the ingestion of an
acute overdosage (>10 μg/ml) and (2) they were inherently nonspecific,
since structurally related metabolites would interfere with the specificity
and accuracy of the analysis.

2. Analyses Following Solvent Extraction

Analysis following solvent extraction of the sample has been reported using
direct and alternating current, cathode ray and differential pulse polarography (see Table 2). Of the various voltammetric methods, DPP is
generally best suited to the analysis of drugs in biological fluids due to its
sensitivity, rapidity, relative straightforwardness, reliability, and amenability to routine analysis. DPP sensitivities as low as 10 ng/ml have
been measured in conjunction with a micro sample cell (see Fig. 6b) [11].

Solvent extraction* of the drug and/or its major metabolites at a specific
pH can separate them from interfering endogenous materials. Further
sample clean-up can be effected after consideration of the proper pK_a
values by acid or base washing of the solvent extract to remove endogenous
impurities. Back-extraction of the compounds of interest can be effected
into the aqueous phase with retention of endogenous impurities in the solvent extract. This aqueous phase (0.1 N HCl or NaOH) can be then washed
with an extracting solvent and used directly as the supporting electrolyte
for a "total" analysis of drug and metabolites.

Analysis of the sample after solvent extraction can still lack specificity
unless extracted drug and metabolites can be resolved by the analysis of
different functional groups in their respective molecules. For example,

---

*See chapter "Liquid Extraction and Isolation" to be published in a future
volume of this series.

de SILVA and BROOKS

TABLE 2

Voltammetric Parameters for the Analysis of

Generic Name	Systematic Name	Structure	Pharmacological Activity	Electro-phore	
Acenocoumarol	3-(α-acetonyl-p-nitrobenzyl)-4-hydroxycoumarin	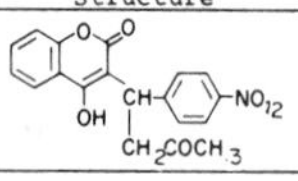	Anticoagulant	$-NO_2$	
Bromazepam	7-bromo-5-(2-pyridyl)-1,3-di-hydro-2H-1,4-benzo-diazepine-2-one	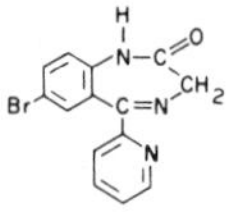	Anxiolytic	$>$C=N-	
Chlorbutanol	1,1,1-trichloro-2-methyl-2-propanol	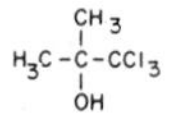	Anesthetic, Antiseptic	$-\overset{\mid}{\underset{\mid}{C}}-Cl$	
Chlordiazepoxide	7-chloro-2-methyl-amino-5-phenyl-3H-1,4-benzodiazepine-4-oxide	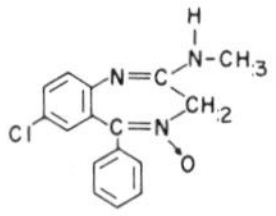	Anxiolytic	$>$C=N-	
Chlorpromazine	2-chloro-10-(3-di-methylaminopropyl)phenothiazine	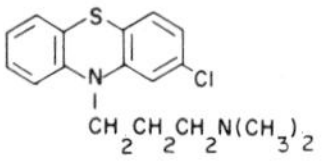	Antipsychotics	S→O	
				S·O N→O	
Clonazepam	7-nitro-5-(2-chloro-phenyl)-1,3 dihydro-(2H)-1,4-benzodiazepin-2-(1H)-one	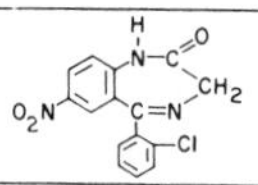	Anticonvulsant	$>$C=N-	
Dantrolene	1-{[5-(p-nitrophenyl)furfurylidene]amino}hydantoin	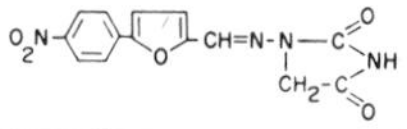	Muscle Relaxant	$-NO_2$ $>$C=N-	
Diazepam	7-chloro-1,3-dihydro-1-methyl-5-phenyl-2H-1,4-benzodiazepin-2-one	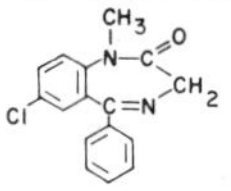	Anxiolytic	$>$C=N-	

Electroactive Drug Substances in Biological Fluids

Supporting Electrolyte	$E_{1/2}$ or E_p [a]	Concentration	Isolation [b]	Notes	Reference
Britton-Robinson Buffer (pH 10)	$-0.70V$[1]	20-100 µg/ml blood	D	Toxicological Procedure; blood levels in rat following 50 mg/kg dose; DC	Fidelus et al. (1971) [41]
Phosphate Buffer, 1M (pH 5.5)	$-0.535V$[1]	0.05-10 µg/ml urine	E	Urinary excretion following 12 mg dose; DPP	de Silva et al. (1974) [53]
Phosphate Buffer, 1M (pH 7.0)	$-0.610V$[2].	0.01-1.0 µg/ml blood	E	Blood levels following 4 mg dose; DPP	Brooks and Hackman (1975) [11]
Phosphate-Borate Buffer (pH 7.0) 5% DMF	$-0.35V$[2]	⟩0.05 µg/ml blood	E	Cathode Ray	Senguen & Oelschlager (1975) [62]
0.05M benzethonium chloride & 0.072 M sodium sulfite	$-1.0V$[1]	5-500 µg/ml serum	S	DC	Birner (1961) [100]
N HCl	$-0.67V$[1]	⟩10 µg/ml	E	Toxicological Procedure for blood, urine, gastric contents; DC	Cimbura & Gupta (1965) [57]
0.1N H_2SO_4	$-0.61V$[1]	2.5×10^{-3} to $10^{-6}M$	D	Toxicological Procedure; DC	Jacobsen & Jacobsen (1971) [42]
0.1N H_2SO_4	$-0.60V$[1]	0.05-10 µg/2 ml plasma	E	Plasma levels following 30 mg oral dose; also det'n of N-desmethyl & lactam metabolites; DPP	Hackman et al. (1974) [58]
0.5N HCl	$-0.93V$[3]	2-10 µg/ml urine	C	As sulfoxide derivative-Br$_2$ oxidation; urinary assay following 100 mg dose; cathode ray	Porter & Beresford (1966) [48]
0.5N HCl	$-0.74V$[1]	10^{-5} to $5 \times 10^{-8}M$	E	Biological fluids also determines N-oxide and N-oxide, sulfoxide; cathode ray	Beckett et al. (1973) [49]
0.1N HCl	$-0.1, -0.6V$[1]	⟩0.5 µg/ml urine	E	Urinary excretion following 2 mg dose; also metabolites; DPP	de Silva et al. (1974) [55]
0.2M Acetate Buffer (pH 4)- 4% DMF	$-0.26V$[1] $-0.86V$[1]	⟩0.1 µg/ml urine & plasma	E	Determination of total and reduced metabolites; DPP	Cox et al. (1969) [51]
N HCl	$-0.7V$[1]	⟩10 µg/ml	E	Toxicological Procedure for blood, urine and gastric contents; DC	Cimbura & Gupta (1965) [57]
0.1N HCl sat'd with sodium tetraborate	$-1.22V$[1]	0.02-10 µg/ 5 ml plasma	E	Plasma levels following 10 mg i.v. and oral doses; cathode ray	Berry (1971) [59]
Britton-Robinson buffer (pH 2.8) in 20% methanol	$-0.82V$[1]	⟩20 µg/ml blood	D	Toxicological Procedure; DC	Fidelus et al. (1972) [40]
0.1N HCl	$-0.64V$[1]	0.2-10 µg/ml blood	E	Therapeutic & toxicological levels; also det'n of N-desmethyl metabolite; DPP	Brooks et al. (1973) [61]
0.1N H_2SO_4	$-0.61V$[2]	⟩0.03 µg/ml serum	E	Therapeutic levels; total of diazepam and N-desmethyl metabolite; DPP	Jacobsen & Jacobsen (1973) [60]
1N HCl	$-0.7V$[2]	⟩0.1 µg/ml urine	E	Urinary levels following 100 mg dose; evaluation of urinary metabolites; DC	Dugal et al. (1973) [52]

TABLE 2

Generic Name	Systematic Name	Structure	Pharmacological Activity	Electro-phore
Dimetridazole	1,2-dimethyl-5-nitroimidazole		Histamonastat	$-NO_2$
Diphenylhydantoin	5,5-diphenyl-2,4-imidazoline-dione		Anticonvulsant	$-NO_2$
Disulfiram	Bis(diethylthio-carbamoyl)disulfide	$(C_2H_5)_2\overset{S}{\overset{\|}{N}}C\text{-}SS\text{-}\overset{S}{\overset{\|}{C}}N(C_2H_5)_2$	Anti-alcoholic	$-S-S-$
Dopa	3-(3,4-dihydroxy-phenyl)-L-alanine		Anti-Parkinson	$-OH$
Ethioniamide	2-ethyl-4-thio-carbamido-pyridine		Anti-Tuberculant	$>C=S$
Flurazepam	7-chloro-1-(2-di-ethylaminoethyl)-5-(2-fluorophenyl)-1,3-dihydro-2H-1,4-benzodiazepin-2-one		Sedative	$>C=N-$
Glibornuride	1-[(1R)-2-endo-hydroxy-3-endo bornyl]-3-(p-tolyl-sulfonyl) urea		Hypoglycemic	$-NO_2$
Haloperidol	4-[4-(p-chloro-phenyl)-4-hydroxy-piperidino]-4'-fluorobutyro-phenone		Antipsychotic	$>C=O$
Ipronidazole	1-methyl-2-iso-propyl-5-nitro-imidazole		Histamonastat	$-NO_2$
Isoniazid	isonicotinic acid hydrazide		Antituberculant	$>N-N<$ $>C=N-$
Lorazepam	7-chloro-3-hydroxy-1,3-dihydro-5-(2'-chlorophenyl)-2H-1,4-benzodiazepin-2-one		Anxiolytic	$>C=N-$

(Continued)

Supporting Electrolyte	$E_{1/2}$ or E_p [a]	Concentration	Isolation [b]	Notes	Reference
2M KOH	-0.5V [4]	～0.1 ppm	E	Analysis of tissues (turkeys); sampled DC	Kane (1961) [39]
0.2N NaOH	-0.65V [1]	～2 µg/g tissue ～0.1 µg/ml urine & plasma	D,E	Blood & tissue levels following 250 mg/kg to guinea pigs; DC	Allen & McLoughlin (1972) [66]
2N KOH	-0.75V [2]	0.1-10 µg/g tissue	E	Pig tissue; DC	Parnell (1973) [67]
0.1N NaOH	-0.625V [1]	～1 µg/ml blood	E	Nitro derivative; therapeutic levels; DPP	Brooks et al. (1973) [79]
Britton-Robinson Buffer (pH 3.5): DMF: 0.1% gelatin (60:30:10)	-0.378V [2]	≳2.5 µg/ml plasma	E	Nitro derivative; therapeutic levels; DC	Wiegrebe & Wehrhahn (1975) [80]
0.6M HCl: Ethanol (1:1)	-0.5V	0.5-2.0 µg/ 20 ml urine	E	Cathode ray	Porter & Williams (1972) [50]
0.01M H$_2$SO$_4$ & 0.04M Na$_2$SO$_4$	+0.72V [2]	≳10 ng/ml serum	E	LC with carbon paste voltammetric detection; Vydac bonded phase cation exchange resin; also determine dopamine	Kissinger et al. (1974) [86] Riggin et al. (1976) [75]
Analysis in body fluid	-0.78V [1]	≳0.2 µg/ml serum, cerebrospinal fluid & urine	D	Therapeutic levels; identification of sulfoxide metabolite; DC	Kane (1959) [8] Kane (1962) [39]
2M Borate Buffer (pH 8.2)	-1.2V [2]	50 µg/ml urine	D	Urinary excretion following 1 gram administration; AC	Bieder & Brunel (1971) [47]
Phosphate Buffer (pH 4.0)	-0.8V [1]	0.5-20 µg/ml urine	E	Urinary excretion following 90 mg dose; DPP in man	de Silva et al. (1974) [56]
Britton-Robinson buffer (pH 4.0) - 10% Methanol	-0.79V [1]	≳0.03 ng	E	Plasma level determination of N-desalkyl & hydroxyethyl metabolite; DPP in dogs	Clifford et al. (1974) [63]
Phosphate Buffer (pH 4.0)	-0.725V [2]	0.01-1 µg/ml	E	Blood levels of N-desalkyl-metabolite following 30 mg dose; DPP in man	Brooks & Hackman (1975) [11]
0.1N NaOH	-0.490V [1]	≳0.1 µg/2 ml blood	E	Determined as nitro-derivative; blood levels following 50 & 100 mg doses; DPP	de Silva & Hackman (1972) [77]
				Determined as nitro-derivative; blood levels following 50 mg chronic administration; DPP	Dubach et al. (1975) [78]
Britton-Robinson Buffer (pH 4.6): Methanol (2:3)	-1.32V [1]	10-50 µg/ml blood	E	Toxicological assay; blood levels following 80 mg/kg dose to the rat; also det'n of haloperidid; DC	Mikolajek et al. (1974) [73]
Basic (pH 11)		1-10 ppb tissue	E	Confirmatory test in turkey tissues; DPP	MacDonald et al. (1973) [68]
0.1N HCl	-0.54V [1] -0.72V [1]	30 µg/ml	D,E	Toxicological procedure for tissues, blood, serum & urine; DC	Lauermann & Otto (1968) [45]
0.1N HCl	0.62V [1]	0.2-1 µg/ml urine	E	Urinary excretion following 4 mg of 7-chloro-1,3-dihydro-5-(2'-chlorophenyl)-2H-1,4-benzodiazepin-2-one; DPP	de Silva et al. (1974) [54]

TABLE 2

Generic Name	Systematic Name	Structure	Pharmacological Activity	Electro-phore
Mephenytoin	5-ethyl-3-methyl-5-phenylhydantoin		Anticonvulsant	$-NO_2$
Methyldopa	L-3-(3,4-dihydroxy-phenyl)-2-methyl-alaline		Antihypertensive	$-OH$
Metronidazole	1-(2-hydroxyethyl)-2-methyl-5-nitro-imidazole		Trichomonacide	$-NO_2$
Nicarbazin	An equimolar complex of 4,4'-di-nitrocarbanilide and 2-hydroxy-4,6-dimethylpyrimide		Coccidiostat	$-NO_2$
Nitrazepam	7-nitro-5-phenyl-1,3-dihydro-(2H)-1,4-benzodiazepin-2-(1H)-one		Hypnotic	$-NO_2$
Nitrofurantoin	N-(5-nitro-2-fur-furylidene)-1-amino-hydantoin		Antibacterial	$-NO_2$
Ornidazole	1-(3-chloro-2-hydroxypropyl)-2-methyl-5-nitro-imidazole		Amoebicide Trichomonacide	$-NO_2$
Oxazepam	7-chloro-1,3-dihydro-3-hydroxy-5-phenyl-2H-1,4-benzodiazepin-2-one		Anxiolytic	$>C=N-$
Phenidione	2-phenyl-1,3-indan-dione		Anticoagulant	$>C=O$
Phenobarbital	5-ethyl-5-phenyl-barbituric acid		Sedative	$-NO_2$
Primaclone	5-ethyl-dihydro-5-phenyl-4,6(1H,5H)-pyrimidinedione		Anticonvulsant	$-NO_2$

(Continued)

Supporting Electrolyte	$E_{1/2}$ or E_p [a]	Concentration	Isolation [b]	Notes	Reference
Britton-Robinson Buffer (pH 3.5); DMF:0.1% gelatin (60:30:10)	$-0.402v$ [1]	>3.5 µg/ml plasma	E	Determined as nitro derivative; therapeutic levels; DC	Wiegrebe & Wehrhahn (1975) [80]
1N HCl	$+0.55v$ [1]	$>10^{-4}$M plasma, blood or urine	C	Tubular carbon electrode; DC	Stewart et al. (1974) [74]
0.01M H_2SO_4 & 0.04M Na_2SO_4	$+0.72v$ [2]	>10 ng/ml	E	LC with carbon paste electrode; Zipaz SCX column	Riggin et al. (1976) [75]
2M KOH	$-0.6v$ [4]	>0.05 µg/ml serum	D	Determination in serum & urine following 200 mg dose; Sampled DC	Kane (1961) [39]
				Following doses 4-15 g; DC	Deutsch et al. (1975) [71]
0.1N NaOH	$-0.625v$ [1]	>0.1 µg/ml serum	E	Therapeutic levels; DPP	Brooks et al. (1975) [70]
0.1M tetraethyl-ammonium per-chlorate & 2 x 10^{-3}M benzoic acid in dimethyl-sulfoxide	$-0.95v$ [1]	$>0.2-0.3$ ppm tissue	E	Determination in chicken muscle, liver, kidney and skin fat	Michielli & Downing (1974) [99]
Phosphate Buffer (pH 6.9)	$-0.38v$ [2]	$0.5-80$ µg/ml serum	D	Toxicological procedure; DC	Halvorsen & Jacobsen (1972) [43]
Ammonia Buffer	$-0.32v$ [3]	>1 µg/ml urine	D	Therapeutic urine levels fol-lowing repeated administration of 100 mg; also determination of NF 246; DC	Jones et al. (1965) [46]
0.1 N NaOH	$-0.59v$ [1]	$>0.2-0.3$ µg/ml blood	E	Therapeutic levels; DPP	de Silva et al. (1970) [69]
	$-0.62v$ [1]	>0.1 µg/ml plasma	E	Therapeutic levels in dog and man; DPP	Brooks et al. (1976) [70]
0.1N H_2SO_4	$-0.660v$ [1]	>0.25 µg/ml urine	E	Urinary excretion fol-lowing therapeutic levels; DPP	Brooks & de Silva (1975) [64]
0.15M citrate buffer (pH 4.9)-5% ethanol	$-0.948v$ [2]	$4-500$ µg/ml serum	D	DC	Jacobsen & Klevan (1972) [44]
Phosphate Buffer (pH 7.0)	$-0.38v$ [1]	$1-100$ µg/ml blood	E	Nitro derivative; blood levels following thera-peutic doses; DPP	Brooks et al. (1973) [79]
Britton-Robinson buffer (pH 3.5); DMF:0.1% gelatin (60:30:10)	$-0.39v$ [2]	>3.5 µg/ml plasma	E	Nitro derivative; plasma levels following therapeutic doses; also determination of methylphenobarbital; DC	Wiegrebe & Wehrhahn (1975) [80]
Britton-Robinson buffer (pH 3.5); DMF:0.1% gelatin (60:30:10)	$-0.408v$ [2]	>4 µg/ml plasma	E	Nitro derivative; plasma levels following therapeutic doses; DC	Wiegrebe & Wehrhahn (1975) [80]

TABLE 2

Generic Name	Systematic Name	Structure	Pharmacological Activity	Electro-phore	
Prothonamide	2-propylthioiso-nicotinamide	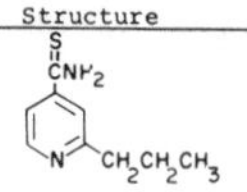	Antituberculant	$>C=S$	
Ro 7-0582	1-(3-methoxy-2-hydroxypropyl(-2-nitroimidazole	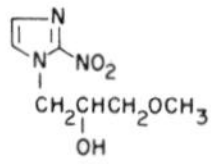	Radiosensitizer	$-NO_2$	
Trifluperidol	4'-fluoro-4-[hydroxy-4-(α,α,α-trifluoro-m-tolyl)piperidino]butyrophenone	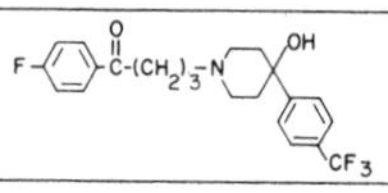	Antipsychotic	$>C=O$	
Trimethoprim	2,4-diamino-5(3,4,5-trimethoxybenzyl)-pyrimidine	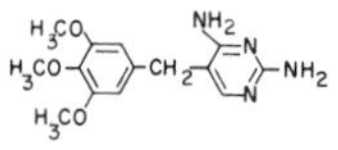	Antibacterial	$>C=N-$	
Vitamin C	L-ascorbic acid	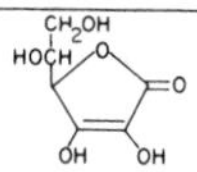	Vitamin	$-OH$	

^{a} Reference Electrodes ^{b} Isolation Technique
  1 - SCE   C - Chromatographic
  2 - Ag/AgCl   D - Direct (No Isolation)
  3 - Hg pool   E - Extraction
  4 - Ag wire   S - Steam Distillation

three structurally dissimilar compounds which contain either a nitro, azo-methine, or carbonyl group in their respective molecules can be polar-ographically resolved by scanning the sample in 0.1 N HCl from 0.0 V to (-) 1.20 V vs. SCE, where by DPP three peaks would be noted at approximately (-) 0.1 V ($-NO_2$) at (-) 0.5 V (azomethine) and at (-) 0.6 V (carbonyl). However, such a fortuitous set of conditions is rare.

Specificity and further clean-up can be ensured by TLC* of the organic extract followed by elution of the drug from the chromatoplate and subsequent voltammetric analysis. Quantitative elution from the TLC plate may require the use of an organic solvent, the residue of which is dissolved in the supporting electrolyte prior to analysis. DPP procedures in conjunction with TLC separation can be used for quantitation in the nanogram (10^{-9} g) concentration range with sensitivity limits comparable to GLC with

—————————

*See chapter "Thin Layer Chromatography" to be published in a future volume of this series.

(Continued)

Supporting Electrolyte	$E_{1/2}$ or E_p [a]	Concentration	Isolation [b]	Notes	Reference
2M borate buffer (pH 8.2)	$-1.2v^2$	50 µg/ml urine	D	Urinary excretion following 1 gram administration, AC	Bieder & Brunel (1971) [47]
0.1N NaOH	$-0.50v^1$	$>0.2-0.3$ µg/ml blood	E	Therapeutic levels after single dose; DPP	de Silva et al. (1970) [69]
	$-0.52v^1$	>0.1 µg/ml plasma	E	Therapeutic levels; DPP	Brooks et al. (1976) [70]
--	--	--	D	Levels in man following 3 g dose using method of Kane [39]; DC	Foster et al. (1975) [72]
Britton-Robinson buffer (pH 4.6): methanol (2:3)	$-1.32v^1$	10-50 µg/ml blood	E	Toxicological assay: blood levels following 80 mg/kg. dose to the rat; DC	Mikolajek et al. (1974) [73]
0.1N H_2SO_4	$-1.07v^1$	>0.5 µg/ml blood & urine	E	Blood and urine levels in man following 80 mg dose; DPP	Brooks et al. (1973) [76]
1M phosphate buffer (pH 3.0)	$-1.190v^1$	>0.5 µg/ml urine	E	Study of metabolic formation of N_1- and N_3-oxides in rat, dog and man	Brooks et al. (1973) [89]
0.07M acetate buffer (pH 4.75)	$+0.800v^2$	>15 µg/ml serum & urine	D	LC with carbon paste voltammetric detection; Zipax SAX column	Pachla & Kissinger (1976) [88]

flame ionization detection, HPLC with UV detection or spectroluminescence methods [37].

The analysis of urine is convenient in clinical pharmacokinetic studies since concentration is not usually as limited as in plasma. If 10 mg of a drug were administered and 50% were recovered in 1,000 ml of urine voided over the 0 to 24 h excretion period, the resulting concentration in the urine would be approximately 5 µg/ml. Cathode ray and differential pulse polarography are ideally suited for quantitation in this concentration range. Chlorpromazine and its sulfoxide metabolite have been determined by CRP in the urine of patients receiving 100 mg of the drug [48]. Endogenous interfering constituents were removed by an Amberlite resin [IRA-400 (C1)] column, followed by polarographic determination of the sulfoxide at -0.75 V vs. a mercury pool electrode. Chlorpromazine was oxidized to the sulfoxide using bromine, and the total sulfoxide content was also determined. The concentration of chlorpromazine was then calculated by difference. Beckett et al. [49] used CRP for the determination of chlorpromazine and its metabolites in biological fluids following extraction.

Disulfiram was determined by CRP following selective extraction into chloroform from urine buffered to pH 8.0 [50]. Polarography was performed in ethanolic-hydrochloric acid in the concentration range of 0.5 to 2.0 μg/ml. Recovery ranged from 85 and 95%, respectively, at the above limits of quantitation.

Dantrolene-sodium and its nonreduced and reduced metabolites were determined in urine after ethyl acetate extraction using DPP [51]. The residue of the ethyl acetate extract was analyzed for dantrolene sodium plus the reduced and nonreduced metabolites using the reduction of the azomethine group at -0.86 V vs. SCE in dimethylformamide-acetate buffer (pH 4.0). The nitro compounds were simultaneously quantitated in the same medium as dantrolene equivalents using the reduction of the nitro group at -0.26 V vs. SCE. The difference between the two determinations represented the reduced metabolites. Concentrations as low as 0.1 μg/ml were determined for either functional group.

Polarographic methods have been extensively used for the determination of the urinary excretion of 1,4-benzodiazepines, due mainly to the facile reduction of the azomethine ($>C_5=N_4-$) group in the molecule. Diazepam and its major metabolites, nordiazepam and oxazepam, were analyzed following acid hydrolysis to their respective benzophenones which were extracted and used to measure the urinary excretion of diazepam [52]. DPP analysis was used to measure the urinary excretion of bromazepam and its major metabolites in man following a single 12-mg dose [53]. Selective extraction of the conjugated metabolites (3-hydroxybromazepam and 2-amino-3-hydroxy-5-bromobenzoyl pyridine) and the unconjugated metabolites (bromazepam and 2-amino-5-bromobenzoyl pyridine) into separate diethyl ether fractions was used in the assay. The residues of the respective extracts were dissolved in phosphate buffer (pH 5.4) and analyzed by DPP which yielded two distinct well-resolved reduction peaks for the 4,5-azomethine functional group of the benzodiazepine-2-one and for the carbonyl functional group of the benzoyl pyridine in each fraction, (Fig. 9). DPP assays have also been reported for the determination of the urinary excretion of 7-chloro-1,3-dihydro-5-(2'-chlorophenyl)-2H-1,4-benzodiazepin-2-one as the 3-hydroxy metabolite; lorazepam [54], clonazepam [55], flurazepam [56], and their respective major metabolites.

The assay for flurazepam involved analysis of the three major metabolites using a combination of selective extraction, TLC separation, and DPP analysis to measure urinary excretion following a 90-mg oral dose. A direct assay with phosphate buffer (pH 7.0) was also described as a rapid means of measuring total benzodiazepines to confirm ingestion of flurazepam. The DPP assays [53-56] for the 1,4-benzodiazepin-2-ones typically had sensitivity limits of 0.1 to 0.2 μg/ml, which were more than sufficient to determine the urinary excretion of these compounds.

A toxicological assay for chlordiazepoxide or diazepam using DC polarography was described [57]. It required a large volume of blood (10 ml)

to confirm the ingestion of an overdosage of either drug. The blood sample
was made alkaline with Na_2CO_3 solution and extracted into diethyl ether.
The compound was back-extracted into 3 ml of 1.0 N HCl and analyzed by
DC polarography ($E_{1/2}$ = -0.67 and -0.70 V vs. SCE for chlordiazepoxide
and diazepam, respectively). The assay was relatively insensitive with a
limit of detection 10 μg/10 ml sample.

Chlordiazepoxide and its plasma metabolites were determined by DPP
[58]. The assay involved the extraction of chlordiazepoxide and its metabolites from plasma buffered to pH 9.0 followed by a TLC separation, elution, and determination of the three compounds in 0.1 N H_2SO_4. The sensitivity limit of the assay was 0.05 to 0.1 μg for each compound per ml of
plasma with a 2-ml sample. The assay was used to measure plasma levels
of parent drug and metabolites following a single 30-mg i.v. and oral dose
and following multiple oral administration of 30-mg doses.

The determinations of diazepam in plasma by CRP [59] and by DPP [60]
with sensitivity limits of 0.03 and 0.2 μg/ml have been described. A specific
DPP assay for diazepam [61] differed from the other polarographic assays
[59, 60] in that the more polar solvent diethyl ether was used to ensure
quantitative extraction along with a TLC separation step for the determination of both diazepam and N-desmethyldiazepam the major blood metabolite.

Voltammetric assays for the determination of bromazepam [11, 62] and
flurazepam [11, 63] in blood with nanogram sensitivity by DPP or CRP have
been reported. The determination of 1,4-benzodiazepines in biological
fluids using DPP has recently been reviewed [64].

The nitroimidazole class of antibacterial compounds were among the
first to be analyzed by DC polarography directly in biological samples [39].
The nitro group is an excellent electrophore and can be determined with
nanogram sensitivity using DPP. Solvent extraction followed by analysis
with or without TLC separation was utilized effectively in bioavailability
studies. Compounds of the 5-nitroimidazole class such as dimetridazole
(histamonostat) [39, 65-67], ipronidazole (histamonostat) [68], metronidazole (trichomonicide) [39, 70], ornidazole (amoebicide) [69, 70], and the
use of metronidazole [71] and a 2-nitroimidazole analog (Ro7-0582) (radio-
sensitizer in cancer chemotherapy) [69, 70, 72], have been reported. They
have all been analyzed following solvent extraction with sensitivity in the
range of 0.1 to 0.2 μg/ml of blood or plasma. The analysis of ornidazole
in plasma following a single oral dose of 10 mg/kg in a dog did not show
any serious interference due to the presence of metabolites [70] as determined by direct analysis compared to analysis following TLC separation.
The absence of interfering metabolites may have been due to the poor
recovery of the more polar metabolites from plasma. However, chronic
dosing may reveal the presence of significant amounts of metabolites which
may be extracted in sufficient amounts requiring TLC separation prior to
quantitation to ensure specificity.

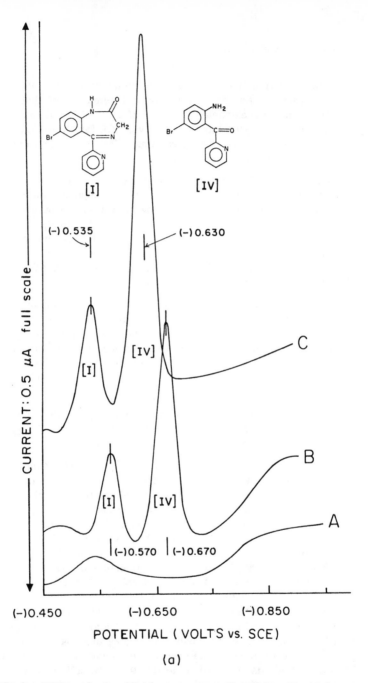

FIG. 9. DPP analysis of (a) bromazepam (I) and 2-amino-5-bromo-benzoylpyridine (IV) and (b) 3-hydroxybromazepam (II), and 2-amino-3-hydroxy-5-bromo-benzoylpyridine (V) in 1.0 M pH 5.5 phosphate buffer:

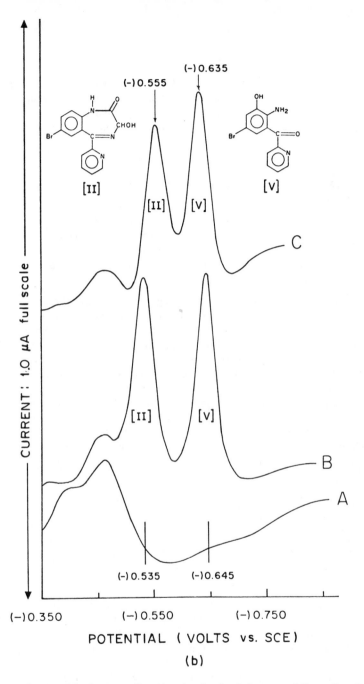

A, control urine blank; B, authentic standard mixture; and C, authentic compounds recovered from urine. (Reprinted from Ref. 53 by permission of the American Pharmaceutical Association.)

Other types of functional groups that have been used for voltammetric analysis include the reduction of the carbonyl group in the butyrophenones, such as haloperidol and triflurperidol [73], the oxidation of the phenolic hydroxy group in methyl dopa [74, 75], and the pyrimidine-azomethine group in trimethoprim [76].

B. Analyses Following Chemical Derivatization

Compounds that do not possess functional groups having electrochemical activity can be derivatized to yield electroactive compounds. The generally used derivatization reactions have been discussed previously. Aromatic phenyl compounds can be nitrated using 10% KNO_3/H_2SO_4; the nitro derivatives are extracted and analyzed.

Glibornuride, a tolylsulfonylurea hypoglyceamic agent [77, 78], phenobarbital and diphenylhydantoin [79, 80], and mephenytoin and primaclone [80] have all been determined after extraction from blood as their nitro derivatives. Blood levels of glibornuride were measured following the administration of single 50- and 100-mg doses [77] and following multiple oral doses of 25 mg [78]. The recovery of the assay was $80.7\% \pm 8.0$ (S. D.) with a sensitivity limit of 0.05 to 0.10 $\mu g/ml$ using a 2-ml sample/assay [77]. The determination of phenobarbital and diphenylhydantoin from blood with recoveries of $72.3\% \pm 6.5$ (S. D.) and $76.7\% \pm 2.3$ (S. D.), respectively had a sensitivity limit of 1 to 2 $\mu g/ml$, using a TLC separation step for specificity [79]. The utility of voltammetric methods in the analysis of drugs in biological fluids is therefore well documented (Table 2).

VII. ANCILLARY TECHNIQUES USING VOLTAMMETRIC
        METHODS

A. Voltammetric Detectors for High Performance
     Liquid Chromatography*

Differential pulse polarography has an absolute sensitivity limit of approximately 10^{-8} M, and thus sensitive determinations of drugs in biological fluids [11] are only possible when the volume of the final solution to be assayed is reduced. A working volume of 0.5 ml is probably the smallest feasible with the conventional three electrode assembly due to the build-up of mercury in the cell and the resultant shorting of the electrodes during

---

*See chapter "High Performance Liquid Chromatography" to be published in a future volume of this series.

analysis. Consequently, much effort has been directed towards the construction of microcells (volume ~50-100 μl) which will employ a DME with a continuous flow to remove the build-up of mercury [81, 82]. Others have employed solid electrodes in micro flow cells of volumes of less than 10 μl to attain sensitivities for solid electrode voltammetry which approach the sensitivity of DPP.

These micro flow cells can be placed "on-line" with the effluent of a high performance liquid chromatograph to serve as a detector with high sensitivity and selectivity [83, 84]. Specificity is extremely important in the analysis of drugs from biological fluids where the compound of interest must be separated from metabolites and endogenous interferences derived from the biological matrix. The feasibility of the use of the electrochemical detectors in high performance liquid chromatography (HPLC) for compounds of biological importance was demonstrated by Kissinger et al. [85] who designed a carbon paste voltammetric detector for liquid chromatography having a dead-volume of less than 1 μl capacity. Detection was feasible in the 50 to 100 pg range. The detector was used for the oxidative analysis of biogenic amines such as dopamine, 6-hydroxydopamine, and L-dopa [75, 86, 87]. Compounds such as uric acid, ascorbic acid, catecholamines, and related tyrosine metabolites could also be measured in serum and urine [88]. The use of electrochemical detectors for HPLC shows promise for sensitive and specific quantitation of a variety of compounds [31].

B. Metabolism Studies

Functional group analysis by DPP can be a useful ancillary technique in structure elucidation of metabolites isolated either from in vitro incubates or from biological specimens. The loss of a predominant functional group such as the nitro group by reduction to the amine, a carbonyl group to an alcohol, or the introduction of a new functional group such as an N-oxide can be readily determined [89] (Fig. 10).

C. Protein Binding Studies*

The binding characteristics of a drug can modify the pharmacological response exerted by a therapeutic agent. The strength and extent to which a drug binds to plasma albumin may markedly affect its distribution, metabolism, and excretion characteristics as well as its onset and duration of activity. Several studies have been reported which measure steady-

*See also Volume 1, Chapter 5: Protein Binding.

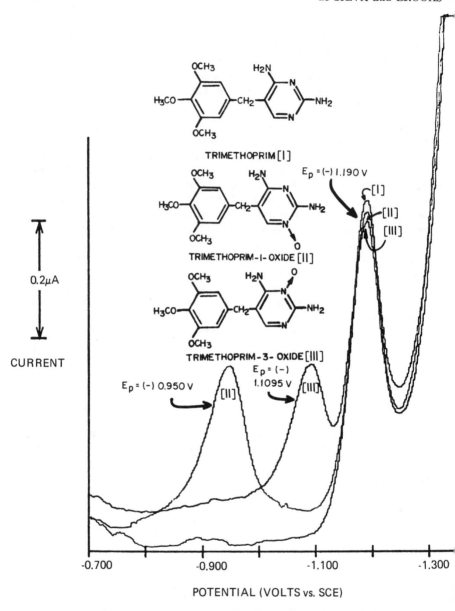

FIG. 10. DPP of trimethoprim and its N-oxide metabolites in 1 M phosphate buffer (pH 3). (Reprinted from Ref. 89 by permission of the American Pharmaceutical Association.)

state and nonsteady-state transport through membranes and the binding
of drugs to macromolecules using rotating disc electrode polarography
[90, 91]. A recent study on the binding of 1,4-benzodiazepines using DPP
showed correlations between the extent of binding and the lipophilicity of
the compound [92].

D. Physicochemical Studies

The facile reduction of the $(>C_5=N_4-)$ azomethine of the 1,4-benzodiazepine
class of compounds has led to an extensive study of these compounds.
Correlations between the $E_{1/2}$ or E_p (half-wave or peak potential) with
different substituent groups on the molecule have been used to predict the
reduction mechanisms involved [93, 94] and the relationship of E_p of a
compound to Hammett constants for the substituent groups involved [95].

E. Permeability Studies

Transport of drugs across the lipoidal intestinal mucosa, e.g., a segment
of the everted rat intestine, is a viable means of assessing the permeability
characteristics of drugs during their biopharmaceutical evaluation [96].
DPP analysis is readily amenable to the analysis of drug concentrations
that traverse the lumen of the intestine [97]. Such a study on the permeability of several 1,4-benzodiazepines was recently reported [61].

F. Automated Polarographic Analysis

Automated analysis of discrete samples using the Technicon Auto Analyzer
principle is widely used in chemical, pharmaceutical, and clinical chemical analysis. The design of polarographic flow through cells for this type
of analysis was recently reported [98].

G. Tissue Analysis

The analysis of drugs in tissues is pertinent to forensic toxicology for the
identification of the drugs ingested in cases of death due to either accidental

or intentional overdosage. It is also required in trace residue level
analysis for therapeutic agents used in veterinary medicine to establish
the clearance of a drug and its metabolites from edible organs and the car-
cass before it can be certified as fit for human consumption prior to mar-
keting. Trace residue analysis of veterinary products involves such
compounds as coccidiostats used in the poultry industry, antibiotics such
as sulfonamides, antihelminthics used against intestinal parasites, and
other agricultural products such as insecticides and herbicides which can
be ingested by grazing farm animals. The FDA has established stringent
specifications for low residue levels in the part per million (ppm), i. e.,
10^{-6} g to part per billion (ppb), i. e., 10^{-9} g range before the animal product can be marketed. All edible organs have to be analyzed for concentrations in the μg to ng/g range depending on the drug. DPP has been used
successfully in residue level analysis of a number of coccidiostats such as
the nitroimidazoles [39, 65-68] and nicarbazin, an equimolar complex of
(4, 4'-dinitrocarbanilide and 2-hydroxy-4, 6-dimethylpyrimide) [99].

VIII. CONCLUSION

Voltammetric techniques have been shown to be applicable to the analysis
of drugs in biological materials. Differential pulse polarography, in particular, is a most sensitive technique for the analysis of subnanogram concentrations of drugs in biological fluids. A very attractive feature of its
use in trace-level analysis is specificity of detection. Analyses can be
performed with a simple extract, protein-free filtrate, a dilution of the
original specimen (e.g., urine), or after TLC separation of an extract
with a minimum of sample clean-up or preparation. This is possible
because of the low electroactive background obtained from biological specimens in relation to the electroactive species to be analyzed. Thus, small
amounts of a drug can be detected specifically and with high sensitivity
(especially those possessing a nitro, carbonyl, azomethine, or azo-dye
electrophore) against a larger background of a nonelectroactive sample
matrix. In principle the phenomenon is analogous to that occurring in
electron capture detection in GLC. The technique is thus superior to
absorptiometric analysis in the UV or visible regions which are normally
affected by high "blanks" or interference from extracted materials present
in the matrix to be analyzed. The sensitivity and specificity of modern
polarographic techniques and instrumentation are well documented and
warrant their use in the development of submicrogram level analytical
methods.

REFERENCES

1. P. Zuman and M. Brezina, in Progress in Polarography, Vol. II
    (P. Zuman and I. M. Kolthoff, eds.), Wiley (Interscience), New
    York, 1962, pp. 687-701.
2. R. J. Gajan, in Methods in Pharmacology, Vol. II: Physical
    Methods (C. F. Chignell, ed.), Appleton-Century-Crofts, New York,
    1972, pp. 443-463.
3. J. E. Page, J. Pharm. Pharmacol., 4, 1 (1952).
4. W. F. Smyth, Proc. Soc. Anal. Chem., 10, 9 (1973).
5. K. Stulik and J. Zyka, Chemist-Analyst, 55, 120 (1966).
6. M. A. Brooks, in Laboratory Techniques in Electroanalytical Chem-
    istry (P. T. Kissinger, ed.), Dekker, New York, to be published.
7. H. Hoffmann and J. Volke, in Advances in Analytical Chemistry
    and Instrumentation, Vol. 10: Electroanalytical Chemistry
    (H. W. Nurnberg, ed.), Wiley, New York, 1974, pp. 287-334.
8. P. O. Kane, Nature, 183, 1674 (1959).
9. H. Oelschläger, Arch. Pharm. (Weinheim), 296, 396 (1963).
10. H. Oelschläger, J. Volke, and E. Kurek, Arch. Pharm. (Weinheim),
    297, 431 (1964).
11. M. A. Brooks and M. R. Hackman, Anal. Chem., 47, 2059 (1975).
12. J. Heyrovsky, Chem. Listy, 16, 256 (1922).
13. M. Shikata, Trans. Faraday Soc., 21, 42, 53 (1925).
14. P. Zuman, Organic Polarographic Analysis, Pergamon Press,
    Oxford, 1964, pp. 1-313.
15. P. Zuman, in Advances in Analytical Chemistry and Instrumentation,
    Vol. 2 (C. N. Reilly, ed.), Wiley (Interscience), New York, 1963,
    pp. 219-253.
16. J. B. Flato, Anal. Chem., 44, 75A (1972).
17. D. Ilkovic, Collect. Czech. Chem. Commun., 6, 498 (1934).
18. I. M. Kolthoff and J. J. Lingane, Polarography, Vol. I, 2nd ed.,
    Wiley (Interscience), New York, 1965, pp. 3-184.
19. L. Meites, Polarographic Techniques, 2nd ed., Wiley (Interscience),
    New York, 1965, pp. 95-331.
20. D. R. Crow and J. V. Westwood, Polarography: Metheun's Mono-
    graphs on Chemical Subjects, Methuen and Co. Ltd., London, 1968,
    pp. 1-61.
21. J. Heyrovsky and P. Zuman, Practical Polarography, Academic
    Press, New York, 1968, pp. 1-42.
22. A. Weissberger, Physical Methods of Chemistry: Techniques of
    Chemistry, Vol. 1, Part IIA, Wiley (Interscience), New York,
    1971, pp. 297-421.
23. G. C. Barker and A. W. Gardner, Anal. Chem., 173, 79 (1960).

24. R. A. Osteryoung and E. P. Parry, J. Electroanal. Chem., 9, 299 (1965).

25. E. P. Parry and R. A. Osteryoung, Anal. Chem., 36, 1366 (1964).

26. E. P. Parry and R. A. Osteryoung, Anal. Chem., 37, 1634 (1965).

27. H. Oelschläger, J. Volke, H. Hoffmann, and E. Kurek, Arch. Pharm. (Weinheim), 300, 250 (1967).

28. H. Schmidt and M. von Stackelberg, Modern Polarographic Methods, Academic Press, New York, 1963, pp. 29-51.

29. B. Breyer and H. U. Bauer, Alternating Current Polarography and Tensammetry, Wiley (Interscience), New York, 1963, pp. 1-94.

30. J. Heyrovsky and J. Foreyt, Z. Phys. Chem. (Leipzig), 193, 77 (1943).

31. B. Fleet and C. J. Little, J. Chromatogr. Sci., 12, 747 (1974).

32. P. T. Kissinger, C. Refshauge, R. Dreiling, and R. N. Adams, Anal. Lett., 6, 465 (1973).

33. Modern Analytical Polarography Workshop Manual (G. W. O'Dom and H. Siegerman, eds.), Princeton Applied Research Corporation, Princeton, 1973, Section V, pp. 6-14.

34. C. K. Mann, in Electroanalytical Chemistry, Vol. 3 (A. J. Bard, ed.), Dekker, New York, 1969, pp. 57-134.

35. B. Brodie and W. M. Heller (eds.), Bioavailability of Drugs, Karger, Basle, 1972, pp. 1-213.

36. J. A. F. de Silva, in Current Concepts in the Pharmaceutical Sciences: Biopharmaceutics (J. Swarbrick, ed.), Lea and Febiger, Philadelphia, 1970, pp. 203-264.

37. M. A. Brooks, "The Polarographic Determination of Psychotropic, Hypnotic and Sedative Drugs," in Polarographic Determination of Compounds of Biological Significance (W. F. Smyth, ed.), MacMillan, New York, 1977, in press.

38. P. O. Kane, Nature, 195, 495 (1962).

39. P. O. Kane, J. Polarogr. Sci., 7, 58 (1961).

40. J. Fidelus, M. Zietek, A. M. Kolajek, and Z. Grochowska, Mikrochim. Acta (Wien), 1972, 84.

41. J. Fidelus, M. Zietek, and A. M. Kolajek, Z. Anal. Chemie, 256, 131 (1971).

42. E. Jacobsen and T. V. Jacobsen, Anal. Chim. Acta, 55, 293 (1971).

43. S. Halvorsen and E. Jacobsen, Anal. Chim. Acta, 59, 127 (1972).

44. E. Jacobsen and K. H. Klevan, Anal. Chim. Acta, 62, 405 (1972).

45. I. Lauermann and L. Otto, Wiss. Z. Martin-Luther-Univ., Halle-Wittenberg, Math.-Naturwiss, Reihe, 17, 56 (1968); and Anal. Abstr., 19, 4146 (1970).

46. B. M. Jones, R. J. M. Ratcliffe, and S. G. E. Stevens, J. Pharm. Pharmacol., Suppl., 17, 52S (1965).

47. A. Bieder and P. Brunel, Ann. Pharm. Fr., 29, 461 (1971).

48. G. S. Porter and J. Beresford, J. Pharm. Pharmacol., 18, 223 (1966).

49.   A. H. Beckett, E. E. Essein, and W. F. Smyth, J. Pharm. Pharmacol., 26, 399 (1973).
50.   G. S. Porter and A. Williams, J. Pharm. Pharmacol., Suppl., 24, 144P (1972).
51.   P. L. Cox, J. P. Heotis, D. Polin, and G. M. Rose, J. Pharm. Sci., 58, 987 (1969).
52.   R. Dugal, G. Caille, and S. F. Cooper, Un. Med. Can., 102, 2491 (1973).
53.   J. A. F. de Silva, I. Bekersky, M. A. Brooks, R. E. Weinfeld, W. Glover, and C. V. Puglisi, J. Pharm. Sci., 63, 1440 (1974).
54.   J. A. F. de Silva, I. Bekersky, and M. A. Brooks, J. Pharm. Sci., 63, 1943 (1974).
55.   J. A. F. de Silva, C. V. Puglisi, and N. Munno, J. Pharm. Sci., 63, 520 (1974).
56.   J. A. F. de Silva, C. V. Puglisi, M. A. Brooks, and M. R. Hackman, J. Chromatogr., 99, 461 (1974).
57.   G. Cimbura and R. C. Gupta, J. Forensic Sci., 10, 228 (1965).
58.   M. R. Hackman, M. A. Brooks, J. A. F. de Silva, and T. S. Ma, Anal. Chem., 46, 1075 (1974).
59.   D. J. Berry, Clin. Chim. Acta, 32, 235 (1971).
60.   E. Jacobsen, T. V. Jacobsen, and T. Rojahn, Anal. Chim. Acta, 64, 473 (1973).
61.   M. A. Brooks, J. A. F. de Silva, and M. R. Hackman, Amer. Lab., 5, (9), 23 (1973).
62.   F. I. Sengün and H. Oelschläger, Arch. Pharm. (Weinheim), 308, 720-723 (1975).
63.   J. M. Clifford, M. R. Smyth, and W. F. Smyth, Z. Anal. Chemie, 272, 198 (1974).
64.   M. A. Brooks and J. A. F. de Silva, Talanta, 22, 849 (1975).
65.   P. C. Allen, J. Assn. Offic. Anal. Chem., 55, 743 (1972).
66.   P. C. Allen and D. K. McLoughlin, J. Assn. Offic. Anal. Chem., 55, 1159 (1972).
67.   M. J. Parnell, Pestic. Sci., 4, 643 (1973).
68.   A. MacDonald, E. Castro, G. Chen, and P. Hopkins, Poultry Sci., 48, 1837 (1969).
69.   J. A. F. de Silva, N. Munno, and N. Strojny, J. Pharm. Sci., 59, 201 (1970).
70.   M. A. Brooks, L. D'Arconte, and J. A. F. de Silva, J. Pharm. Sci., 65, 112 (1976).
71.   G. Deutsch, J. L. Foster, J. A. MacFadzeam, and M. Parnell, Brit. J. Cancer, 31, 75 (1975).
72.   J. L. Foster, I. R. Flockhart, S. Dische, A. Gray, I. Lenox-Smith, and C. E. Smithen, Brit. J. Cancer, 31, 679 (1975).
73.   A. Mikolajek, A. Krzyzanowska, and J. Fidelus, Z. Anal. Chem., 272, 39 (1974).

74. J. T. Stewart, H. C. Lo, and W. D. Mason, J. Pharm. Sci., 63,
     956 (1974).
75. R. M. Riggin, R. L. Alcorn, and P. T. Kissinger, Clin. Chem.,
     22, 782 (1976).
76. M. A. Brooks, J. A. F. de Silva, and L. D'Arconte, Anal.
     Chem., 45, 263 (1973).
77. J. A. F. de Silva and M. R. Hackman, Anal. Chem., 44, 1145
     (1972).
78. U. C. Dubach, A. Korn, and J. Raaflaub, Arzneim.-Forsch., 25,
     1967 (1975).
79. M. A. Brooks, J. A. F. de Silva, and M. R. Hackman, Anal. Chim.
     Acta, 64, 165 (1973).
80. W. Wiegrebe and L. Wehrhahn, Arzneim.-Forsch., 25, 517
     (1975).
81. J. G. Koen, J. F. K. Huber, H. Poppe, and G. den Boef,
     J. Chromatogr. Sci., 8, 192 (1970).
82. R. Stillman and T. S. Ma, Mikrochim. Acta, (Wien), 1973, 491.
83. P. L. Joynes and R. J. Maggs, J. Chromatogr. Sci., 8, 427 (1970).
84. A. MacDonald and P. D. Duke, J. Chromatogr., 83, 331 (1970).
85. P. T. Kissinger, C. Refshauge, R. Dreiling, and R. N. Adams,
     Anal. Lett., 6, 465 (1973).
86. P. T. Kissinger, L. J. Felice, R. M. Riggin, L. A. Pachla, and
     D. C. Wenke, Clin. Chem., 20, 992 (1974).
87. P. T. Kissinger, R. M. Riggin, R. L. Alcorn, and L. D. Rau,
     Biochem. Med., 13, 299 (1975).
88. L. A. Pachla and P. T. Kissinger, Anal. Chem., 48, 364 (1976).
89. M. A. Brooks, J. A. F. de Silva, and L. D'Arconte, J. Pharm.
     Sci., 62, 1395 (1973).
90. Y. W. Chen, C. L. Olson, and T. Sokoloski, J. Pharm. Sci.,
     62, 435 (1973).
91. Y. W. Chen, T. Sokoloski, C. L. Olson, D. T. Witiak, and
     R. Nazareth, J. Pharm. Sci., 62, 440 (1973).
92. R. W. Lucek and C. B. Coutinho, Mol. Pharmacol., 12, 612 (1976).
93. J. M. Clifford and W. F. Smyth, Z. Anal. Chem., 264, 149 (1973).
94. J. Barrett, W. F. Smyth, and J. P. Hart, J. Pharm. Pharmacol.,
     26, 9 (1974).
95. M. A. Brooks, J. J. Bel Bruno, J. A. F. de Silva, and M. R.
     Hackman, Anal. Chim. Acta, 74, 367 (1975).
96. S. A. Kaplan, in Current Concepts in the Pharmaceutical Sciences:
     Dosage Form Design and Bioavailability (J. Swarbrick, ed.), Lea
     and Febiger, Philadelphia, 1974, pp. 1-30.
97. S. A. Kaplan and S. Cotler, J. Pharm. Sci., 61, 1361 (1972).
98. W. Lund and L. N. Opheim, Anal. Chim. Acta, 79, 35 (1975).
99. R. F. Michielli and G. V. Downing, J. Agr. Food Chem., 22, 449
     (1974).
100. J. Birner, Anal. Chem., 33, 1955 (1961).

Chapter 2

GAS-LIQUID CHROMATOGRAPHY

W. J. A. VandenHeuvel

Department of Animal Drug Metabolism and Radiochemistry
Merck Sharp & Dohme Research Laboratories
Rahway, New Jersey

and

A. G. Zacchei

Department of Drug Metabolism
Merck Sharp & Dohme Research Laboratories
West Point, Pennsylvania

I. INTRODUCTION

An analysis by gas-liquid chromatography (GLC) yields two types of data:
the retention times of the sample components and the responses the latter
evoke from the detection system employed. Although the chromatographic
process occurs only in the column, the detector (whether it be a simple
system designed to respond to pH changes, the experienced nose of an
organoleptic analyst, an insect responding to an eluted hormone, or a
sophisticated electronic device) is an integral component of a GLC system
and is usually regarded as such. The separation aspects of GLC are exemplified in the biological area by the multicomponent analyses or "metabolic profiles" reported by Horning and Horning [1] and Zlatkis and coworkers [2] using high efficiency columns and temperature programming.
Another use of a GLC column, equally valid in the appropriate circumstances, is as a simple delivery system to a selective detector without
regard for separation of the components of interest from anything but perhaps the injection solvent.

Regardless of the detection system employed in GLC, the chemical
nature of the sample must be such that it possesses a suitable vapor pressure under the column conditions and is not subject to significant adsorption or "loss on the column." Thanks to the use of thin films of stationary
phases [3], the column temperatures required for compounds of moderate
molecular weight (300-600) are not so great as to cause thermal degradation of most compounds [4]. Deactivated supports (the packing or capillary
column surfaces) facilitate the successful GLC of submicrogram samples;
this is true, however, only for those compounds not possessing multiple
"polar" functional groups. Many drugs and especially their metabolites
are polar organic compounds and cannot be analyzed directly by GLC.
Indeed, it appears in many instances that desirable GLC properties are
inversely proportional to the pharmacological activity of compounds. Thus
if GLC methodology is to be widely employed in drug metabolism studies,
derivatization -- organic chemistry at the microgram level -- must be
employed to convert polar functional groups to less polar moieties. Once
reproducible and quantitative conversion to derivatives amenable to gas
phase analysis can be achieved, GLC can be brought to bear upon quantification and metabolite structure problems, allowing an understanding of
the fate of drugs. Furthermore, it can be assumed that GLC methods
will increasingly provide pharmaceutical chemists, clinical pharmacolo-
gists, pharmacists, and other health professionals with the bioavailability
data necessary for the evaluation of drugs. Lest GLC be extolled in too
one-sided a fashion, it should be stated that the rapidly developing field of
high-performance liquid chromatography (HPLC) offers much to drug
metabolism, especially because certain polar compounds may be analyzed
without derivatization and the mobile phase can be varied. Another tech-

nique, polarography, can serve as a highly sensitive and selective quantitation approach with drugs possessing reducible functional groups. But at least for the next few years, or until HPLC is successfully combined with the remarkable array of detectors now coupled with GLC (e.g., hydrogen flame ionization, electron capture, nitrogen-selective, radioactivity monitoring, mass spectrometric) it will be methods of gas phase analysis that will be employed most extensively in drug metabolism studies. A compilation of literature references to the GLC of various drugs is presented in Table 1.

TABLE 1

Literature References to the GLC of Various Drugs

Drug	Reference
Alprenolol	[25]
Amitriptyline	[121-124, 127, 175, 176, 242]
Amphetamine metabolites	[206]
Anticonvulsants	[177]
Antiepileptics	[53, 64]
Atenolol	[30]
Barbiturates	[30, 40, 49, 52, 67, 71, 112, 178]
Benzodiazepines	[117]
1, 2-Bis(3, 5-dioxopiperazinyl)propane	[36]
Bromazepam	[16]
3-Bromo-5-cyanobenzenesulfonamide	[113]
Bumetamide	[62]
Cambendazole	[78]
Camphor metabolites	[21]
Cannabinol	[168]
Carbamazepine	[80, 115, 181]
Chloral hydrate	[185]
Chlordiazepoxide	[201]
Chlorooxazepam	[80]
Chlorphenesin carbamate	[76]
Chlorpromazine and metabolites	[209]
Chlorpropamide	[42, 63]
Chlorthalidone	[69]
Clonazepam	[14]
Cocaine	[56]

TABLE 1 (Continued)

Drug	Reference
Cortisone	[97]
Cyclophosphamide	[169]
Cyproheptadine metabolites	[155]
Dapsone	[77, 126]
Desimipramine	[175]
Diethylhexylphthalate	[219]
Diftalone	[244]
1', 2'-Dihydro-(-)-zearalenone and metabolites	[216]
Diisopyramide	[173]
Dimethisterone metabolite	[223]
1-(2, 6-Dimethylphenoxy)-2-aminopropane	[147]
Dimethyltryptamine	[192, 193]
Diphenylhydantoin and metabolites	[50, 51, 55]
Ecdysones	[143]
Ethosuximide	[68]
N-Ethyl-N-methylaniline and metabolites	[207]
5-Ethyl-5-phenylhydantoin	[53]
Fenoprofen	[75]
Fenfluramine and metabolites	[208]
Floropipamide	[80]
Flurbiprofen	[109]
Furosemide	[72]
Flunitrazepam	[14]
Flurazepam	[31]
Fomocaine metabolite	[220]
Glucuronide conjugates	[48, 86-93, 95]
Glutethimide	[34, 40, 52, 112, 229, 230]
Heroin (diacetylmorphine)	[179]
Hydrochlorothiazide	[61]
Ibuprofen	[45, 129, 130]
Imipramine	[121-123, 175]
Indomethacin	[8]
Lidocaine	[180]
Lorazepam	[140, 141]
Lorazepam glucuronide	[95]
Mephenytoin	[53]
Mephobarbital	[53]
Meprobamate	[34]
Mesoridazine metabolite	[225, 226]

TABLE 1 (Continued)

Drug	Reference
Methapyrilene	[170]
2-Methyl-4-(5-nitro-2-furyl)thiazole	[210]
Methylphenidate	[118, 119]
Methylphenobarbitone	[66]
Methyprylon	[34]
Mitotane metabolites	[234]
MK-196	[184]
MK-251	[146]
MK-647 metabolites	[222]
Morphine	[15]
Nitrazepam	[70]
Nitrooxazepam	[80]
Norethindrone	[100]
Norethisterone	[223]
Nortriptyline	[175, 176]
Oxazepam	[80]
Oxazepam glucuronide	[95]
α-[4-(1-Oxo-2-isoindolinyl)phenyl] propionic acid	[47, 130]
Oxprenol	[25]
Perphenazine	[28]
Pethidine	[243]
β-Phenethylbiguanide and metabolite	[240]
Phenmetrazine	[145]
Phenobarbital	[53, 59, 60, 66]
Phenothiazines	[23]
Phenylbutazone	[54]
Phenylbutazone metabolites	[58]
Phenytoin	[53]
Pilocarpine	[182]
Practolol	[25, 144]
Primidone	[53]
Probenecid	[43, 44]
Pronethalol	[25]
Propranolol	[25]
Propranolol glucuronides	[91]
Propoxyphene and metabolite	[233]
Prostaglandin Es and metabolites	[101-104, 159-162]
Prostaglandin $F_{2\alpha}$	[105, 108, 157, 158]
Pyrimethamine	[183]

TABLE 1 (Continued)

Drug	Reference
Quinidine	[57]
Rafoxanide	[81]
Ro5-3027	[140]
Ronidazole	[77]
Sotalol	[25]
Sulfaquinoxaline	[96]
Sulindac metabolite	[232]
Sulfate conjugates	[83-85]
Δ^9-Tetrahydrocannabinol	[27, 168]
Thioridazine metabolite	[225, 226]
Tilidine	[231]
Tolbutamide	[41, 42, 235]
Tolmetin	[241]
Triethylammonium cyclamate	[142]
Warfarin	[26, 37]

II.   ISOLATION PROCEDURES

The analysis of drugs and their metabolites in biological matrices usually cannot be accomplished solely by GLC techniques. It is essential in most instances to utilize one or more preliminary purification steps to isolate the material from the biological specimen. Typical procedures employed in this initial "clean-up" step involve solvent partitioning under pH control and column and/or thin-layer chromatographic (TLC) approaches. * Isolation and clean-up methods, although of obvious importance, will be discussed only with respect to providing an isolate which is amenable to GLC analysis. The extent to which preliminary separation is required depends upon the concentration of the compound to be analyzed and the degree to which endogenous substances lead to possible interference. Only the most rudimentary sample isolation procedures are necessary when the concentration of drug and/or metabolites is high (>20 μg/ml). However, extensive purification may be necessary when one is trying to analyze nanogram levels of drug, especially if closely related in GLC properties to endogenous components. In some instances the need for extensive purification

---

*See chapters "Liquid Extraction and Isolation," "Liquid Chromatography," and "Thin-Layer Chromatography" to be published in future volumes of this series.

may be eliminated if one can employ a selective detector (e.g., electron capture, selective ion, etc.).

During the process of isolation or concentration care must be exercised to prevent volatilization or adsorption of the compound when low levels (< 1 μg) of drug or metabolite are analyzed. To prevent such volatilization, basic or acidic compounds can be converted to salts by the addition of trace amounts of acid or base, respectively. The deleterious effects of such losses are minimized by the addition of an internal standard/carrier at the initial step in the isolation procedure.

The authors have previously described some of the techniques used in sample isolation and preparation prior to GLC analysis [5]. Sohn et al. [6] discuss the methods currently employed in the clean-up procedures in drug screening. They state that solvent partitioning followed by TLC and/or GLC are the most commonly employed methods. A few examples from the 1974-75 literature are presented to illustrate the techniques currently employed. Injection of a crude organic extract into GLC columns has succeeded in a number of instances [7-13]; however, in some cases undesirable biological components are concomitantly injected, thereby causing a high base line and occasionally resulting in interfering peaks (from the same and possibly previous injections). Cleaner preparations are usually obtained when the initial organic extract is subjected to additional solvent partitioning at selected pH values (back extraction techniques). Numerous investigations have used this approach [14-24]. Extensive purification and derivatization were required in other analyses [14,25-31]. The use of salt-solvent pairs for the isolation of drugs and metabolites has been proposed by Horning et al. [32]. Nonionic resins such as XAD-2 and XAD-4 have provided extremely clean samples [6,33] and allow an approach for obtaining intact sulfate or glucuronide conjugates. Subsequent acid or enzyme hydrolysis prior to solvent extraction would give intact drug or metabolite. Care must be exercised when using acid hydrolysis, however, since partial or total destruction of the compound may result. Enzyme hydrolysis, although slower, is generally preferred.

Shipe and Savory [34] used an extremely simple isolation method for the determination of 21 drugs including all the barbiturates, methylprylon, glutethimide, meprobamate, etc. The method involves the extraction of the biological sample (containing the internal standard) with chloroform at a pH of 4.9 or 8.3. The drugs in the organic extract are concentrated and then identified and quantitated by GLC on a 3% OV-17 column. Analysis times are kept below 7 min using temperature programming techniques. All calculations were based upon the peak area ratio method. Care should be exercised when employing chloroform as the solvent, since it has been demonstrated by Leeling et al. [35] that secondary amines react with chloroform in a variety of ways including dimerization, and formyl and chlorocarbonyl addition.

The use of an internal standard in the isolation procedure was also employed by Sadee et al. [36] in the analysis of (±)-1,2-bis(3,5-dioxopiperazinyl)propane in rat, rabbit, and human plasma. The drug was extracted from the plasma into an ether - isopropyl alcohol solution following saturation of the aqueous phase with ammonium sulfate. After concentration, the residue was treated with diazomethane (methylated secondary amino group) prior to injection into the column.

Kaiser and Martin [26], in contrast, used a somewhat elaborate method to isolate low levels of warfarin from plasma. Two μg of an internal standard (p-chloro analog of warfarin) was added to the biological specimen followed by extraction of the compounds into ethylene chloride from an acidic medium. The organic phase was subsequently concentrated and subjected to TLC. The respective regions of drug and internal standard were eluted, the material concentrated, and then allowed to react with pentafluorobenzylbromide for 1 h at 60°C. The resulting derivatives were extracted into hexane and subjected to analysis using an electron capture detector (ECD) and a 1% OV-17 column. The method provides a low limit of detection, 20 ng/ml. Midha et al. [37] used a simpler approach which involves extraction of the drug and the internal standard (phenylbutazone) into ethylene chloride followed by back extraction into alkali and then reextraction into an organic solvent. The residue was treated with diazomethane and injected directly into the GLC equipped with a flame ionization detector (FID). The method is sensitive enough to detect 250 ng/ml, a factor of 10 poorer than the method of Kaiser and Martin [26].

III.   CHROMATOGRAPHIC BEHAVIOR AND DERIVATIZATION

The successful GLC of steroids and alkaloids reported in 1960 [3,4,38] silenced those voices which proclaimed that vapor phase separation of compounds possessing moderately high molecular weights and polarity was impossible because of the unacceptably high temperatures thought to be required. The contention that a high boiling point at atmospheric pressure

---

*Throughout this chapter, parenthetical numbers in reactions refer to reference numbers.

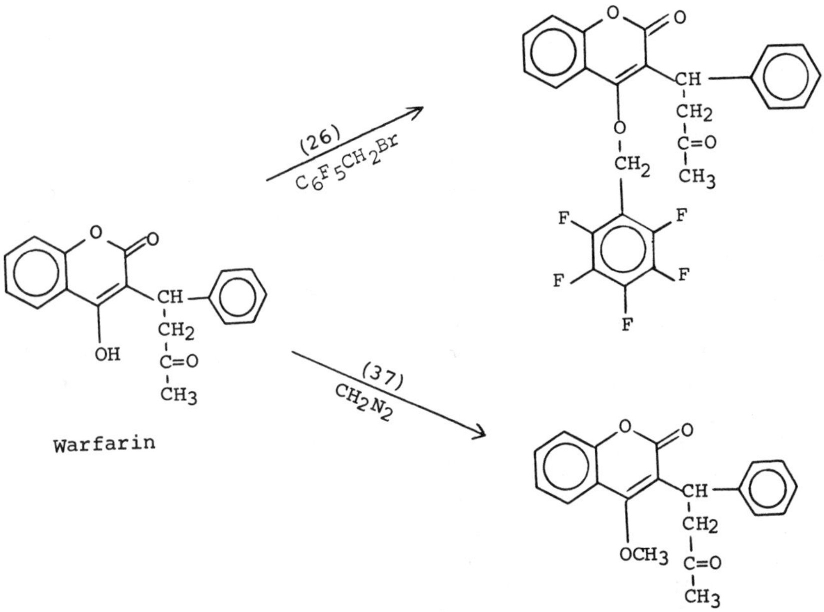

(26)
$C_6F_5CH_2Br$

CH
CH_2
$C=O$
CH_3
O
CH_2
F F
F F
F

CH
CH_2
OH $C=O$
CH_3

Warfarin

(37)
CH_2N_2

CH
CH_2
OCH_3 $C=O$
CH_3

would inevitably lead to an unreasonably long retention time was based on the assumption that analogous intermolecular forces are involved in GLC and in the escape of molecules from an environment of similar molecules (i.e., distillation of a pure liquid). In the latter case with polyfunctional compounds, strong intermolecular forces indeed must be overcome, but interactions in GLC occur in the liquid phase between solute (sample) and solvent (liquid phase), not between solute molecules. Stationary phases, especially the "nonselective" polysiloxanes, are usually less polar than the solute, and as a result solute-solvent interactions are much weaker than might be expected, and less thermal energy (lower column temperatures) is required to achieve a sufficient vapor pressure. Even at temperatures of 250°C or above, most compounds are stable, as the GLC separation takes place in a dark, inert (e.g., helium, nitrogen, argon) environment. Thermally induced structural alterations, analogous to those observed in classical organic chemistry, are occasionally noted [3-5].

The vast majority of GLC analyses in drug metabolism are carried out using thermally stable polysiloxane stationary phases such as SE-30, OV-1, OV-17, OV-210, and OV-225. SE-30, the dimethylpolysiloxane used in the first practical separations of steroids, alkaloids, and other biologically important compounds [3,4], probably remains the most widely used stationary phase for work with drugs, and Moffat [39] has reviewed the SE-30 retention behavior of more than 400 drugs. OV-1, another dimethylpolysiloxane, is virtually identical to SE-30 in partitioning properties; OV-17 is a methylphenylpolysiloxane, and exhibits greater polarity or selectivity [3,4] with respect to functional groups present on solute molecules. Less frequently used, but possessing greater selectivity, are OV-210 and OV-225 (trifluoropropyl and cyanopropylphenyl methylpolysiloxanes, respectively) and Carbowax 20M (a polyethyleneglycol). The great advantage of SE-30, OV-1, and OV-17 is that they can be employed at the temperatures (e.g., 225-275°C) often required for the elution (10-15 min retention time) of high molecular weight drugs.

The use of thin films of stationary phase results in increased volatility at a given temperature, thus allowing reduction in column temperatures. Perhaps the major problem in GLC is the lack of a truly nonadsorptive or inert support for thin film coatings of stationary phase useful at elevated temperatures. Adsorptive columns can be tolerated when sample sizes are large (i.e., >10 μg) and/or the sample does not possess polar functional groups. But work in drug metabolism and related fields often involves the assay or analysis of nanogram quantities of polar substances, and under such conditions unsatisfactory GLC is often the rule. The use of capillary columns prepared from deactivated glass rather than packed columns may be one solution to this problem. Certainly with packed columns means must be found to reduce the polarity or "deactivate" the sample molecules. This approach, best known as derivatization, has resulted in an array of techniques involving functional group alteration at the microgram and nanogram level, both prior to and during injection. It has permitted the successful GLC of compounds otherwise possessing insufficient volatility at all, and has resulted in greatly improved results at low levels with compounds which otherwise would exhibit significant adsorption. Since drugs and their metabolites fall into these two categories more often than not, it is no wonder that derivatization is widely employed in the field of drug metabolism. Some of the more frequently employed derivatization approaches are listed in Table 2.

A. Methylation

Methylation of polar compounds, e.g., sugars, was employed in classical organic chemistry many years before the advent of GLC, and thus it is not surprising that this approach should have been incorporated into many GLC methods. Dimethylsulfate has been employed, for example, in GLC methods for barbiturates and glutethimide [40], tolbutamide [41,42], and chlorpropamide [42]; however, methyl derivatives of sulfonylureas may be thermally labile. Diazomethane (CH_2N_2) is a useful reagent for the methylation of carboxyl and phenol groups. It has been employed in GLC determinations of probenecid [43,44] and warfarin [39].

$$CH_3CH_2CH_2)_2NSO_2-\underset{\text{Probenecid}}{\bigcirc}-\overset{O}{\underset{\|}{C}}-OH \quad \xrightarrow[\text{CH}_2\text{N}_2]{(43)} \quad (CH_3CH_2CH_2)_2NSO_2-\bigcirc-\overset{O}{\underset{\|}{C}}-OCH_3$$

As use of CH_2N_2 for conversion of indomethacin to its methyl ester (R_1 = R_2 = CH_3) to allow GLC analysis might convert a known phenolic metabolite (R_1 = R_2 = H) and the drug to the same compound, Helleberg [8] employed the reagent diazoethane for alkylation of the carboxyl group.

Indomethacin (R_1 = CH_3; R_2 = H)

An assay for (+)-1,2-bis(3,5-dioxopiperazinyl)propane in plasma involves N-methylation by diazomethane [36]. Sensitivity limits are 5 ng/ml by flame ionization detection and 0.2 ng/ml by mass fragmentography (vide infra).

A GLC assay for ibuprofen [(+)-2(p-isobutylphenyl)propionic acid] in human plasma suitable for drug absorption studies has been developed by Kaiser and Vangiessen [45]; 1,1'-carbonyldiimidazole is used to convert this acid to its methyl ester.

Ibuprofen

TABLE 2

Derivatization Approaches Frequently Employed in GLC for Commonly Occurring Functional Groups

Functional group	Derivative	Reagent	Illustrative references
Amido $R-\overset{\overset{O}{\|}}{C}-NH_2$	Dimethyl N-DMAM[b] Mono-TMSi[d]	TMAH[a] DMFDMA[c] BSTFA[e]	See p. 73 cambendazole metabolite [115]; see p. 82, carbamazepine [77] cambendazole metabolite
$R-\overset{\overset{O}{\|}}{C}-\overset{\overset{H}{\|}}{N}-R_1$	TMSi	BSA[f]	[81] Rafoxanide
Amino RNH_2	Alkyl, perfluoroalkyl aryl, perfluoroaryl amides	Corresponding anhydrides and acyl chlorides	[96, 118], [132–138] Sulfaquinoxaline
	Schiff base	Reactive ketones	
	TMSi	BSA, BSTFA	[73, 74]
	Carbamates	Corresponding chloro-formates	[74] Amitriptyline
	N-DMAM	DMFDMA	[111] Octopamine
$\overset{R}{\underset{R_1}{>}}NH$	Amides as above	e.g., Pentafluoropropionic anhydride	[25, 118]
	Carbamates	e.g., Pentafluorobenzyl chloroformate;	[122], [123] Amitriptyline

Functional group	Derivative	Reagent	References / Compounds
		trichloroethyl chloroformate	[120], [124] Amitriptyline
$RN(CH_3)_2$	Methyl	Diazomethane TMAH	[36], [95] Oxazepam glucuronide [155], [224] Cyproheptadine metabolite
	Carbamates of desmethyl amine	See above	[120–124] Amitriptyline
	Hydrolysis of above carbamates to secondary amine followed by acylation	Anhydrides and acyl chlorides	[121] Amitriptyline, imipramine
Imidazole NH	TMSi Methyl	BSA TMAH	[78] Cambendazole See p. 73, cambendazole and metabolite
Indole NH	TMSi	BSTFA	[193] Dimethyltryptamine
Carbamoyl $R\text{-}O\text{-}\overset{\overset{\displaystyle O}{\|}}{C}\text{-}\overset{\overset{\displaystyle H}{\|}}{N}\text{-}R_1$	Methyl	TMAH	See p. 73, cambendazole and metabolite
		BSA	[76,78] Cambendazole, chlorphenesin carbamate
Carbonyl $\dfrac{R}{R_1}\!\!>\!\!C{=}O$	Methoxime	Methoxylamine · HCl	[97–104,216,223] Cortisone, prostaglandin E_2, dimethisterone

TABLE 2 (Continued)

Functional group	Derivative	Reagent	Illustrative references
Carboxyl R—C—OH (O=)	Methyl	Diazomethane	[43, 44, 95, 110, 111], [182] Probenecid
		TMAH	[62] Bumetamide
	TMSi	BSA, BSTFA	[73–75] Fenoprofen
	Pentafluorobenzyl	Pentafluorobenzylbromide	[26], [108] Prostaglandin $F_{2\alpha}$
	α-Phenylethylamide	Thionyl chloride; α-phenylethylamine	[129–131] Ibuprofen
Guanido	Cyclization product	Hexafluoroacetylacetone	[139]
Hydroxyl R—CH$_2$OH, RCHOHR$_1$	Alkyl, perfluoroalkyl aryl, perfluoroaryl esters	Corresponding anhydrides and acyl chlorides	[25, 27, 74, 79, 91, 118], [132–138] Propanolol
	Permethyl	Methyl iodide/sodium DMSO	[48] Glucuronides
	TMSi	BSA, BSTFA	[73, 74, 100–105], [206] Prostaglandins
phenol	Methyl	Diazomethane/methanol	[37], [74] Warfarin
	TMSi	BSA, BSTFA	[81], p. 77 Rafoxanide, Aldomet

Functional group	Derivative	Reagent	Reference / Compound
N-oxide $R-N{\overset{\underset{\uparrow}{O}}{\diagdown}}{\overset{R_1}{\underset{R_2}{}}}$	Tertiary amine	TiCl$_3$/HCl	[207]
Sulfonamide RSO$_2$NH$_2$	Dimethyl	TMAH Methyl iodide/base	[61], [62] Hydrochlorothiazide [69] Chlorthalidone
	N-DMAM	DMFDMA	[113] 3-Bromo-5-cyanobenzene-sulfonamide
	Perfluoroacyl	Perfluoroacyl anhydride	[114] Benzenesulfonamide
RSO$_2$NHR$_1$	Methyl	TMAH Diazomethane Methyl iodide/base	[61] Hydrochlorothiazide [96] Sulfaquinoxaline [69] Chlorthalidone
Vicinal dihydroxyl, amino hydroxyl, and hydroxylcarboxyl	Cyclic boronates	n-Butyl boronic acid Phenyl boronic acid	[105-107] Prostaglandin F$_{2\alpha}$ [106-107] Salicylic acids

[a] Trimethylanilinium hydroxide.

[b] N-dimethylaminomethylene.

[c] Dimethylformamide dimethylacetal.

[d] Trimethylsilyl.

[e] Bis(trimethylsilyl)trifluoroacetamide.

[f] Bis(trimethylsilyl)acetamide.

[g] Dimethylsulfoxide.

This method has been employed by Kaiser and Glenn [46] to correlate plasma ibuprofen levels with biological activity. A different route of esterification has been employed by Tosolini et al. [47] for the GLC determination of plasma and urine levels of dl-α[4-(1-oxo-2-isoindolinyl)-phenyl]propionic acid. These authors convert this drug to its 2, 2, 2-trifluoroethyl ester by reaction with 2, 2, 2-trifluoroethanol · BF_3 and employ flame ionization rather than electron capture detection.

Thompson et al. [48] have reported a method for the methylation of glucuronides and other polar drug metabolites found in bile. The total bile is permethylated using methyl iodide and the sodium salt of dimethylsulfoxide.

Alkylation at the time of injection, the technique known as flash or on-column alkylation, has become a widely used approach for the analysis of polar drugs such as various antiepileptics, barbiturates, and sulfonamides. Trimethylanilinium hydroxide (TMAH) in methanol, first employed by Brochmann-Hanssen and Oke [49], is perhaps the most widely used reagent for this purpose.

Phenobarbital

Tetramethyl and tetraethylammonium hydroxides (either aqueous or methanolic) have also proven useful for a number of workers. MacGee [50] employed the former to achieve on-column methylation of diphenylhydantoin in plasma, and Estas and Dumont [51] used this approach to determine this drug and its metabolite p-hydroxyphenylphenylhydantoin in serum, urine, and tissues. Tetraethylammonium hydroxide was utilized by MacGee [52] for the identification and quantification of barbiturates and glutethimide in blood.

Diphenylhydantoin

More recently Friel and Troupin [53] reported on the flash heater (on-column) ethylation of some antiepileptic drugs (mephenytoin, 5-ethyl-5-phenyl hydantoin, phenobarbital, primidone, mephobarbital, and phenytoin) using triethylanilinium hydroxide in ethanol.

The GLC determination of plasma levels of phenylbutazone and its phenolic metabolite oxyphenbutazone utilizing flash methylation with TMAH has been reported by Midha et al. [54]. Both compounds yielded two methylated products [as demonstrated by combined GLC-MS (MS = mass spectrometry)] but the major, shorter retention time peaks were used for quantitation. Evidently the parent drug forms two separable isomeric monomethyl derivatives, whereas the metabolite yields a mixture of mono and dimethyl products (the latter possessing the shorter retention time). The authors state that this derivatization approach offers several advantages: extracts need not be completely moisture-free, the reagent is stable for long periods of time, and the reaction is readily carried out (in the injection port of the chromatograph at 300°C). Hammer and co-workers [55] have commented earlier on the advantages of flash methylation vis-a-vis trimethylsilylation; these authors employ TMAH for the analysis of diphenylhydantoin and its p-hydroxyphenyl metabolite in plasma and urine. Hammer et al. [56] used this derivatization approach to prevent the misidentification of cocaine; the authors state that underivatized cocaine can be erroneously reported as pentazocine, levophenol, or methaqualone when using a 7% OV-17 column. At least seven peaks were detected if the reagent was allowed to react with the drug for 24 h prior to GLC analysis. The quantitation of quinidine in biological fluids using the internal standard (cinchonidine) method and on-column derivatization with TMAH was reported by Midha and Charette [57]. The derivatization reaction was carried out in the injection port (350°C). The limit of detection was 0.05 μg/ml. A linear response was obtained in the 0.2 to 12.0 μg/ml range. Midha et al. [58] used the same approach for the analysis of γ-hydroxy metabolite of phenylbutazone. The plasma samples, to which an internal standard was added, were subjected to solvent partitioning at selected pH values to remove interfering components. Upon GLC analysis, γ-hydroxyphenylbutazone and oxyphenylbutazone (another metabolite of phenylbutazone) give rise to four and two peaks, respectively, following flash methylation. The authors used one peak from each set for calculation of the amounts of metabolites using the peak height method, as they showed that the peak height was proportional to the concentration of material added to plasma. The overall recovery from plasma was low (~20%) in the range examined. The appearance of multiple peaks is not highly uncommon with on-column derivatization.

As concentrated solutions of TMAH are strongly basic in nature, it is not surprising that base hydrolyzable drugs might undergo chemical alteration during exposure to this and similar reagents. Osiewicz et al. [59] observed this phenomenon with the on-column methylation of phenobarbital, and identified two products, the expected N,N-dimethylphenobarbital plus N-methyl-α-phenylbutyramide.

The authors found that factors influencing formation of the latter are the concentration of the reagent and the length of time the drug is exposed to it prior to injection. They deliberately employed 1.8 M TMAH and 10 min exposure time to convert phenobarbital via hydrolysis and methylation to N-methyl-α-phenylbutyramide and use this peak for the assay of the parent drug. An aliquot of the reaction solution was injected slowly (over a period of 10 sec) into the chromatograph with the injector port at 260°C.

This slow introduction of the solution into a "hot tube" may help to account for the chemistry observed. A more recent paper on the simultaneous determination of these three drugs in human serum states that the conversion of phenobarbital to N-methyl-α-phenylbutyramide is negligible if contact time of the drug with 50% TMAH is less than 10 min [60]. As the authors failed to state otherwise, one can assume that samples are injected over a normal 1 to 2 sec period. It is clear from these two papers that certain drugs cannot be dissolved in the strongly basic reagents and then be allowed to await analysis for relatively long periods of time in an automatic injection tray or turntable.

A GLC method for hydrochlorothiazide in human blood, plasma, and urine based upon on-column methylation with 0.005 to 0.01 M TMAH has been developed for use with individuals on therapeutic dosage levels of this drug [61]. The drug and internal standard (the bromo analog) are converted to the tetramethyl derivatives which possess satisfactory chromatographic behavior allowing successful GLC of nanogram quantities of these compounds.

Hydrochlorothiazide

The chromatogram in Figure 1 results from the assay of blood from a patient 3 h post dose; the tetramethylhydrochlorothiazide peak at 15 min retention time (the retention time of the methylated internal standard is 20 min) corresponds to 0.62 μg drug/ml blood. At 24 h post dose the peak corresponding to the drug is greatly diminished (Fig. 2), corresponding to 0.11 μg/ml. Another diuretic, bumetamide, has been determined in human urine by employing on-column methylation; a mixture of tetramethyl-ammonium hydroxide and TMAH were employed as the derivatization reagent [62]. The compound which eluted from the column has been shown to possess the structure given below. It has been proposed by the authors that the methylation occurs concomitantly with a Smiles rearrangement. This is one example of the thermally induced structural alterations mentioned earlier. Another structural transformation has been observed by Aggarwal and Sunshine [63] in their work on the GLC determination of sulfonyl ureas in human plasma. Injection of chlorpropamide dissolved in TMAH results in the elution of N,N-dimethyl-p-chlorobenzenesulfonamide. The authors hypothesize that the drug is converted to the primary

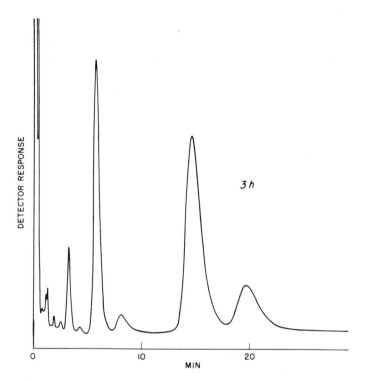

FIG. 1. Electron capture GLC analysis of an isolate [from the blood (3 h post dose) of a patient treated with hydrochlorothiazide] which had been subjected to on-column methylation with TMAH. Column conditions: 4 ft × 2.5 mm i.d. glass column packed with 1% 6:1 OV-1/CHDMA two component stationary phase on 80 to 100 mesh acid-washed and silanized Gas-Chrom P; 235°C; 60 ml/min carrier gas. (Reprinted from Ref. 61 by courtesy of the American Pharmaceutical Association.)

sulfonamide in the injector port and immediately methylated. Neither this transformation nor the Smiles rearrangement precludes obtaining useful

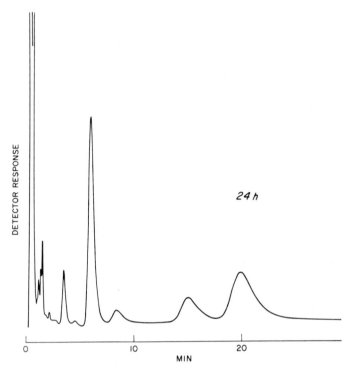

FIG. 2. Electron capture GLC analysis of an isolate [from the blood (24 h post dose) of a patient treated with hydrochlorothiazide] which had been subjected to on-column methylation with TMAH. Column conditions as Figure 1. (Reprinted from Ref. 61 by courtesy of the American Pharmaceutical Association.)

data from the GLC method. On-column methylation in the GLC analysis of antiepileptic drugs in multiple drug therapy is the subject of a recent article by Solow et al. [64]. MacGee [65] reviewed the chemistry and techniques of on-column alkylations.

On-column methylation is not a suitable approach for the simultaneous assay of methylphenobarbitone and phenobarbitone since they yield the same dimethyl derivatives. Hooper et al. [66] have reported an on-column butylation method using tetrabutylammonium hydroxide which obviates this problem for assay of these barbiturates in human plasma and serum. The authors observed that blood stored in glass for weeks, or freshly collected in plastic bags and sampled immediately, contains no interfering peaks (OV-101 column). A component with the same retention time as butylated phenobarbitone was found, however, from blood stored (refrigerated) in the plastic bags for two weeks. This phenomenon was not observed with polypropylene tubes.

A technique for the formation of N-alkyl derivatives of barbiturates suitable for GLC analysis and not involving on-column alkylation has been reported by Greeley [67], who claims that reagents for on-column butylation caused rapid deterioration of GLC columns. * He found that butylation allowed the simultaneous assay of several barbiturates which are not separated either underivatized or methylated. Greeley's off-column alkylation approach involves the addition of alkyl iodides (e.g., n-butyl iodide) to a solution of the barbiturate (from an extract of blood) in a mixture of methanol, N,N-dimethylacetamide, and a strong organic base, tetramethylammonium hydroxide. As the derivative is prepared prior to injection, the flash heater need not be at the high temperature (300-350°C) usually recommended for on-column alkylation. Further, the tetramethylammonium iodide resulting from the reaction precipitates during derivatization and is not injected into the column. An aliquot of the supernatant liquid is assayed after 10 min reaction time (at room temperature). The Greeley method of butylation has been used by Least et al. [68] in a quantitative GLC determination of the anticonvulsant ethosuximide. This approach is favored by the authors over on-column methylation for the reasons listed above, and over trimethylsilylation because of the instability of trimethylsilyl (TMSi) derivatives in the presence of moisture.

Another related off-column approach to the derivatization of polar drugs prior to their assay by GLC is "extractive alkylation" [69] or "extractive methylation" [70]. Ervik and Gustavii [69] converted chlorthalidone to its tetramethyl derivative by reaction with methyl iodide in a mixture of methylene chloride, aqueous sodium hydroxide, and tetra-n-hexylammonium hydroxide. The anionic form of the polar drug (A^-) is extracted into the methylene chloride as an ion pair with the quaternary tetra-n-hexylammonium ion (Q^+), where it is methylated. After centrifugation an aliquot of the organic layer is taken to dryness and the residue dissolved in a suitable solvent (e.g., hexane, in which tetra-n-hexylammonium iodide is insoluble) for GLC analysis. Extraction of the drug from body

---

*This has been disputed by Hooper et al. [66].

Chlorthalidone

$$A^- + Q^+ \rightleftharpoons QA_{org}$$

$$QA_{org} + CH_3I_{org} \rightleftharpoons CH_3A_{org} + QI_{org}$$

fluids prior to the extractive alkylation derivatization is, of course, a key step; these authors employed methylisobutyl ketone for chlorthalidone in plasma. The rate of methylation depends upon the concentration of the various species and the reaction time and temperature. Ehrsson has published methods for the GLC determination of nitrazepan [70] and barbiturates [71] utilizing extractive methylation. The former method involves the extraction of plasma with benzene and alkylation of an aliquot of the resulting solution using methyl iodide as the methyl source and the tetra-n-butylammonium ion as the counter ion. An aliquot of the benzene phase is then taken to dryness and the residue dissolved in ethyl acetate prior to GLC. As carbon disulfide causes a very small solvent front with a FID, this solvent, rather than methylene chloride, was employed as the reaction solvent in the barbiturate method. An aliquot of the organic phase from the mixture is injected directly into the gas chromatograph rather than employing an evaporation step. Furosemide was determined in plasma by Lindström and Molander [72] using an extractive methylation technique and an ECD. The residue which resulted from extraction of the drug from plasma with ether and subsequent evaporation of the solvent was dissolved in 0.2 M NaOH, 0.1 M tetra-n-hexylammonium hydrogen sulfate, and methyl iodide in methylene chloride. Derivatization was completed in 10 min at 50°C; the organic phase was taken to dryness, and the residue dissolved in hexane and injected directly into the GLC.

B.   Trimethylsilylation and Related Approaches

Trimethylsilylation* was one of the earliest derivatizing approaches for polar compounds of biological interest, e.g., steroids, sugars, and other compounds containing hydroxyl groups. Formation of TMSi derivatives

---

*A number of reagents and derivatization conditions are employed [73, 74], but the most frequently used of the former are bis-trimethyl-silylacetamide (BSA), bis-trimethylsilyltrifluoroacetamide (BSTFA), and hexamethyldisilazane (HMDS).

has been much less frequently employed with drugs, probably because
many drugs contain functional groups other than hydroxyl groups, e.g.,
amino and amido, which do not readily form stable products. TMSi derivatives of these and, to a lesser extent, carboxyl groups are sufficiently
labile so that at low levels a significant proportion may revert to the
parent functional group during GLC. Trimethylsilylation of carboxylic
acids can be an attractive alternative to methylation with diazomethane,
and Nash and coworkers [75] have developed a method involving formation
of a TMSi ester for the GLC determination of fenoprofen, dl-2(3-phenoxy-
phenyl)propionic acid, in human plasma. The method has clinical utility
and is quantitative above 0.25 μg/ml using FID.

The GLC determination of chlorphenesin carbamate in serum using trimethylsilylation has been reported by Kaiser and Shaw [76].

The chromatogram resulting from analysis of the trimethylsilylated drug
contains an intense peak (the expected di-TMSi derivative) plus three small
peaks; these are the mono-TMSi derivatives of chlorphenesin carbamate
[presumably the O-TMSi ether (?)], and the mono- and di-TMSi derivatives
of the thermal degradation product of this drug, the corresponding primary
alcohol. Thermal degradation was minimized by maintaining the flash
heater at the same temperature as the column. Conversion of another
carbamate drug to the TMSi ether of the parent alcohol has been reported
by VandenHeuvel and associates [77]; in this case the conversion apparently

occurred during the derivatization. GLC of the underivatized drug resulted in elution of the alcohol. As the latter is a metabolite of the drug, the lack of appreciation of such a thermally induced transformation could have serious repercussions.

Although trimethylsilylation is generally thought to retard the thermal breakdown of carbamates, GLC of the di-TMSi derivative of cambendazole has been reported to yield only one peak, the mono-N-TMSi derivative of the corresponding isocyanate, whereas GLC of cambendazole itself shows two peaks: cambendazole and its isocyanate [78].

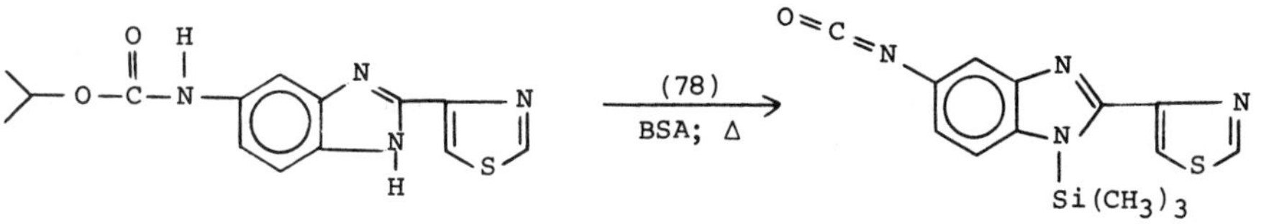

Thus in this case derivatization facilitates an on-column transformation. No conversion to the isocyanate is observed if the drug is injected dissolved in TMAH; the compound eluted is the dimethylated drug. Isocyanate formation also occurs with a trimethylsilylated metabolite of cambendazole [77], but on-column derivatization of this amide using TMAH results in conversion to the tetramethyl product:

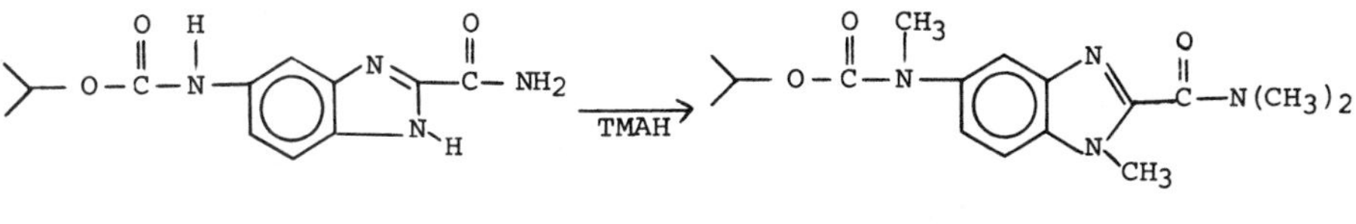

A hydroxylated methyl group metabolite of cambendazole undergoes on-column conversion to the same isocyanate as from cambendazole. This is another instance of when data from GLC (or even GLC-MS) alone could be misleading. The major carbinol metabolite [79] of the antiarrhythmic agent MK-251 undergoes slight dehydration at elevated temperatures; however, the trifluoroacetyl derivative of the carbinol is quantitatively converted to the olefin.

Frigerio et al. [80] studied the GLC behavior of several drugs and their metabolites, particularly with regard to decomposition and, hence, errors in identification. Compounds examined included oxazepam (OXA), N-methyloxazepam (MOXA), nitrooxazepam (NOXA), o-chlorooxazepam (COXA), carbamazepine, carbamazepine-10,11-epoxide, 10,11-dihydroxy-carbamazepine, and floropipamide. A number of drugs, OXA, COXA,

R = CF$_2$CF$_2$C$_6$H$_5$

and NOXA underwent decomposition to give 4-phenylquinazaline-2-carbox-aldehyde derivatives, whereas MOXA was stable.

The same reaction occurred upon heating the compounds to 200°C. In the presence of methanol, carbamazepine partly decomposed to give imino-stilbene and 9-methylacridine. The 10,11-epoxide (a) of carbamazepine decomposed completely to 9-acridine-carboxaldehyde (b); the same degra-dation product was obtained from the 10,11-dihydroxycarbamazepine (c). Both reactions are catalyzed by the slightly acidic conditions of the column. Floropipamide undergoes thermal dehydration of the amide to give the corresponding nitrile.

The anthelmintic agent rafoxanide must be converted to a less polar compound prior to its analysis by GLC [81]. Treatment with BSA yielded

(a)   (b)   (c)

the di-OTMSi derivative which possessed good chromatographic properties
at the microgram level.

The ECD response for this halogenated species at the nanogram level was
found to be dependent upon its column residence time, strongly suggesting
the occurrence of irreversible adsorption. This phenomenon probably involves exchange of one of the TMSi groups with a hydrogen atom from an
active site on the packing to form a more polar mono-TMSi drug. A system involving use of a short column containing only 4 in. of packing allowed
satisfactory quantitation down to the injection of 0.2 ng of drug from animal plasma. Isolates from control plasma spiked with rafoxanide and
from on-drug plasma both show a peak with a shorter retention time than
the di-TMSi derivative of the drug. This has been identified as the di-TMSi
derivative of 3-desiodorafoxanide, the product of a photolytic, not metabolic,
retention. Two metabolites have been found in the bile of monkeys dosed
with this drug [82]. These compounds can be chromatographed as their
tri-TMSi derivatives and were shown by MS to be isomers in which an
iodine atom was replaced by a hydroxyl group. The chromatogram result-

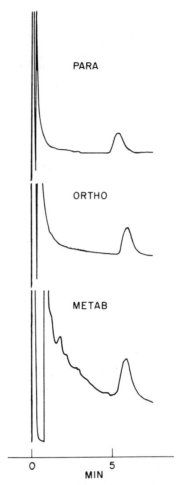

FIG. 3. GLC comparison of 3'-chloro-4'-(p-chlorophenoxy)-3-hydroxy-
5-iodosalicylanilide and 3'-chloro-4'-(p-chlorophenoxy)-5-hydroxy-3-
iodosalicylanilide and a biliary metabolite of Rafoxanide as their trimethylsilylated derivatives. Column conditions: 3 ft × 2.5 mm i.d. glass column
packed with 1.8% OV-17 on 60 to 80 mesh Gas-Chrom P; 250°C; 30 ml/min
carrier gas.

ing from analysis of the authentic ortho and para dihydroxy desiodo compounds and one of the metabolites (as TMSi derivatives) is shown in Figure
3. The isomers exhibited slightly different retention times on this 3 ft
column of 1.8% OV-17, and the retention time of the derivative of the
metabolite corresponded to that of the ortho reference compound. The
second metabolite was identified as the para isomer.

Phenolic drugs or metabolites are often excreted in urine as their ethereal sulfates. It is possible to prepare TMSi derivatives of these conjugates [83], but they are thermally labile species and readily lose sulfur trioxide to form the TMSi ether of the parent phenol when subjected to GLC at elevated temperatures.* The chromatogram resulting from analysis of the trimethylsilylated O-sulfate of α-methyldopa (Aldomet) is seen in Figure 4. The major peak is the tetra-TMSi derivative of Aldomet, and the minor peak is the tri-O-TMSi derivative of this amino acid, as demonstrated by combined GLC-MS. No evidence is found for the elution of the derivatized intact conjugate. Derivatization of dopa under the same conditions yields the tetra-TMSi derivative only; evidently the methyl group of α-methyldopa hinders trimethylsilylation of the amino group. Conversion

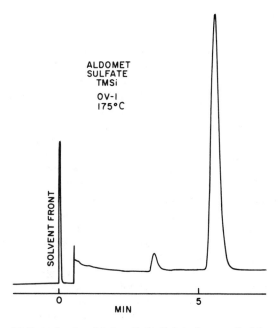

FIG. 4. GLC analysis of trimethylsilylated α-methyldopa O-sulfate. The two eluted component are the tri-O-TMSi derivative of α-methyldopa (small peak) and the tetra-TMSi derivative of α-methyldopa. Column conditions: 5 ft $\times$ 3 mm i.d. glass column packed with 3% OV-1 on 80 to 100 mesh acid-washed and silanized Gas-Chrom P; 175°C; 30 ml/min carrier gas.

---

*Methylated derivatives of O-sulfates undergo the analogous reaction to form the phenolic methyl ether [84].

of O-sulfates to the corresponding O-acetyl derivatives with acetic anhydride prior to GLC has been investigated [85].

Many drugs and their metabolites containing carboxyl, amino, and hydroxyl groups are excreted as urinary glucuronides. Their relatively high molecular weights and polarity preclude direct GLC analysis, and GLC of glucuronides has usually been performed indirectly after acid or enzymatic hydrolysis. Intact glucuronides can undergo chromatography successfully when converted to the appropriate derivatives, and a number of investigators have reported on the GLC analysis of intact glucuronides after conversion to methyl-TMSi [86-88], methylacetyl [89, 90], methyltrifluoroacetyl [91], per-TMSi [92], and per-methyl [48, 93] derivatives. MS was carried out in most instances for structure confirmation of the derivatives (see especially [88]). Although the derivatives possess significantly increased molecular weights, the reduction in polarity resulting from converting the carboxyl and hydroxyl groups to, for example, TMSi derivatives, makes GLC possible at column conditions not radically different from those used for steroid analysis. Chromatography of the trimethylsilylated glucuronide of 5-hydroxythiabendazole, an ovine urinary metabolite of thiabendazole [94], gave the results shown in Figure 5. Rather than trimethylsilylation of both the hydroxyl and carboxyl groups, some workers prefer to form the methyl ester prior to trimethylsilylation. Marcucci et al. [95] used this approach in their GLC assay of the intact urinary glucuronides of oxazepam (a metabolite of diazepam) and of lorazepam, another benzodiazepine. The methylation step (CH_2N_2 in ethereal methanol) also resulted in formation of the N_1-methyl derivative. Trimethylsilylation was carried out in pyridine using a 5:1 (v/v) mixture of hexamethyldisilazane and trifluoroacetic anhydride. Ehrsson et al. [91] describe a method for the analysis of intact ether glucuronides as methyltrifluoroacetyl derivatives using an FID-GLC method. The authors first form the methyl ester, followed by acylation with trifluoroacetic anhydride in ethyl acetate. The β-D-glucuronic acid conjugates of 1-naphthol and androsterone were used as the model compounds. Removal of excess

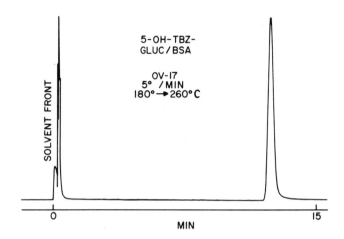

FIG. 5. GLC analysis of the TMSi derivative of 5-hydroxythiabenda-zole glucuronide. Column conditions: 3 ft × 3 mm i.d. glass column packed with 2% OV-17 on 800 to 100 mesh acid-washed and silanized Gas-Chrom P; temperature programmed from 180 to 260°C at 5°C/min; 30 ml/min flow rate (Reprinted from Ref. 82 by courtesy of Plenum Press.

Oxazepam glucuronide

reagent by evaporation or solvent extraction resulted in rapid decomposition of the derivatives. The technique has been employed successfully in the identification of glucuronide conjugates of propranolol.

Multi-step derivatization is often utilized with compounds of biological interest. Daun [96] has employed an imaginative two-step derivatization for the conversion of sulfa drugs (e.g., sulfaquinoxaline) to less polar compounds. Reaction with CH_2N_2 forms the N-methyl sulfonamide, and then heptafluorobutyrylation yields the amide; not only does this derivative exhibit excellent GLC properties, but the heptafluorobutyramide moiety confers electron capture properties.

Formation of methoximes as an analytical derivatization method was first reported by Fales and Luukkainen [97], and employed shortly thereafter for the stabilization of the dihydroxyacetone side chain of adrenocortical steroids (in combination with trimethylsilylation) by Gardiner and Horning [98]. The Baylor group has successfully employed methoxime (and other substituted oximes) formation with many types of carbonyl group-containing compounds of biological interest [99].

Conversion of the keto and hydroxyl groups of norethindrone to methoxime and TMSi ether groups has been employed by Cook and associates [100] to achieve satisfactory GLC behavior in their assay for this drug in human plasma. Sensitivity down to 1 ng/ml of plasma has been achieved by using mass spectrometric detection. Three separate derivatization steps including trimethylsilylation have been employed by several groups of workers in developing GLC-based assays for prostaglandins of the E-type. The β-ketol system in the cyclopentane ring of these compounds is particularly labile during GLC but, as demonstrated by Vane and Horning [101], can be stabilized by formation of the methoxime-TMSi ether, analogous to the stabilization of the dihydroxyacetone side chain of adrenocorticoid steroids.

Samuelsson et al. [102] developed a GLC-MS method for PGE$_1$ by conversion to the methyl ester-methoxime-di-TMSi derivative. Hamberg [103] has used this derivatization approach in converting 7α-hydroxy-5,11-diketotetranorprostane-1,16-dioic acid, the major human urinary metabolite of PGE_1 and PGE_2, to its dimethyl ester-dimethoxime-TMSi ether, and has established a GLC-MS assay for this compound in human urine. He has demonstrated that drugs such as aspirin, sodium salicylate, and indomethacin sharply reduce the urinary output of this metabolite, probably because they inhibit prostaglandin synthesis. Horodniak and coworkers [104] have studied the inhibitory effects of aspirin and indomethacin on PGE_2 biosynthesis from archidonic acid by bovine seminal vesicles in vitro. PGE_2 was also converted by methylation, methoxime formation, and trimethylsilylation to a derivative suitable for GLC analysis (FID). Determination of the effect of drugs upon levels of endogenous compounds in human body fluids would appear to be a natural area of application for sensitive and selective GLC-based assays, assuming suitable derivatives can be prepared.

Several other GLC derivatization approaches for the analysis of prostaglandins in biological fluids involve trimethylsilylation. Kelly [105], for example, has converted $PGF_{2\alpha}$ to its methyl ester 9, 11-butylboronate-15-TMSi ether.

The use of cyclic boronate derivatives in GLC studies has been pioneered by Brooks and MacLean [106]. Rabinowitz et al. [107] have used this approach to develop a specific assay for sorbitol, a humectant and sweetner. The author discusses the advantages of cyclic boronate over TMSi derivatives. Wickramasinghe et al. [108] have employed the pentafluorobenzyl ester TMSi ether for GLC of $PGF_{2\alpha}$ in biological fluids using an ECD. The introduction of electron capturing moieties by derivatization of carboxyl groups has also been explored by Kaiser et al. [109] in their method on the GLC determination of dl-2-(2-fluoro-4-biphenylyl)propionic acid or flurbiprofen. The lower limit of sensitivity is 0.05 $\mu g/ml$ of human plasma, suitable for successful applications to drug absorption studies resulting from various dosage formulations for up to 24 h post dose (10 mg). A TLC step is necessary to separate an interfering plasma component from the internal standard (the 2-methoxy analog).

C. Miscellaneous Approaches

Thenot and coworkers [110, 111] have reported that dimethylformamide dimethylacetal is a useful reagent for converting fatty acids to their methyl esters, and amino acids to the N-dimethylaminomethylene (N-DMAM) methyl ester derivatives.

$$
\underset{\substack{| \\ NH_2}}{\overset{\overset{\displaystyle O}{\parallel}}{R - CHC}} - OH \quad \xrightarrow[\text{DMFDMA}]{(111)} \quad \underset{\substack{| \\ N = CHN\,(CH_3)_2}}{\overset{\overset{\displaystyle O}{\parallel}}{R - CHC}} - OCH_3
$$

Venturella et al. [112] have employed this reagent for converting barbiturates and glutethimide to their acetals. VandenHeuvel and Gruber [113] have found that primary sulfonamides react with dimethylformamide dimethylacetal to form N-DMAM derivatives possessing good GLC properties.

As these can be prepared at the microgram level, they should be useful derivatives for metabolism studies involving determination of levels of sulfonamide group-containing drugs in body fluids. This is demonstrated by the data reported in Figure 6, which shows the blood and plasma levels of 3-bromo-5-cyanobenzene-sulfonamide in a sheep dosed with this compound. The chromatogram resulting from the assay of an aliquot of the isolate from sheep plasma 21 days post dose is seen in Figure 7 (the internal standard is the analogous dibromo compound). The N-DMAM moiety possesses a large retention factor (causes long retention times), and thus drugs possessing several primary sulfonamide groups and/or primary amino groups may possess volatilities too low for GLC analysis under normal conditions. Their formation can be demonstrated by direct probe MS, however, as each condensation results in an increase of 55 mass units in the m/e of the molecular ion, and these derivatives may prove useful for MS characterization. Perfluoroacyl anhydrides have been reported to react with primary and secondary sulfonamide group-containing compounds to form derivatives with good GLC properties [114].

A recently published method for the determination of carbamazepine in human plasma (cyheptamide serving as the internal standard) employs dimethylformamide dimethylacetal as the derivatization agent [115]. The authors indicated that the structures of the products resulting from the derivatization were not known. Based on the work of Thenot and Horning [111] and VandenHeuvel and Gruber [113] and the patent by Weinberg [116]

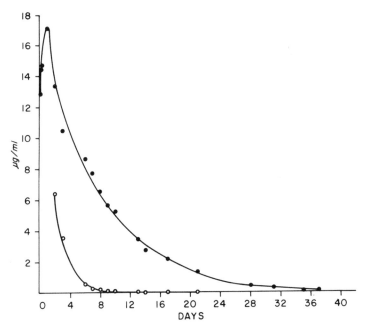

FIG. 6. Plot of ovine blood (•—•) and plasma (o—o) levels of 3-bromo-5-cyanobenzenesulfonamide vs. days post dose. (Reprinted from Ref. 113 by courtesy of Elsevier Publishing Company.)

(reporting that dimethylformamide dimethylacetal reacts with amides to form N-DMAM derivatives), it can be speculated that carbamazepine and its internal standard also form N-DMAM derivatives.

The genius of derivatization for GLC purposes has often been to simply recognize potentially useful transformations from classical organic chemistry and adapt them to biological isolates at the microgram level. In the absence of adequate electron capturing properties per se, or normally derivatizable functional groups, specific derivatization techniques have been employed. For example, hydrolysis of benzodiazepines has yielded benzophenones [117]. Reduction of esters to the alcohols followed by perfluoroacylation has been employed [118]. Blake et al. [119] have described similar methods for reductive fragmentation to an alcohol and subsequent derivatization. Dealkylation of tertiary amines by conversion to the corresponding carbamates using chloroformate esters, followed by hydrolysis to the secondary amine, has been practiced for several years. Montzka et al. [120], for example, recommend 2, 2, 2-trichloroethyl chloroformate for demethylation of tertiary amines. Although tertiary amines exhibit significantly better GLC properties than primary and secondary amines

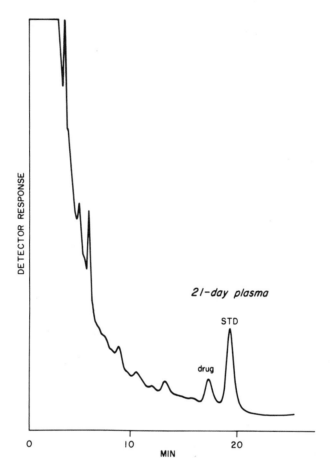

FIG. 7.   Electron capture GLC analysis of an aliquot of an isolate from
ovine plasma 21 days post dose (3-bromo-5-cyanobenzenesulfonamide).
Column conditions: 8 ft × 3 mm i.d. glass column packed with 1% OV-17
on 80 to 100 mesh Chromosorb WHP; 250°C; 40 ml/min carrier gas.
(Reprinted from Ref. 113 by courtesy of Elsevier Publishing Company.)

(i.e., better peak shape, less adsorption), the latter can be derivatized
with the appropriate alkylating agents to form derivatives with high electron affinity.

Hartvig and Vessman [121] converted the cyclic antidepressants imipramine and amitriptyline to their demethyl heptafluorobutyramides by
the use of carbamate formation (using methylchloroformate) and hydrolysis
followed by reaction with heptafluorobutyric anhydride. They extended
their work by using pentafluorobenzylchloroformate as the demethylating

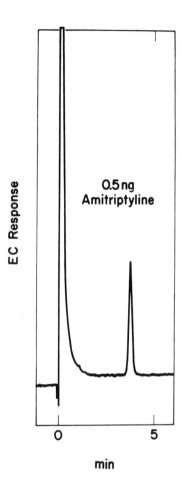

FIG. 8. Electron capture GLC analysis of 0.5 ng amitriptyline as the
1,1,1-trichloroethyl carbamate of the corresponding secondary amine.
Column conditions: 4 ft × 2.5 mm i.d. glass column packed with 1%
W-98 on 80 to 100 mesh Chromosorb WHP; 240°C; 40 ml/min carrier gas.

agent and subjecting the resulting carbamate directly to electron capture
GLC [122, 123]. * There would appear to be no reason why the trichloroethyl carbamates formed using the approach of Montzka et al. [120] could
not also be subjected to GLC analysis. The chromatogram resulting from
GLC with an ECD of 0.5 ng of amitriptyline as the demethyl trichloroethyl
carbamate is seen in Figure 8 [124].

---

*Demethyl metabolites would, of course, form the same derivative.

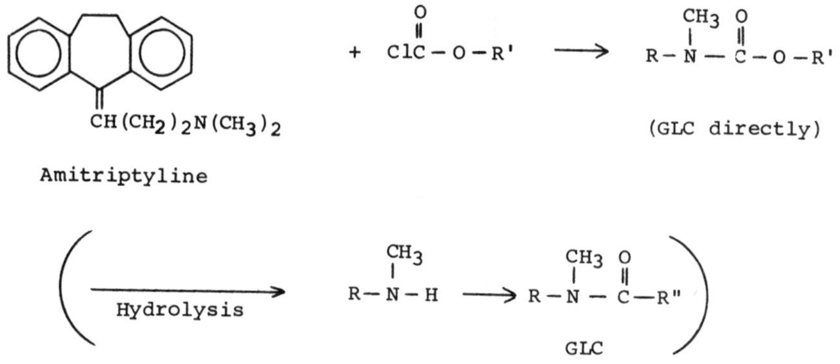

Amitriptyline

$$+ \quad ClC-O-R' \quad \longrightarrow \quad R-N-C-O-R'$$

(GLC directly)

$$\xrightarrow[\text{Hydrolysis}]{} \quad R-N-H \quad \longrightarrow \quad R-N-C-R''$$

GLC

Friedel-Crafts acylation techniques for aromatic compounds were described by Blake et al. [119] in their procedures for drug screening. More recently, Walle [125] has reported trifluoroacetyl substitution in the aromatic ring (C-acylation) of tertiary aromatic amines to yield trifluoroacetophenone derivatives suitable for ECD. This approach may be applicable to drugs and their metabolites.

Burchfield and coworkers [126] converted Dapsone, 4,4'-diaminodiphenylsulfone, to the corresponding 4,4'-diiodo compound in order to introduce improved electron capture properties. The chemistry involves diazotization of the amino groups followed by reaction with a solution of iodine in aqueous potassium iodide. Dapsone has also been analyzed by electron capture GLC as its diheptafluorobutyramide [77]. Hamilton et al. [127] have found that amitriptyline can be analyzed by GLC as its ceric sulfate - sulfuric acid oxidation product, anthraquinone, which exhibits a high electron capture response. This product can also be determined spectrophotometrically. The authors suggest that related compounds containing the benzocycloheptadine system might also be amenable to this type of derivatization.

The GLC separation of closely related compounds can usually be achieved by the use of high efficiency columns and/or the judicious choice of stationary phases and derivatives. Enantiomeric forms of a compound cannot be separated using normal GLC techniques. As the optical antipodes of a drug may differ in pharmacological activity, their separation and individual quantification is highly desirable. Certain drugs are administered in a racemic form (d,l mixture), and the ability to quantify the levels of each

of the enantiomeric forms in plasma, urine, etc. would be helpful in
establishing the contributions of each to the biological effects of the drug.
Such separations can be achieved by the use of optically active stationary
phases [128] or by transformation of the d, l pair into diastereoisomers
(which do differ in physical properties) by reaction with an optically active
reagent (e.g., base or acid chloride). This special type of derivatization
is an extension of the classical approach to the resolution of optical isomers but is carried out on the microgram rather than milligram-gram
scale. Several recent papers have described the determination of the
enantiomeric composition of drugs in human urine and plasma following
administration of the drug in its racemic form. Brooks and Gilbert [129]
investigated the enantiomeric composition of 2-(4-isobutylphenyl)propionic
acid (ibuprofen) excreted in human urine. The drug was converted to its
acid chloride (with thionyl chloride) and then reacted with R-(+)-α-phenyl-
ethylamine to form the diastereoisomeric amides, and separation carried
out using a 5-m column of OV-17. GLC analysis of ibuprofen isolated from
urine following derivatization gave the results shown in Figure 9.

The amide from (-)-ibuprofen exhibited a shorter retention time than that
from the (+)-enantiomer, and it is clear that excreted drug is highly en-
riched in the latter. Vangiessen and Kaiser [130] carried out the GLC
determination of the enantiomeric forms of ibuprofen in human plasma as
well as urine and found that the (+)- or d-enantiomer predominated in the
latter but that nearly equal amounts of the d and l forms were present in
plasma (1 h post dose) (see Fig. 10). The d:l concentration ratio in plasma
and urine increased with time; the authors suggested that this indicates
stereospecific metabolic transformations, excretion, or isomer inversion.
These authors used (-)- or l-α-phenylethylamine rather than the (+) form
used by Brooks and Gilbert [129] to form the diastereoisomeric amides,
with the result that on an OV-17 column it is the amide from the (+)- or
d-enantiomer which possesses the shorter retention time.

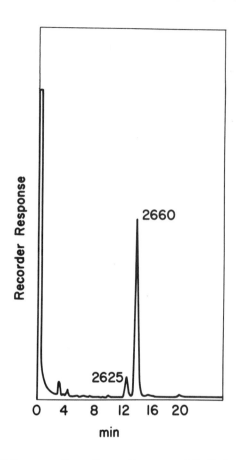

FIG. 9. GLC separation of enantiomers of 2-(4-isobutylphenyl)-
propionic acid, isolated from the urine of a patient treated with racemic
drug, as the diastereomeric amides from (+)-α-phenylethylamine. The
Kovats retention indices of the two amides are indicated. Column
conditions: 5 m × 3.5 mm i.d. glass column packed with 1% OV-17
on 100 to 120 mesh Gas-Chrom Q; 245°C. (Reprinted from Ref. 129
by courtesy of Elsevier Publishing Company.)

The GLC determination of plasma levels of the enantiomers of
α-[4-(1-oxo-2-isoindolinyl)phenyl]propionic acid has been carried out
by Tosolini et al. [131] utilizing the same chiral reagent as Vangiessen
and Kaiser [130]. At 1 h post dose, approximately equal amounts of
the d and l isomers were found in plasma, but by 6 h post dose the
d:l ratio had increased to greater than 2.

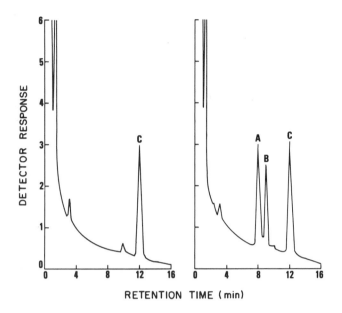

FIG. 10. Right panel: GLC separation of enantiomers of 2-(4-isobutyl-
phenyl)propionic acid, isolated from the plasma of a patient treated with
racemic drug, as the diastereomeric amides from (-)-α-phenylethylamine;
A and B are the diastereomeric amides, C is the internal standard. Left
panal: result from control plasma. Column conditions: 1.5 m × 3 mm
i.d. glass column packed with 3% OV-17 on 60 to 80 mesh Gas-Chrom Q;
220°C; 90 ml/min carrier gas. (Reprinted from Ref. 130 by courtesy of
the American Pharmaceutical Association.)

IV. DETECTION

A. Electron Capture Detection*

As stated earlier, because of the chemical nature of some drugs and their
metabolites, derivatization of the isolated components is essential prior
to GLC analysis. Other drugs can undergo successful chromatography
directly; however, it is often advantageous to prepare one of a variety of
derivatives to reduce column adsorption, and thereby minimize tailing.
This is especially important for analyses at the nanogram level, and facilitates the quantitative aspects of assay for drugs and their metabolites.

---

*See also chapter "Electron-capture Gas-Liquid Chromatography" to
be published in a future volume of this series.

The introduction of moieties possessing high coefficients of electron affinity allows selective analysis of low levels of many drugs by ECD [5, 123, 132-136]. Pellizzari [137] discussed in detail the use of ECD in GLC analysis. The functional groups usually derivatized include primary and secondary amino, phenolic, and hydroxyl groups. Introduction of heptafluorobutyryl, chloroacetyl, pentafluorophenyl, trifluoroacetyl, and pentafluoropropyl-containing moieties is usually employed. As a chapter on ECD appears in this series [138], we will discuss only a limited number of recent GLC results using this detection method.

The reagent hexafluoroacetylacetone was employed for the detection of guanido-containing drugs (via a cyclization reaction) by Erdtmansky and Goehl [139] using a GLC method with an ECD. The method has the advantage of using plasma or urine directly without prior extraction of drug and provides sensitivity down to the 25 ng/ml level.

An ECD method for the analysis of low levels of the tranquilizer Ro5-3027 and its metabolite, lorazepam, in blood and urine was used by de Silva et al. [140]. (A previously published method [141] which involved the hydrolysis of lorazepam to the corresponding benzophenone was not applicable since both Ro5-3027 and its metabolite would yield the same benzophenone, thereby resulting in nonspecificity.) The method requires the direct injection of the isolate into a 3% OV-17 column. The procedure employs an internal standard, and all calculations were made using the peak area ratio method. The sensitivity of analysis for either compound was in the 2 to 5 ng/ml range.

Clonazepam and its metabolite, flunitrazepam, two drugs which exhibit marked anticonvulsant properties, were determined in blood and urine using an electron capture method described by de Silva et al. [14]. The assay for clonazepam uses flunitrazepam as an internal standard and vice versa. Selective extraction of the drugs by ether at pH 9 followed by acid hydrolysis to the respective benzophenones permits quantitation by electron capture GLC. The levels of sensitivity are about 1 ng/ml. The authors state that the clean-up procedure is essential for the quantitative determination of the drugs prior to GLC analysis. The one drawback with this method is the fact that any metabolite which yields the same benzophenone would interfere with the assay.

The electron capture approach has also been applied to the analysis of methylphenidate, an antidepressant drug in humans, in horse blood [119]. This drug is reputed to be an equine stimulant and hence is a drug of abuse in racing. As the drug is usually administered at a dose of 50 to 200 mg intramuscularly (I. M.), plasma levels in the order of 100 ng/ml or less are commonly encountered. Consequently, the ECD method was utilized, especially since the drug is amenable to derivatization. Two approaches were employed by Huffman et al. [118], namely, acylation of the secondary amine and reduction of the ester to the alcohol followed by acylation with pentafluoropropionic anhydride (PFPA). The reaction sequences are illustrated below:

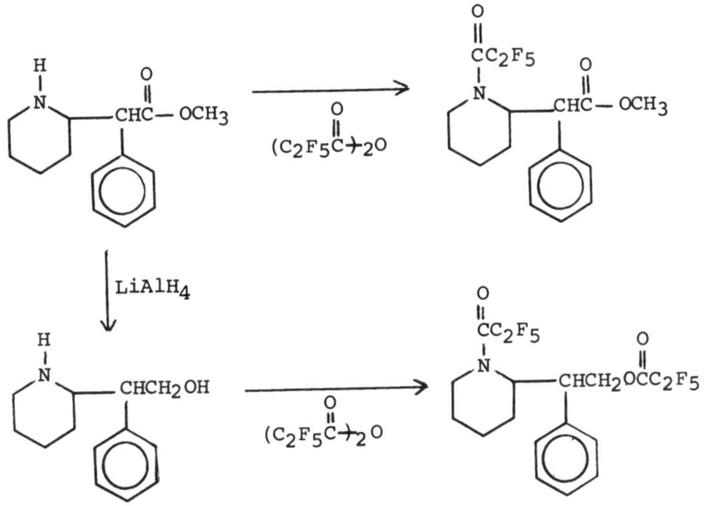

Using the reductive-acylation technique the authors were able to obtain drug plasma profile curves in six horses. A rapid rate of drug elimination was observed ($T_{1/2} \sim 1$ h).

Fenimore et al. [27] devised an ECD method for Δ^9-tetrahydrocannabinol, the major active component in marijuana, in an attempt to correlate blood levels of this pharmacologically-active drug with its physiological and behavioral effects of the drug. The authors found the heptafluorobutyryl derivative to be most effective and permitted determinations as low as 0.1 ng/ml of plasma.

Recent (1974-75) electron capture GLC methods have been reported for a number of drugs and their metabolites, namely, morphine [15], bromazepam (an antianxiety agent) and its 3-hydroxymetabolite [16], perphenazine (a neuroleptic drug) and its sulfoxide metabolite [28], the new cerebral vasodilator 2,6-dimethyl-4-(3-nitrophenyl)-1,4-dihydropyridine-3,5-dicarboxylic acid 3-(2-N-benzyl-N-methylamino)1-ethyl ester, 5-methyl ester [29], triethylammonium cyclamate [142], ecdysone hormones [143], phenmetrazine [145], indomethacin [8], atenolol [30], practolol [144], flurazepam [31], and the antiarrhythmic drug, α,α-dimethyl-4-($\alpha,\alpha,\beta,\beta$-tetrafluorophenethyl)benzylamine [146].

In general, electron capture GLC has been utilized for the quantitative analysis of low levels of drugs ($< 1 \mu$g/ml). In almost all instances an internal standard was employed and the drug and its metabolites, when applicable, were isolated usually by solvent partitioning under acidic or alkaline conditions. Most drugs are not detected by the ECD at the sensitivity required without conversion to compounds that possess electron capturing properties. Hydroxyl and amino moieties were the most commonly derivatized functional groups, usually by the introduction of the heptafluorobutyryl or trifluoroacetyl moiety. A few instances of reduction followed by acylation have been reported. In the preparation of a derivative one must be sure that: (1) the derivative is formed quantitatively, even in the presence of often massive amounts of extraneous material, (2) no loss occurs as a function of time due to lack of stability of the derivative or unexpected side reactions, and (3) no abnormal functional group alterations occur during the reaction. The last point is extremely critical when one is using this technique for structure elucidation.

Electron capture detectors which employ ^{63}Ni as the source of β-radiation exhibit a greater linear range than detectors which employ ^{3}H sources, and afford greater stability at the higher temperatures required in some assays. Unlike the FID, however, the ECD is one of the most difficult detectors to use successfully; unless extreme care is exercised to establish proper operating conditions, disappointing and misleading results, and considerable frustration, are inevitable. ECDs should be cleaned frequently as they tend to decrease in sensitivity with extensive use. The internal standard method using either peak area or peak height ratios is highly recommended for accurate, reproducible results.

Not in every situation, however, does the EC-GLC method provide the best condition for the analysis of low levels of drugs. Perchalski et al. [147] presented a comparison on the determination of 1-(2,6-dimethylphenoxy)-2-aminopropane using FID and ECD methods. The authors state that the ECD method was found to give no advantage. Relative standard deviations of replicate samples extracted for the FID method were less than 7% with a limit of detection of 7 ng/ml. Of great importance was the fact that the commonly used anticonvulsants including ethosuximide, primidone, carbamazepine, and diphenylhydantoin do not interfere with the method (which involves derivatization of the amino group with trifluoroacetic anhydride to form the corresponding acetamide).

B. Radioactivity Monitoring

The use of radiolabeling is highly desirable in any serious drug metabolism study. This is because metabolic transformations can dramatically alter physicochemical properties (e.g., solvent extractibility, pK, chromatographic mobility), with the result that a metabolite may behave very

differently in a given isolation procedure than the parent drug. It is
possible to compare fractions from biological fluids from normals with
those from drug-treated individuals. This approach does not, however,
possess the benefits of tagging the drug so that the presence of a
drug-related substance can be recognized immediately in a fraction or
aliquot, and procedures designed to effect its isolation, purification,
and identification. GLC analyses are usually carried out on zones
from TLC plates, cuts from LC columns, or solvent extracts. If the
parent drug were radiolabeled, the presence of a metabolite in one of
the abovementioned fractions could be readily ascertained. There is
no guarantee that the isolate would be single component in nature. Indeed, a feature of GLC analysis is that qualitative and quantitative information can be obtained from nonhomogeneous samples. Thus a detection system capable of indicating which of numerous components is
radioactive, and hence drug-related, becomes imperative. The simplest
approach for determining this is to follow the GLC separation via a
mass detector (e.g., FID) and to collect or trap the observed components and subject them to radioactivity assay in a liquid scintillation
spectrometer. This procedure permits long-term counting of components containing low levels of radioactivity, but requires that the compound of interest be trapped. Radioactivity in GLC effluents can be
monitored continuously by flow-through detectors, but this approach has
several drawbacks [148-150]. Combustion (yielding $^{14}CO_2$ from ^{14}C-
labeled compounds) of the column effluent prior to delivery to the radioactivity detector has been strongly recommended by Karmen [149].
Several groups of workers [151, 152] have advocated trapping the CO_2
from each GLC component in an organic base and subjecting these
fractions to radioassay. An example of this combustion/collection approach in a drug metabolism project is seen in Figure 11. A radioactive fraction containing a neutral metabolite of [^{14}C] cambendazole
was obtained via liquid chromatographic techniques. When an aliquot
was subjected to GLC with combustion and collection of the effluent
corresponding to the individual peaks (the column effluent was split
between an FID and the combustion/collection system [152]), more than
85% of the injected radioactivity was found to be associated with the
major peak in the lower chromatogram. With the drug-related component
of the sample thus recognized, combined GLC-MS was employed to
demonstrate that the metabolite possessed the structure given below [153].

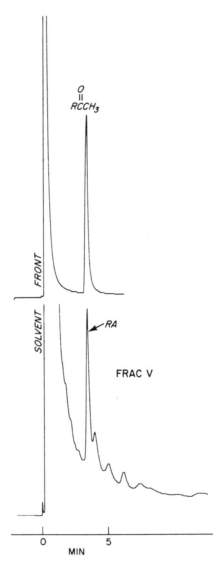

FIG. 11. Lower chromatogram: GLRC of a urinary isolate from a cow dosed with [^{14}C] cambendazole. The component "RA" was shown to contain a radioactive metabolite, identified as 2-(4'-acetyl)-5-isopropoxycarbonyl-aminobenzimidazole. Upper chromatogram: GLC analysis of a sample of authentic 2-(4'-acetyl)-5-isopropoxycarbonylbenzimidazole. Column conditions: 6 ft × 3 mm i.d. glass column packed with 1% OV-17 on 100 to 120 mesh acid-washed and silanized Gas-Chrom P; 200°C; 60 ml/min carrier gas.

In another study, an acidic urinary metabolite isolated from a wether lamb dosed with [^{14}C] bis(chloromethyl)sulfone was obtained in a partially purified state via TLC. No volatile radioactive component was found (using the combustion/collection approach) with the radioactive isolate, but when the analysis was repeated following derivatization with bis(trimethylsilyl)trifluoroacetamide (BSTFA) a radioactive compound was eluted (see Fig. 12). This component was subsequently identified by combined GLC-MS as the ester of chloromethanesulfinic acid [154].

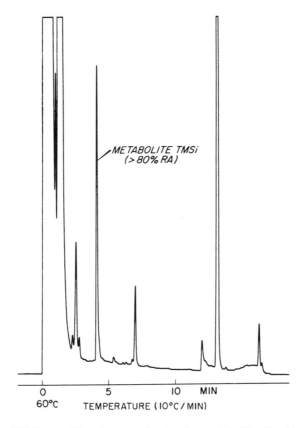

FIG. 12. GLRC resulting from analysis of a metabolite fraction isolate (from the urine of a lamb dosed with [^{14}C] bis(chloromethyl)sulfone) which had been exposed to trimethylsilylating conditions. The component with the 4 min retention time was shown to be radioactive. Column conditions: 6 ft × 4 mm i.d. glass column packed with 5% F-60 on 80 to 100 mesh acid-washed and silanized Gas-Chrom P; temperature program from 60 to 200°C at 10°C/min; initial carrier gas flow rate 75 ml/min. (Reprinted from Ref. 154 by courtesy of Elsevier Publishing Company.)

Continuous assay of the gaseous effluent from the combustion system
by use of a proportional type counter is generally preferred to the discon-
tinuous collection of fractions and subsequent determination of their activity.   The former approach is analogous to collecting an infinite number of
fractions, and although such a dynamic approach requires higher levels of
radioactivity (because of a limited period of time, i.e., 30 sec, for detection) a labeled component is less likely to escape detection.   The use of a
flow-through counter is especially useful when a multicomponent sample is
examined as, for example, in Figure 13.   A radioactive zone obtained by
TLC of a crude urinary isolate from a human treated with [^{14}C] cyrohepta-
dine yielded the lower FID chromatogram.

Cyproheptadine

Temperature programming was employed to yield a "metabolic profile"
from the trimethylsilylated isolate.   Radioactivity was found to be associated with only one of the many components in this rather complex chromatogram.   The metabolite has been characterized by combined GLC-MS as a
hydroxylated N-demethyl cyproheptadine [155].   Collecting and counting the
CO_2 from each component would surely have proven to be a tedious task in
this case.   Even with an isolate containing only a few components (e.g.,
see Fig. 14) the continuous assay of the combustion tube effluent for radioactivity, simultaneous with mass detection via FID, is an attractive approach provided the level of radioactivity is sufficiently great. * The radioactivity monitor (RAM) peak in Figure 14 represents 500 cpm of [^{14}C]-2-
methyl-3'-hydroxyphenylpropionic acid, a monkey urinary metabolite of
carbidopa [156].

^{14}C is the most frequently employed isotope in radiolabeling studies,
but tritium is also used under appropriate conditions.   Sun and coworkers
have used ^{3}H-labeled prostaglandin $PGF_{2\alpha}$ in metabolism studies of this
abortifacient agent in the rat [157] and rhesus monkey [158].   The retention time of each radioactive (and hence drug-related) component in deriv-

---

*Our experience suggests lower limits of 250 and 600 cpm (^{14}C and ^{3}H,
respectively) injected on-column with a RAM/FID split ratio of 3:1.

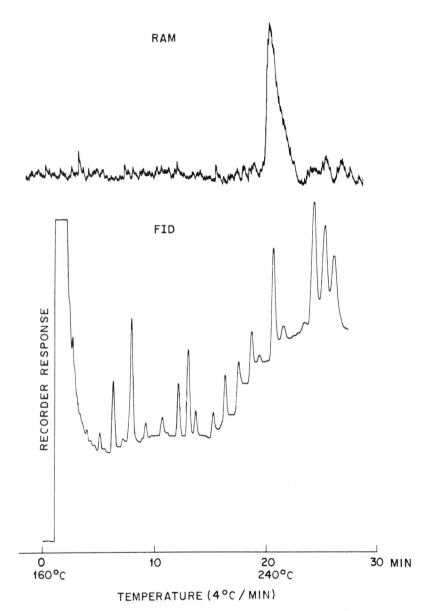

FIG. 13. Simultaneous RAM and FID analysis of an isolate (from the urine of a patient treated with [^{14}C] cyproheptadine) which has been subjected to trimethylsilylation conditions. Column conditions: 6 ft × 4 mm i.d. glass column packed with 3% OV-17 on acid-washed and silanized Gas-Chrom P; temperature program from 160 to 240°C at 5°C/min, then isothermal at the upper temperature; initial carrier gas flow rate, 60 ml/min.

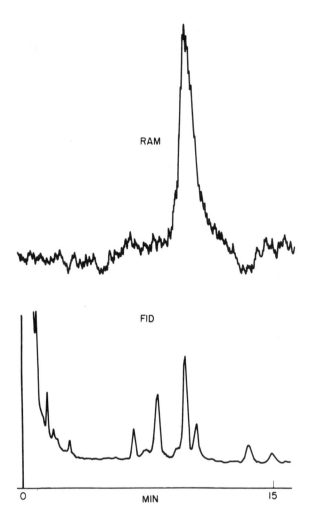

FIG. 14. Simultaneous RAM and FID analysis of an isolate (from the urine of a monkey dosed with [^{14}C] Carbidopa) which had been subjected to trimethylsilylation conditions. Column conditions: 6 ft × 4 mm i.d. glass column packed with 3% OV-1 on 80 to 100 mesh acid-washed and silanized Gas-Chrom P; 165°C; 60 ml/min carrier gas.

atized (methyl ester-methoxime-TMSi ether) isolates was determined by simultaneous monitoring for mass (FID) and radioactivity (combustion to CO_2 and ^3H_2O, followed by reduction of the latter to $^3H_2$). The mass spectrum of each tritium-containing component was then obtained by combined

Carbidopa

GLC-MS. In a similar way we have demonstrated, following the work of Seyberth and coworkers [159] and Hamberg and Samuelsson [160], that ^{3}H- (and ^{2}H)-labeled 15-keto-PGE_0 is converted by the rabbit to several urinary metabolites including 7α-hydroxy-5, 11-diketotetranorprostane-1, 16-dioic acid and 5β, 7α-dihydroxy-11-keto-tetranorprostanoic acid [161]. An isolate containing the first-named metabolite was subjected to gas-liquid radiochromatography (GLRC) as its dimethyl ester dimethoxime-TMSI ether, and the tritium-containing component was found to exhibit the same retention time (on SE-30) as the methyl ester of the C_{24} long chain fatty acid (see Fig. 15), as reported by Hamberg and Samuelsson [162]. The RAM peak represents ~800 cpm of ^{3}H injected.

C. Element Selective Detectors

Although the majority of GLC analyses in drug metabolism utilize FID or ECD, applications involving element selection detectors are becoming more frequent. Good absolute sensitivity (usually at least as great as that for the FID) plus the resulting specificity for a drug or metabolite containing the element for which the detector is selective make this detection approach highly attractive. This is especially true when one considers that, in general, less extensive purification is required to provide a sample suitable for element selective detection. These detectors are also insensitive to increased column bleed resulting from temperature programming. Furthermore, by simultaneously using two detectors with different selectivities and determining their response ratios, specific assays for low levels of drug in tissue or body fluids can be developed. Aue [163] and Natusch and Thorpe [164] have published review articles dealing with these detectors, and Maier-Bode and Riedman [165] recently discussed use of the nitrogen selective FID in the determination of nitrogen-containing pesticides.

McLeod and coworkers [166] have described a GLC system with five types of detectors operating simultaneously—flame ionization; phosphorus,

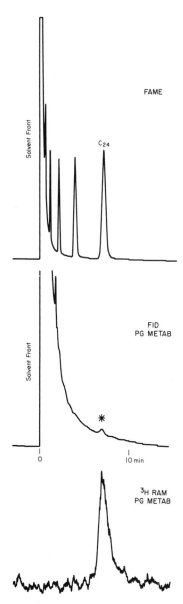

FIG. 15.   Bottom and middle: simultaneous RAM and FID analysis of
an isolate (from the urine of a rabbit dosed with ^{2}H, ^{3}H-labeled 15-keto-
PGE$_0$) which had been subjected to methylation, methoxime formation, and
trimethylsilylation conditions. Top: GLC analysis of a homologous series
of fatty acid methyl esters, including the C$_{24}$ species. Note the starred
peak in the FID chromatogram which yields a RAM peak with the same retention time as the C$_{24}$ fatty acid methyl ester. Column conditions: 6 ft ×
4 mm i.d. glass column containing 1% OV-1 on 80 to 100 mesh Gas-Chrom
P; 220°C; 60 ml/min carrier gas.

sulfur, and nitrogen selective; and electron capture—for pesticide residue analysis. The column is equipped with a three-way effluent splitter, by which approximately one-half of the effluent goes to a Coulson electrolytic detector operated in the nitrogen mode, approximately 45% of the effluent goes to a flame photometric detector which can function in the flame ionization, sulfur and phosphorous modes, and approximately 5% goes to an ECD. Although we have not discussed pesticide residue studies in this chapter, the multidetector approach employed by these authors should be equally applicable in drug residue studies for screening purposes and for establishing confirmatory assays.

A Coulson electrolytic conductivity detector has been employed to study the GLC analysis of medazepam and its metabolites in rat plasma spiked (2 μg/ml) with these compounds [167]. Ether extracts of 25 ml plasma were taken to dryness and 1/100 of the residue analyzed; no further purification was found to be necessary. The response of this detector to benzodiazepams in the oxidative mode is felt to be due to both the chlorine and nitrogen atoms. Optimal detection for the nonhalogen containing nitrazepam (7-nitrobenzodiazepine) would be in the reductive mode.

The flame photometric detector can be operated in the phosphorus-selective or sulfur-selective modes. An example of the former is reported by McCallum [168] on the measurement of cannabinol and Δ^9-THC levels in human blood. Detectability is introduced by an infrequently employed derivatization step: conversion of these phenolic compounds to their diethyl-phosphate ethers. The authors claim a sensitivity of better than 1 ng/ml of plasma when 10 ml of plasma is assayed. Another paper on the use of phosphorus selective detectors is that by Jackson and Reynolds [169] on the determination of cyclophosphamide residues in sheep tissue. This antitumor drug was found to be a potential defleecing agent, and earlier methods were not satisfactory for trace tissue residue studies. The authors reported that using 10 g of sample the GLC approach was quantitative to 0.01 ppm.

Schirmer and Pierson [170] have developed an assay for methapyrilene in plasma and urine using a flame photometric detector in the sulfur specific mode. Sensitivity of the assay was held to be 50 ng/ml of human plasma. Although injection of 10 ng of the drug resulted in GLC detection, none was found in the plasma or urine from patients receiving 20 mg/day i.m. or 50 mg/day p.o. Lamkin et al. [171] have applied the flame photometric detector to the GLC analysis of methylthiohydantoins and their TMSi derivatives.

Palframan et al. [172] have compared the alkali flame ionization and Coulson electrolytic conductivity detectors operating in the nitrogen selective mode for the analysis of N-nitrosamine residues in foods. The two detectors were found to exhibit similar lower limits of sensitivity (approximately 100 pg, calculated as nitrogen, for dibutylnitrosamine), but the electrolytic conductivity detector exhibited greater selectivity.

A GLC method for diisopyramide in serum employing an alkali FID operated in the nitrogen selective mode has been developed by Duchateau et al. [173]. An endogenous compound in serum causes interference with the internal standard peak when a hydrogen flame ionization detector is employed. This serum component causes no response with the nitrogen detector, however, and the latter yields a very small solvent front. Thus, the need for a possibly extensive cleanup if FID were employed is avoided by use of the nitrogen detector, and a simple chloroform extraction of alkalinized urine or serum yields an isolate suitable for analysis.

The major advantage of nitrogen selective detection as opposed to FID, i.e., the suitability of simplified isolation procedures, has been utilized by Cameron [174] in his assay for etidocaine in plasma. Analysis of plasma samples containing 50 ng/ml of drug was possible with no interference from endogenous plasma components or several other anesthetics in current use. The simple ether extraction of 2 ml of plasma followed by partition against base gave an extract which, following evaporation, yielded a residue suitable for assay (dissolved in carbon disulfide).

Several papers have appeared recently which describe the use of nitrogen selective detectors for tricyclic antidepressants in human plasma. Gifford et al. [175] found detection limits of 1 to 5 ng (injected) for imipramine, desimipramine, amitriptyline, and nortriptyline. Six replicate assays of 4-ml plasma samples containing 25 ng of imipramine gave a value of 25.8 ng/ml with a standard deviation of 10%. Jorgensen [176] has studied the assay of amitriptyline and nortriptyline in human serum and found lower limits of detection of 5 ng/ml for the former and 10 to 15 ng/ml for the latter. He has used the method for the quantitative estimation of amitriptyline levels following a single 50-mg dose, and for the determination of this drug and its metabolite nortriptyline after repeated doses (3×50 mg/day for two weeks). An acetylation step is employed to improve the separation of amitriptyline and nortriptyline.

GLC methods using nitrogen selective detection have also been employed for the determination of anticonvulsants and barbiturates in biological samples. Toseland and associates [177] found that 0.2 ml of plasma was a sufficiently large sample size to allow the determination of eight of the former. The residue resulting from taking an ether extract to dryness is dissolved in methanol and approximately 5 to 10% of this solution analyzed. Dvorchik [178] has published a method for several barbiturates involving extraction of whole blood (0.1 ml) with chloroform; a sensitivity of 10 μg/ml blood was reported. This author also speaks glowingly of the simplicity of his method, due in large part to use of the nitrogen selective detector.

A nitrogen detector has been employed by Smith and Cole [179] for the assay of diacetylmorphine and its metabolite monoacetylmorphine in blood. Quantitation of diacetylmorphine was possible at 100 ng/ml level in blood,

and was held to be as low as 20 ng/ml for "illicit preparations." The
author indicates that via FID the detection limit for the latter sample is
50 μg/ml. Blood levels of the two compounds of interest were followed in
an Irish greyhound dosed (i. v.) with diacetylmorphine. The metabolite
was found to display a slower rate of disappearance than parent drug.

A rapid, simple method for the determination of plasma levels of lidocaine in which quantitation is achieved by GLC using nitrogen selective
detection has been reported by Hucker and Stauffer [180]. The detector's
thermionic source is electrically heated, resulting in improved performance
relative to flame-heated systems.

Mashford and coworkers [181] measured carbamazepine in human plasma
using nitrogen selective detection. Plasma levels for patients ranged from
1.2 to 2.4 μg/ml. The authors state that injection of more than 5 μg of
drug results in elution of two peaks of widely different retention times, and
that the component of longer retention time is not observed if less than
5 μg is injected. It would appear that an on-column thermal degradation
could be the source of this phenomenon. At the higher levels both the parent drug and its transformation product are eluted, but at the lower levels
only one, probably the latter, is noted. The GLC degradation of carbamazepine and several related compounds has been discussed by Frigerio
et al. [80].

Plazonnet and Cerdeno [182] determined pilocarpine in the aqueous
humor of rabbits using the nitrogen selective thermionic detector. Fifty-
fold enhancement of the detector signal over that of an FID was achieved.
The authors found it was possible to quantitate as little as 2 ng of drug
in aqueous humor samples (0.2 ml) following topical application of commercial pilocarpine eyedrops.

D. Mass Spectrometric Detection*

An especially valuable application of combined GLC-MS is validation of a
GLC assay for a drug or metabolite from a biological source. Retention
time and peak shape with an FID or ECD are useful indications, but no
guarantee, of identity and homogeneity. Combined GLC-MS, however, is
a method offering a much higher level of confidence for the identification
of GLC components and indication of peak homogeneity. We have used this
approach for recently developed electron capture GLC methods for the
coccidiostat pyrimethamine, 2,4-diamino-5-p-chlorophenyl-5-ethylpyrim-
idine [183], for the antiarrhythmic agent, MK-251 [146], and for the

---

*See chapters "Gas Chromatography-Mass Spectrometry-Computer
Techniques" and "Mass Fragmentography" to be published in future volumes of this series.

uricosuric agent, MK-196 [184]. Combined GLC-MS demonstrated conclusively that the components exhibiting the appropriate retention times
were indeed the unchanged drugs. A mass spectrometer can also serve
as a selective GLC detector. Repetitive scanning over a narrow mass
range across a GLC peak is an attractive approach to the characterization
and quantification of trace amounts of compounds. The characteristic pattern and high intensity of the signals in the molecular ion region of the mass
spectrum of pyrimethamine (Fig. 16) make this drug particularly well
suited to this type of analysis. A comparison of the GLC-MS response
(repetitively scanned from m/e 247 to 250) to 20 ng of pyrimethamine and
to an aliquot (20 ng on the basis of ECD-GLC) of an isolate gave practically
superimposable results, and confirmed the specificity and accuracy of the
ECD-GLC assay.

As reported earlier, Sadee et al. [36] have published a GLC method for
the determination of plasma levels of (±)-1, 2-bis(3, 5-dioxopiperazinyl)-
propane in several species including man. The sensitivity of their GLC
assay using an FID was only 5 μg/ml because of an interfering component
with the same retention time as the derivatized (methylated) drug. An increase in the sensitivity limit to 0.2 μg/ml was achieved by use of a mass
spectrometer, operating in the selective single ion detection mode, as the
detector. Monitoring of the ion of m/e 155 permitted the measurement of
the drug in plasma following therapeutic doses.

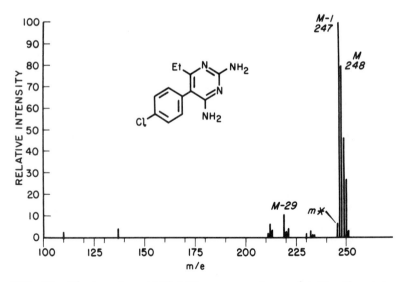

FIG. 16. Electron impact 70 (eV) mass spectrum of pyrimethamine.
(Reprinted from Ref. 183 by courtesy of the American Chemical Society.)

The mass spectrometer can also serve as a multichannel selective GLC detector by simultaneously monitoring several characteristic ions. This approach was employed by Cole et al. [185] to confirm electron capture data suggesting chloral hydrate as a transient metabolite of trichloroethylene in man. Because chloral hydrate is thermally labile, injection of this compound results in the elution of chloral. The latter compound yields a mass spectrum with characteristic chlorine isotope clusters at m/e 111, 113 (M-Cl) and 146, 148 (M). These ions are monitored during GLC-MS of (1) reference chloral hydrate, (2) a plasma extract spiked with the former, and (3) plasma extracts from patients treated with chloral hydrate. With all three samples the intensities of the four ions were seen to maximize at the same retention time and exhibited the same relative intensity relationships, thus fulfilling the mass fragmentographic requirements [186] for demonstrating the elution of chloral from the column. This evidence clearly indicated that chloral hydrate was present in the plasma of the individuals treated with trichloroethylene.

Internal standards are frequently employed in quantitative GLC. As suggested by Gaffney et al. [187], the internal standard of choice for a GLC-MS assay is probably the isotopically-labeled compound of interest. The use of such internal standards provides highly sensitive and selective assays for compounds of biological interest [188-191]. Kaplan and associates [192] have employed a mass fragmentographic assay developed by Walker et al. [193] for the determination of blood levels of N,N-dimethyltryptamine following administration of psychoactive doses of this hallucinogen to human subjects. Deuterated N,N-DMT is employed as the internal standard, and the compounds are analyzed as TMSi derivatives. A plot of mean whole blood concentration vs. time after injection (i.m.) is presented in Figure 17. The blood N,N-DMT levels and the subjective "highs" experienced by the subjects followed a similar time course.

Hamberg [103] has reported on the effect of several anti-inflammatory agents upon urinary excretion of 7α-hydroxy-5,11-diketotetranorprostane-1,16-dioic acid, the major human urinary metabolite of PGE_1 and PGE_2, using a GLC-MS isotope assay. Derivatization steps include methylation, conversion of the keto groups to methoximes, and trimethylsilylation of the hydroxy group. The ditrideuteromethoxime of the tetranorprostane diacid is employed as an internal standard and is introduced partway through the assay procedure. The analogous ions of m/e 365 [M - (31 + 90)] from

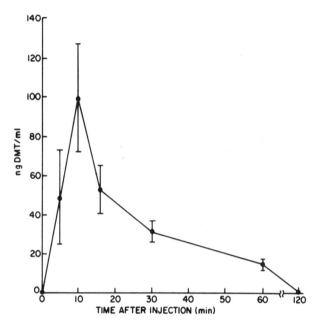

FIG. 17. Plot of mean whole blood concentrations vs. time for a group of subjects following administration of N, N-dimethyltryptamine. (Reprinted from Ref. 192 by courtesy of Springer-Verlag.)

the endogenous metabolite and 368 [M - (34 + 90)] from the internal standard are monitored and their intensity ratio compared to a calibration curve for quantitation. An internal standard is ideally added to the sample prior to initiation of the assay procedure. Preparation of a labeled internal standard is a frequently encountered problem in quantitative GLC-MS. Seyberth and coworkers [159] prepared the prostaglandin metabolite labeled with ^{2}H and ^{3}H by dosing a rabbit with the appropriate precursor. We have also prepared this labeled metabolite [161] * (in approximately 1.5% yield, based on radioactivity in a partially purified isolate) by dosing a rabbit with $[^2H, ^3H]$-15-keto-PGE_0, as suggested by Hamberg and Samuelsson [160]. The most intense signals in the spectrum of the desired compound (as its dimethyl ester dimethoxime TMSi ether) are those of m/e 367 and 368, as the most common isotopic species in this labeled compound contain 2 and 3 deuterium atoms. The ion of m/e 367 was chosen for monitoring in the GLC assay. This internal standard, in an underivatized state, was added to aliquots of urine from a normal adult male collected before and after

*We are grateful to Drs. Oates and Seyberth for their many helpful suggestions on the dosing and isolation procedures.

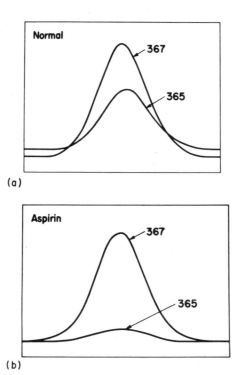

(a)

(b)

FIG. 18. Mass fragmentographic analysis in the determination of the
major human urinary metabolite of PGE_1 and PGE_2 in isolates from a normal male (a) before and (b) after the administration of aspirin. The ions
monitored are m/e 365 from the endogenous metabolite and m/e 367 from
the deuterium-labeled internal standard; the compounds are run as their
dimethyl ester-dimethoxime-TMSi ether derivatives. Column conditions:
5 ft × 2.5 mm i.d. glass column containing 1.5% SE-30 on 80 to 100 mesh
acid-washed and silanized Gas-Chrom P; 222°C; 30 ml/min carrier gas;
20 eV ionizing potential used with accelerating voltage alternater of mass
spectrometer.

his taking 12 5-grain aspirin tablets (over a two-day period). This drug
has been reported by Hamberg [103] to suppress output of the major urinary metabolite in man. Comparison of the mass fragmentograms in Figure
18 (before and after aspirin) shows that the m/e 365 to 367 intensity ratio
is markedly reduced, presumably reflecting suppression by the drug of
PG synthesis. The samples injected were equivalent to approximately 1
ml of urine.

The practical sensitivity of a GLC-MS assay is determined by the intensity of the ion being monitored, the inherent sensitivity of the mass spec-

trometer serving as the detector, and other factors.   As pointed out in
the original paper by Hammar and coworkers [186] on mass fragmentography, adsorption of samples during the GLC process is a potential
source of error (although compensated for by the use of heavy atom labeled carriers).   The sensitivity of the detector is of little value if the sample does not reach it.   Thus judicious choice of derivatives to improve GLC
properties with respect to adsorption and the development of nonadsorptive
column systems appear to be important areas of research.   Indeed, this is
certainly true for any GLC technique, regardless of the detection limit
employed.

V.   QUANTITATION

Both qualitative and quantitative information can be obtained from GLC
analyses.   The qualitative aspects of GLC have been reported in detail
[3,4,194-197].   Qualitative analysis is based primarily on retention time
or more often on the retention time relative to that of a reference standard.
The final identification is usually the result of a comparison of the retention
data of the unknown with those of authentic reference compounds.   The
Kovats retention index [198,199] and the "methylene unit" approach [200]
are the most frequently employed techniques since these values are independent of changes in GLC operating parameters.   Additional qualitative
information may be obtained upon analysis of the sample with selective
detectors.   The quantitative aspects of drug and metabolite concentration
is extremely relevant to clinical pharmacology.   The authors have previously discussed the methods of calibration, peak measurement, and com-
puter data acquisition and analysis [5].   In the GLC analysis of drugs and
their metabolites, the areas under the eluting peaks are dependent upon the
amounts of emerging sample components; therefore, those peak areas after
proper calibration can be quantitatively related to the amount of the individual components present.   The external and internal methods of calibration
are commonly used.   The external calibration approach involves the construction of a calibration curve following the injection of known amounts of
the drug to be analyzed.   The peak area (or height) data are plotted vs.
weight of compound injected.   Although the method is simple, it requires
that: (1) precise amounts of sample are injected and (2) the detector sensitivity remain constant during the analyses.   This approach has produced
good results with the stable FID; however, difficulties can arise with the
ECD because of its instability.   In the analysis of chlordiazepoxide, Zingales
[201] used the external standard approach and obtained a 90 ± 3% recovery
of drug added to control plasma in the 0.03 to 10 μg range (FID).

The internal standard technique obviates some of the stringent requirements of the external method.   The former approach compensates for small

changes in operating conditions and for inaccuracies in injection volumes.
McNair and Bonelli [197] have discussed the quantitative aspects of analysis
in detail. The best calibration curves are obtained when the appropriate
weight ratios of drug to be assayed vs. internal standard are added to the
control biological specimen (plasma, urine, etc.) and then carried through
the entire procedure. For best performance the internal standard should
be structurally similar to the drug being analyzed (to provide similar
chromatographic properties), added to the initial biological specimen before sample manipulation (this compensates for losses due to inaccurate
and nonquantitative steps), and clearly separated from all other peaks in
the chromatogram. The standard curve should cover the entire range in
the analysis to eliminate any error which may arise due to nonlinearity in
the system. By far the most impressive quantitative data are obtained
when an internal standard is added to the initial biological specimen and
carried through the isolation and derivatization procedures. A few examples illustrating the use of the internal standard technique in out laboratories are discussed. In the analysis of probenecid [43] a linear relationship is observed when the peak height ratio is plotted vs. weight ratio
(Fig. 19). The calibration curve was obtained following the addition of
known weight ratios of probenecid and the internal standard to control
urine, plasma, or water. The mean recovery using the FID method of
detection was $100.5 \pm 6.4\%$ over a 0.2 to 60 μg/ml concentration range.
In the quantitation of an antiarrhythmic drug (MK-251) by electron capture,
a similar approach was used [146]. Table 3 presents a summary on the

TABLE 3

Recovery of MK-251 from Dog Plasma

Amount added (ng)	Amount recovered (ng)						Mean ± S.D.
100	93.8	99.4	--[a]	105.6	99.4	109.2	101.5 ± 6.0
80	78.3	76.1	81.6	91.2	81.6	79.6	81.4 ± 5.2
50	47.3	56.2	59.0	43.9	51.4	47.2	50.8 ± 5.8
25	25.0	28.8	21.9	24.7	25.4	25.4	25.2 ± 0.9
15	16.6	13.7	18.5	15.1	15.8	11.9	15.3 ± 2.3
10	10.6	9.6	11.7	9.6	10.3	7.8	9.9 ± 1.3
5	3.7	3.4	5.5	5.5	4.8	3.5	4.4 ± 1.0

[a]No sample analyzed; data obtained from single injections of standard
recovery tubes.

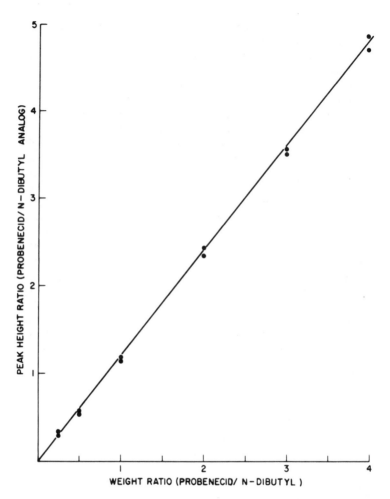

FIG. 19. Relationship between peak height ratio (probenecid/N-dibutyl analog) and weight ratio (probenecid/N-dibutyl analog). Five out of 100 μl were injected in each case. (Reprinted from Ref. 43 by courtesy of the American Pharmaceutical Association.)

recovery of drug added to control dog plasma over a period of several months. The recovery of drug added to control dog plasma was 102.6 ± 13.5% over a range of 5 to 100 ng. Both FID and ECD GLC methods were used for the analysis of the polyvalent saluretic agent (6,7-dichloro-2-phenyl-2-methyl-1-oxo-5-indanyloxy)acetic acid (MK-196) and its metabolite [184]. A typical peak height ratio vs. weight ratio for drug and internal standard is presented in Figure 20. Table 4 summarizes the re-

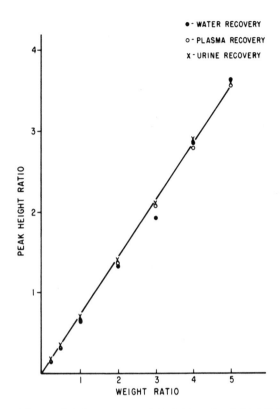

FIG. 20. Relationship between peak height ratio (MK-196/I.S.) and
weight ratio (MK-196/I.S.). Five out of 50 to 100 μl were injected in each
case following recovery of MK-196 (1-50 μg) from water, plasma, or
urine. (Reprinted from Ref. 184 by courtesy of the American Pharmaceutical Association.)

covery results obtained from rat, dog, chimpanzee, monkey, and human
studies. The results were obtained using an FID over a period of one
year. The mean recovery (n = 207) of MK-196 from control plasma was
99.1 ± 4.4% in the 1 to 60 μg/ml range. The mean recovery of MK-196
(n = 163) from control urine was 99.8 ± 4.9% in the same concentration
range. As lower levels of drug were obtained following administration of
drug to man [184], the method was modified to permit detection with a
^{63}Ni ECD rather than an FID. Table 5 summarizes the results obtained
following analysis of various amounts of MK-196 (2.5-100 ng) added to
plasma. The mean recovery of MK-196 from control plasma was 98.8 ±
11.9% (n = 322) over the entire range. Using an ECD-GLC method, similar data were obtained for the analysis of the p-hydroxy metabolite of
MK-196 following trimethylsilylation of the phenolic group. A recovery
of 98.3 ± 6.5% was obtained (n = 62).

TABLE 4

Recovery of MK-196 From Plasma and Urine Using FID Method

MK-196 added (μg)		Amount recovered[a]			
		Plasma		Urine	
		n	Mean ± S.D.	n	Mean ± S.D.
60.0	A	12	60.2 ± 0.75	8	59.1 ± 2.32
	B		100.3 ± 1.3		98.5 ± 3.8
50.0	A	19	50.1 ± 1.13	15	50.2 ± 0.84
	B		100.1 ± 2.2		100.5 ± 1.7
40.0	A	24	40.6 ± 1.07	16	40.5 ± 0.89
	B		101.5 ± 2.7		101.5 ± 2.2
30.0	A	25	30.0 ± 0.70	18	30.2 ± 1.00
	B		100.0 ± 2.3		100.6 ± 3.3
20.0	A	27	19.9 ± 0.77	18	20.0 ± 0.39
	B		99.9 ± 3.8		99.9 ± 1.9
10.0	A	29	9.8 ± 0.38	27	10.0 ± 0.42
	B		98.3 ± 3.8		100.2 ± 4.2
5.0	A	31	4.9 ± 0.22	26	5.0 ± 0.25
	B		98.1 ± 4.4		100.3 ± 4.9
2.5	A	26	2.4 ± 0.13	21	2.5 ± 0.14
	B		97.6 ± 5.3		98.5 ± 5.6
1.0	A	14	1.0 ± 0.09	14	1.0 ± 0.10
	B		96.6 ± 9.1		96.6 ± 11.0
1-60	B	207	99.1 ± 4.4	163	99.8 ± 4.9

[a] Values in A rows represent μg recovered; values in B rows represent percent recovery.

TABLE 5

Recovery of MK-196 From Plasma Using ECD Method

MK-196 added (ng)	n	ng Recovered Mean ± S.D.	% Recovery Mean ± S.D.
100.0	22	98.9 ± 4.3	98.9 ± 4.3
80.0	20	79.0 ± 8.9	98.7 ± 11.1
65.0	21	65.7 ± 5.4	101.1 ± 8.3
50.0	37	48.7 ± 3.4	97.4 ± 6.8
40.0	27	39.4 ± 3.1	98.4 ± 7.7
25.0	42	25.0 ± 2.1	100.1 ± 8.4
20.0	30	19.8 ± 2.3	99.1 ± 11.3
12.5	31	12.9 ± 1.6	103.5 ± 13.0
10.0	26	9.9 ± 1.0	99.1 ± 10.6
6.25	27	5.9 ± 1.1	93.9 ± 17.8
5.0	23	4.9 ± 0.65	97.6 ± 13.0
2.5	16	2.4 ± 0.64	96.2 ± 26.3
2.5-100	322		98.8 ± 11.9

VI. METABOLIC TRANSFORMATIONS

GLC is less frequently employed in the identification of metabolic transformation products than in the measurement of drug or metabolite levels in biological samples. Studies of the former type more often involve GLC in combinations with MS, and there are many excellent examples of the value of this combination of techniques [154-156, 202-204]. (This topic is covered by a chapter in this series [205]). Nevertheless, GLC per se is a valuable tool for metabolite structure elucidation. It has been utilized extensively in drug metabolism to obtain metabolic profiles of drugs. Metabolic inactivation often involves the oxidation of a drug to a more polar species. Metabolites, although at times differing solely by a hydroxyl group, may not be amenable to GLC analysis, especially at the submicrogram level, without prior derivatization to enhance volatility or reduce column adsorption.

GLC is particularly useful for in vitro studies in which an aliquot of a simple extract of the incubation mixture can be examined for parent drug and metabolites, the latter appearing as new peaks when compared to a control sample. Thus Hucker et al. [206] in a study of the oxidative deamination of amphetamine by rabbit liver preparations examined a heptane extraction of the incubation mixture by GLC and observed four peaks with SE-30 (Fig. 21). As no peaks were observed following the incubation of

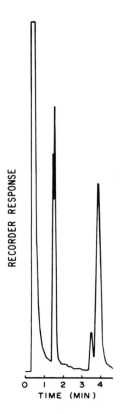

FIG. 21.   GLC analysis of a heptane extract of products from the incubation of amphetamine with rabbit liver preparation.   Column conditions:
6 ft × 4 mm i.d. glass column packed with 3% SE-30 on Chromosorb G;
120°C; 50 ml/min carrier gas.   (Reprinted from Ref. 206 courtesy of
Pergamon Press.)

amphetamine with boiled liver extract, these four peaks corresponded to
metabolites.   The retention time of the major peak was identical to that
of phenylacetone oxime.   Exposure to trimethylsilylation conditions resulted in a shift of the retention time of the major metabolite, demonstrating the presence of a reactive functional group.   The new retention time
was the same as that of the TMSi derivative of phenylacetone oxime.
Preparative GLC was then used to supply sufficient metabolite to further
strenghthen the identification.   The collected material was exposed to
hydrochloric acid which caused conversion to a compound with the same
retention time (1.5 min, SE-30) as another metabolite from the incubation,
the latter possessing the retention time of phenylacetone.   The microchem-
ical and GLC characterization of the major metabolite was confirmed by

mass spectrometric analysis of the collected material; the mass spectrum was identical to that of phenylacetone oxime. Further characterization of the 1.5 min retention time metabolite was achieved by GLC on a selective stationary phase, QF-1; the retention time of this stationary phase matched that of phenylacetone. Use of the two stationary phases demonstrated that the 1.6 min retention time (SE-30) metabolite possessed the same retention behavior as phenyl-2-propanol. This metabolite was found to form a TMSi derivative with the same retention time (QF-1) as the TMSi ether of phenyl-2-propanol.

The in vitro metabolism of N-ethyl, N-methylaniline by rabbit liver microsomes has been studied by Gorrod and coworkers [207] utilizing GLC analysis. A column containing Apiezon L and potassium hydroxide on acid-washed and silanized Chromosorb G was employed to separate the parent drug and internal standard (mesidine, 2,4,6-trimethylaniline) from the desalkyl products, N-ethylaniline and N-methylaniline and the di-desalkyl metabolite (aniline), and was used to quantitate the compounds in ether extracts from alkalinized incubations. The N-oxide of N-methyl, N-ethyl-aniline, not extracted by ether, was reduced with $TiCl_3$/HCl to N-methyl-N-ethylaniline, and the latter then quantified to reflect the amount of N-oxide formed in the incubation. More than 95% of the original substrate was accounted for by these metabolites, demonstrating that ring hydroxylation is a minor pathway. The influence of various incubation parameters upon the metabolism pattern and the tissue distribution of the drug metabolizing activity were also examined by the use of the GLC method.

Other studies in which GLC played a key role in elucidating in vitro transformations include those of Beckett et al. [208] on the metabolism of fenfluramine in which eight products (in addition to the parent drug) were detected, and of Berman and Spirtes [209], in which GLC demonstrated the presence of five metabolites of chlorpromazine in an extract of the incubation mixture. In the latter investigation, the rate of metabolism of chlorpromazine by rabbit liver microsomes was monitored by GLC, and the effect upon metabolism of the addition of Mg^{2+} was estimated.

Wang et al. [210] utilized GLC techniques in their study of the enzymic reduction of 2-methyl-4-(5-nitro-2-furyl)thiazole (MNFT). Anaerobic incubation of this compound with NADPH and NADPH-cytochrome-c reductase led to the formation of metabolite 1 with a retention time of 5 min, whereas incubation of MNFT under the above conditions followed by incubation with mouse liver cytosol led to metabolite 2, with a retention time of 7 min. The latter was identified as 2-methyl-4-(5-amino-2-furyl)thiazole on the basis of its mass spectrum. Chemical reduction (hydrogen) of MNFT was also monitored by GLC; two compounds were initially formed (C1 and C2, retention times of 7 and 9 min, respectively), but after 15 min only the C1 peak was observed. Metabolite 2 and C1, in addition to possessing the same retention times, exhibited identical mass spectra. The spectra of metabolite 1 and C2 were "closely similar . . . except for a slight difference in their relative intensities" [210]. On the basis of such data alone one might be willing to propose the equivalence of two compounds, but the clear difference in retention times demonstrated nonequivalence, again illustrating the value of combining the separating power of GLC with the structure elucidating power of MS.

The use of GLC for preparative purposes has been used in a number of metabolite structural studies. In addition to the report by Hucker et al.

[206] on amphetamine metabolism in vitro, the same laboratory utilized this technique to obtain a sufficient quantity of a halofenate metabolite in dog urine to establish the position of hydroxylation by IR and UV spectrometry [211]. De Leenheer and Heyndrickx [212,213] employed preparative GLC to provide sufficient quantities of purified metabolites of dibenzepine [212] and methotrimeprazine [213] for IR and mass spectrometric analyses. Nelson and coworkers [214] used preparative GLC to collect five drug-related compounds in a metabolism study of lidocaine. The collected fractions were subjected to scintillation counting and high resolution MS. This paper reports condensation of a lidocaine metabolite (an amine) with acetaldehyde, and demonstrated the possibility of reactions between active carbonyl compounds and amines to form artifactually formed species or "metabonates" [215].

Retention time shifts following exposure to various derivatization conditions and the use of stationary phases of differing selectivity are two widely employed GLC techniques for the identification of unknowns. This approach was utilized to identify 1', 2'-dihydro-(-)-zearalenone as the major urinary ovine metabolite of the corresponding 6'-alcohol [216]. Trimethylsilylation and methoxime formation, individually and in combination, were used for derivatization, and the resulting products were examined using columns of the nonselective stationary phase SE-30 and the selective stationary phase QF-1. Excellent correlation was observed between the GLC retention data for the metabolite and the reference standard in an example of functional group chemistry at the microgram scale. The use of derivative formation in the identification of the metabolite is illustrated in Figure 22. The retention time shift associated with exposure to methoxime-forming conditions requires the presence of a reactive carbonyl group such as a ketone.

Diethylhexylphthalate (DEHP), a widely used plasticizer, is often found in biological isolates such as metabolic fractions [217,218]. A frequent source of this compound is contaminated solvents, etc., and plastic storage containers (for blood and other fluids), but its presence in the samples per se is also a real possibility as DEHP is rapidly becoming a ubiquitous environmental contaminant. Albro et al. [219] have studied the metabolism of [^{14}C]DEHP in the rat utilizing a variety of techniques including GLRC and preparative GLC. Methylation of a radioactive urine extract followed by preparative GLC yielded five labeled metabolites. The five metabolites were also isolated as the free acids by TLC techniques; each TLC fraction gave, following methylation, a single radioactive peak of greater than 94% radiochemical purity when assayed by preparative GLC and scintillation counting. The only detectable radiolabeled product resulting from alkaline hydrolysis of the individual metabolites of the total urine extract was identified as o-phthalic acid by TLC and GLRC of the methylated hydrolysis product. Authentic dimethylphthalate was used as carrier in the latter experiments. Mass and NMR spectrometry demonstrated that the five metabolites possess the structures presented below:

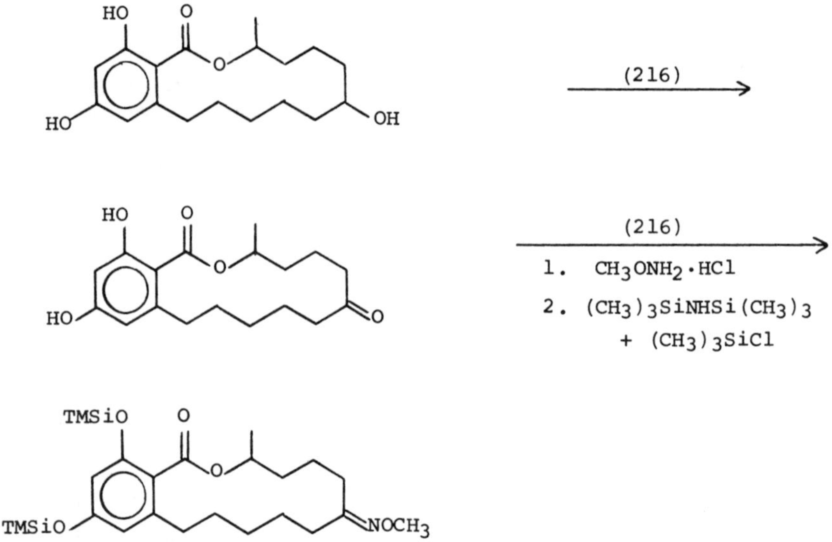

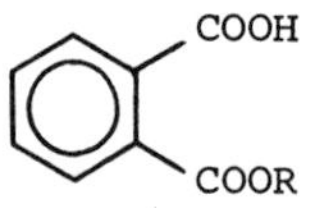

$$R = -CH_2CH(Et)(CH_2)_2COCH_3;$$
$$-CH_2CH(Et)(CH_2)_2CHOHCH_3;$$
$$-CH_2CH(Et)(CH_2)_3COOH;$$
$$-CH_2CH(Et)CH_2COOH;\ H.$$

Another example of the use of different types of stationary phases and derivatives in the identification of a metabolite is found in the paper by Oelschläger et al. [220] on the metabolism of Fomocaine:

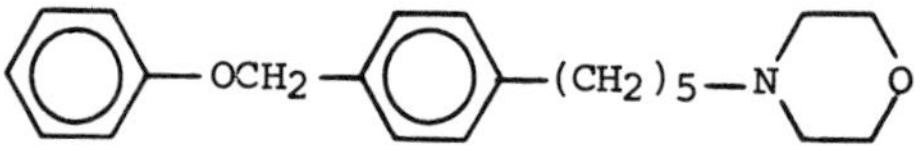

A canine urinary metabolite was characterized by MS as possessing an hydroxyl group in the phenoxy ring. GLC of the metabolite and the three authentic hydroxy isomers on three columns (OV-225, OV-17, OV-1) clearly eliminated the o-isomer from consideration (Table 6). The OV-225 retention data suggested that the p, not the m, isomer was the metabolite;

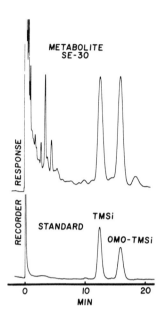

FIG. 22. Comparison of the GLC behavior of the di-TMSi and meth-oxime, di-TMSi derivatives of 1',2'-dihydro-(-)-zearalenone (bottom) with that of the two compounds obtained when the major ovine urinary metabolite of the analogous 6'-alcohol was exposed to the two different sets of derivatizing conditions (i.e., trimethylsilylation alone; methoxime formation followed by trimethylsilylation). Column conditions: 6 ft × 4 mm i.d. glass column packed with 1.7% SE-30 on acid-washed and silanized Gas-Chrom P; 200°C; 25 ml/min carrier gas. (Reprinted from Ref. 216 by courtesy of Marcel Dekker.)

this was demonstrated unequivocally by derivatization techniques (acetylation, trimethylsilylation, and on-column methylation; Table 6).

Liebman and Ortiz [221] were able to separate the 5-keto, 3-endohydroxy, 5-exohydroxy, and 5-endohydroxy metabolites of D-camphor using a 6 ft column containing 20% Carbowax 20M on Chromosorb W, 60 to 80 mesh. The authors studied the metabolism of D-(+) and L-(-) camphor in dog and rabbit and in liver preparations from rats and rabbits. A comparison of the metabolism of the D and L forms of camphor is presented. Zacchei and Wishousky [222] have separated stereoisomers which formed as a result of metabolic hydroxylation of the saluretic agent (6,7-dichloro-2-cyclopentyl-2-methyl-1-oxo-5-indanyloxy)acetic acid (MK-473, II). A chromatogram resulting from analysis of a human urinary extract (methylated) is seen in Figure 23. The sample was analyzed on a 6 ft 0.5% QF-1 column

TABLE 6

Retention Times for Some Hydroxyfomocaine Derivatives
on Gas Chromatography[a]

Compound	Retention time (min)		
	OV-225	OV-17	OV-1
o-Hydroxyfomocaine	7.6	7.7	6.2
o-Acetoxyfomocaine	10.2	12.1	8.2
o-Methoxyfomocaine	7.0	8.0	6.2
o-Trimethylsilyloxyfomocaine	5.5	6.9	17.2
m-Hydroxyfomocaine	18.6	13.5	8.4
m-Acetoxyfomocaine	12.5	13.5	9.6
m-Methoxyfomocaine	7.5	9.8	7.1
m-Trimethylsilyloxyfomocaine	6.2	9.0	9.8
p-Hydroxyfomocaine	17.9	13.5	8.4
p-Acetoxyfomocaine	14.4	15.8	10.4
p-Methoxyfomocaine	7.8	10.1	7.3
p-Trimethylsilyloxyfomocaine	7.0	10.1	9.7
Metabolite III	17.9	13.5	8.4
Metabolite III + (Ac)$_2$O	14.4	15.8	10.4
Metabolite III + TMAH	7.8	10.1	7.3
Metabolite III + BSTFA	7.0	10.1	9.7

[a]Reprinted from Ref. 220 by courtesy of Taylor & Francis Ltd.

operated at 239°C. Components A, B, and C were characterized as
hydroxy metabolites using GLC-MS techniques following derivatization
of the extract with: (a) CH_2N_2; (b) BSA; and (c) CH_2N_2 and BSA. Metabolite D was identified as the corresponding keto analog of metabolite
C [222]. The structures of the metabolites of II are presented below:

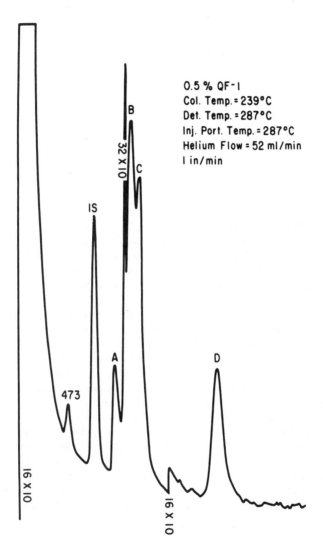

0.5 % QF-1
Col. Temp. = 239°C
Det. Temp. = 287°C
Inj. Port. Temp. = 287°C
Helium Flow = 52 ml/min
1 in/min

FIG. 23. Gas chromatogram resulting from the analysis of an acidic extract of human urine following MK-473 administration. The sample was derivatized with diazomethane prior to GLC analysis.

Stillwell et al. [223] have studied the metabolism of the steroid contraceptives dimethisterone and norethisterone using GLC techniques. Urinary isolates from a normal adult female were subjected to methoxime and TMSi derivative formation and examined by temperature programmed GLC. The chromatogram from the isolate arising from dimethisterone administration contained a peak not found in the corresponding isolate from control urine. Combined GLC-MS demonstrated that this derivative possessed a molecular weight of 488; assuming that this compound was a di-TMSi derivative, the molecular weight of the metabolite itself was thus 244, four mass units greater than that of the parent drug. This suggested that the metabolite was an androstanediol, and the four possible stereoisomeric forms ($5\alpha, 3\alpha$; $5\alpha, 3\beta$; $5\beta, 3\beta$; $5\beta, 3\alpha$) were prepared. The GLC retention data for the metabolite and the four tetrahydro stereoisomers, free and as TMSi derivatives with two different stationary phases, are compared in Table 7. The metabolite is clearly a 5β (A/B cis) androstane on the basis of the retention times of the underivatized compounds. Unequivocal assignment of the stereoisomerism of the 3-hydroxy group is more difficult based on GLC data, although comparison on SE-30 of the TMSi derivatives seems to point to the metabolite being the 3α isomer. The mass spectrometric data also favored this assignment, although again the spectra did not differ greatly.

Comparison of the chromatograms of the isolates from normal urine and urine from a woman treated with norethisterone demonstrated that two peaks were unique to the latter. Both of these were found on the basis of GLC-MS data to possess molecular weights of 446, requiring that if these were di-TMSi derivatives the parent compounds had molecular weights of 302, four mass units greater than those of norethisterone itself. The GLC retention data for the two metabolites and the four isomeric 3-hydroxy estranes (Table 7) clearly demonstrated that the major metabolite was 17α-ethynyl-5β-estrane-$3\alpha, 17\beta$-diol, and the minor metabolite was the $5\beta, 3\beta$ isomer.

TABLE 7

Methylene Unit Values of Reference Steroids and Drug Metabolites[a]

Compound	SE-30		OV-17	
	Free	TMSi	Free	TMSi
6α-Methyl-17α-(1-propynyl)-5α-androstane-3α,17β-diol	26.69	26.80	30.80	28.10
6α-Methyl-17α-(1-propynyl)-5α-androstane-3β,17β-diol	26.78	27.98	31.07	29.10
6α-Methyl-17α-(1-propynyl)-5β-androstane-3α,17β-diol	25.90	26.40	30.25	27.75
6α-Methyl-17α-(1-propynyl)-5β-androstane-3β,17β-diol	25.88	26.70	30.35	27.60
Dimethisterone metabolite	25.98	26.40	30.28	27.62
17α-Ethynyl-5α-estrane-3α,17β-diol	24.00	25.45	27.98	26.43
17α-Ethynyl-5α-estrane-3β,17β-diol	24.17	26.18	28.06	27.32
17α-Ethynyl-5β-estrane-3α,17β-diol	24.14	25.87	28.24	26.95
17α-Ethynyl-5β-estrane-3β,17β-diol	24.13	25.85	28.15	26.77
Norethisterone metabolite (major)	24.14	25.88	28.23	26.98
Norethisterone metabolite (minor)	--	25.50	--	26.46

[a]Reprinted from Ref. 223 by courtesy of Pergamon Press.

Changes in retention behavior resulting from on-column methylation with TMAH have proven valuable in establishing the structures of urinary metabolites of cyproheptadine (see below) in man and the rat. Frigerio and coworkers [224] tentatively identified two rat urinary metabolites of this drug as desmethylcyproheptadine (A) and desmethylcyproheptadine-10,11-epoxide (B) on the basis of TLC and MS data. Confirmation of these assignments was achieved by on-column methylation of a urinary extract containing these two metabolites. The retention times of the peaks corresponding to A and B shifted to those of the parent drug and authentic cyproheptadine-10,11-epoxide, both N-methyl tertiary amines. The identity of the methylated products was verified by GLC-MS. Porter et al. [155] proposed on the basis of GLC-MS data that an aromatic ring hydroxylated desmethylcyproheptadine (C) was a human urinary metabolite of this tricyclic drug. The structure of this metabolite was further substantiated using an on-column methylation approach. GLC of a methanolic solution of desmethylcyproheptadine and TMAH resulted in N-methylation, i.e., cyproheptadine was eluted from the column. When the analogous experiment was carried out with 3-hydroxycyproheptadine, O-methylation resulted in elution of 3-methoxycyproheptadine. If metabolite C indeed possessed the suggested structure, on-column methylation should convert it to a methoxycyproheptadine.

Metabolite

When this experiment was carried out, GLRC demonstrated the formation of a radioactive compound with the same retention time as 3-methoxycyproheptadine. GLC-MS data indicated that this methylated metabolite possessed a mass spectrum compatible with the spectrum of authentic 3-methoxycyproheptadine. Studies such as these demonstrate the close interplay between gas phase analytical techniques such as GLC, GLRC, and GLC-MS and derivatization. It is clear that GLC plays a central role in modern metabolite structure determination work, either per se in retention behavior studies or by serving as a high resolution inlet system for specialized detectors such as RAM systems and mass spectrometers.

Dinovo et al. [225] have employed GLC (and TLC) techniques to demonstrate the presence of a hitherto unrecognized metabolite of thioridazine

and mesoridazine in human plasma. Plasma concentrations of the metabolite and mesoridazine were approximately equal at 1 to 4 h post dose, but
at >8 h the metabolite/drug ratio was increasingly > unity. The retention
time of this metabolite was shown to be different from those of all known
metabolites of these drugs. The unknown metabolite was ultimately identified by Gruenke et al. [226] using TLC, GLC, and chemical ionization MS.
The last technique showed that the molecular formula for the metabolite
corresponded to mesoridazine plus an atom of oxygen. Four isomeric
monooxygenated mesoridazines fit this datum, but two were immediately
eliminated on the basis of the solvent solubility behavior exhibited by the
metabolite. GLC, TLC, and electron impact MS comparison excluded the
authentic ring sulfoxide of mesoridazine (a known metabolite) as the unknown, leaving mesoridazine sidechain sulfone (sulforidazine) as the metabolite structure. This paper again illustrates the value of applying a
variety of methods to metabolite work.

The identification and quantification of drug metabolites in humans is
particularly important if the metabolite is pharmacologically active. In
view of the large variations in response to β-blocking drug therapy it has
been suggested that these variations are a result, in part, to individual
differences in metabolic disposition of these drugs. Walle [25], in an
attempt to shed light on the metabolic variations, developed a highly specific and sensitive electron capture method for a number of β-blocking
drugs which included propranolol, oxprenol, alprenolol, pronethalol,
practolol, sotalol, and several of their metabolites. Analysis of the metabolites is essential since it has been shown that several exhibit important
pharmacological properties [227, 228]. The drugs and their metabolites
were separated and detected as the trifluoroacetyl derivatives. The characteristic β-blocking side chain, which was present in all drugs examined,
yielded the ditrifluoroacetyl derivative

$$R-CHCH_2-N-CH(CH_3)_2$$
$$\quad\ \ |\qquad\ \ |$$
$$\quad OCOCF_3\ \ COCF_3$$

where R represents the remaining portion of the drugs. Minimum detectable amounts ranged from 0.1 to 1.1 pg; however, the lowest detectable
concentration in plasma was 0.1 ng/ml. The propranolol standard curve
(using the internal standard method) was linear in the 0.5 to 500 ng/ml
range. The chemical structures of the derivatives and the metabolites
were confirmed by GLC-MS. The gas chromatogram resulting from analysis of an extract of a dog heart following propranolol perfusion is presented
in Figure 24. It shows evidence for the presence of the two metabolites,
1-(α-naphthoxy)-2, 3-propylene glycol and N-desisopropylpropranolol, as
the trifluoroacetyl derivatives. Similar data were generated for oxprenolol
and its four major urinary metabolites (Fig. 25). The GLC method permits

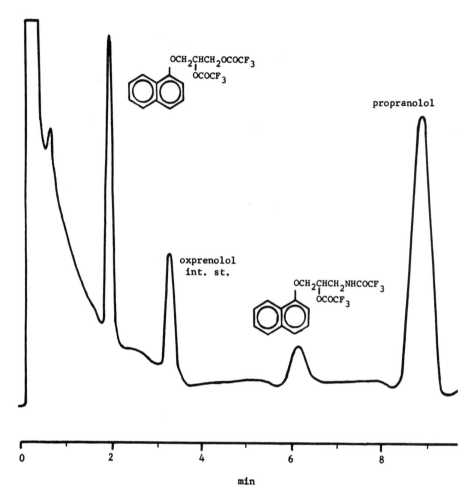

FIG. 24. Gas chromatogram resulting from the analysis of a heart tissue extract obtained from a propranolol-treated, blood-perfused dog heart-lung preparation. Two metabolites, 1-(α-naphthoxy-2,3-propylene)glycol and N-desisopropylpropranolol, are shown. (Reprinted from Ref. 25 by courtesy of the American Pharmaceutical Association.)

accurate terminal half-life determinations, even after low doses, and leads to a better understanding of the complex metabolic disposition and pharmacology of this class of compounds. Hansen and Fischer [229] have used GLC (SE-30) to assay for a biologically active hydroxy metabolite of glutethimide and parent drug in human tissues, plasma, and urine. Specificity of the assay was established by combined GLC-MS and by use of a second

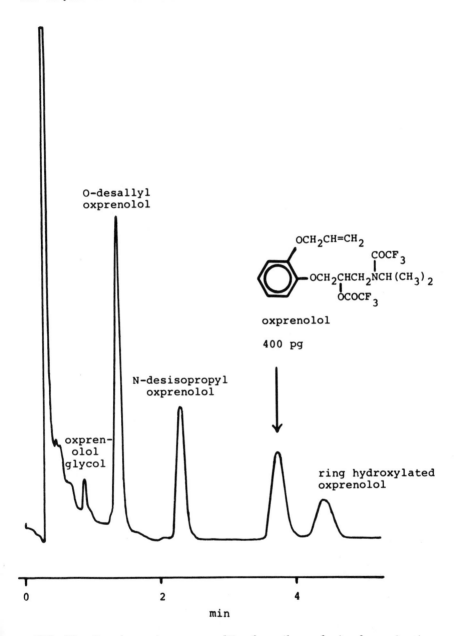

FIG. 25. Gas chromatogram resulting from the analysis of an extract of hydrolyzed urine obtained from a rat administered 10 mg of oxprenolol hydrochloride. (Reprinted from Ref. 25 by courtesy of the American Pharmaceutical Association.)

more selective stationary phase (OV-225) which gave the same quantitative results as the SE-30 columns. Fischer and Ambre [230] had demonstrated earlier by GLC-MS that use of SE-30, OV-1, and OV-17 columns in assays for human urinary glutethimide in patients intoxicated with this drug resulted in overestimation of parent drug because of coelution of the metabolite α-phenyl-2-ethyl-glutaconimide. The two compounds are separable on the selective stationary phases OV-225 and Carbowax 20M, and their use would thus circumvent this error in reported glutethimide levels for such overdose patients. Tilidine and its biologically active N-desmethyl metabolite have been identified and quantified in rat plasma and brain by GLC [231], and Hucker et al. [232] have identified the corresponding sulfide as a biologically active metabolite of cis-5-fluoro-2-methyl-1-[(p-methylsulfinyl)benzylidenyl]indene-3-acetic acid in human plasma.

Nash et al. [233] used an FID-GLC method for the quantitation of propoxyphene and its major metabolite norpropoxyphene (NP) and the minor metabolites, cyclic dinorpropoxyphene and/or dinorpropoxyphene, in plasma of heroin addicts. The assay employed an internal standard, extraction, back-extraction, and quantitation of drug and metabolites using temperature-programmed GLC. No derivatization was required; however, the secondary amine (NP) could not be quantitated unless the extract was treated with strong base which converted NP by intramolecular rearrangement through the O to N shift of the propionyl group to form the stable propionamide (PA).

$$C_6H_5CH_2-\overset{\overset{\displaystyle O}{\overset{\displaystyle \|}{OCC_2H_5}}}{\underset{\underset{\displaystyle C_6H_5}{|}}{C}}\!\!\!-\!\!\!\underset{\underset{\displaystyle CH_3}{|}}{CH_2}-CH_2NHCH_3 \xrightarrow{\ ^-OH\ } C_6H_5CH_2-\overset{\overset{\displaystyle OH}{|}}{\underset{\underset{\displaystyle C_6H_5}{|}}{C}}\!\!\!-\!\!\!\underset{\underset{\displaystyle CH_3}{|}}{CH}-CH_2-\underset{\underset{\displaystyle CH_3}{|}}{N}\overset{\overset{\displaystyle O}{\|}}{C}C_2H_5$$

NP   PA

The metabolism of mitotane in humans was shown by Reif et al. [234] to involve aromatic hydroxylation and alkyl oxidation. The metabolites, after methylation of the extracts, were detected by GLC procedures and identified by comparison of GLC retention times, mass, and IR spectra with those of authentic reference compounds. Following identification of the metabolites, a GLC method was devised which allowed quantitation of the hydroxylated carboxylic acid metabolites. No metabolites with intact alkyl side chains nor the intermediates in the oxidation to the carboxyl group were isolated. The major metabolite resulted from alkyl oxidation and p-hydroxylation. No significance was given to the minor differences noted in the quantities of the various metabolites.

A GLC method was devised by Conway and Melethil [44] for probenecid, a uricosuric agent, and its metabolites in bile and rat urine. The authors showed that 63.8% of an i.v. dose of probenecid (40 mg/kg) was accounted for in the bile (8 h) of normal rats. The metabolites quantitated (GLC method, as percent of dose) included probenecid (10%), probenecid glucuronide (15.7%), glucuronide of the N-2-hydroxypropyl derivative (20.3%), glucuronide of the N-3-hydroxypropyl derivative (14.2%), and unconjugated N-2-carboxyethyl derivative (3.6%). Ligation of the renal pedicles increased the excretion of each metabolite, raising the total to 86.6% of dose.

Highly specific and sensitive ECD-GLC methods have been described by Zacchei and Wishousky [184] for the determination of the polyvalent saluretic agent (6,7-dichloro-2-phenyl-2-methyl-1-oxo-5-indanyloxy)-acetic acid (MK-196) and its major hydroxylated human and chimpanzee metabolite. The procedures involve the addition of an internal standard, an analog of MK-196, to the biological specimens followed by extraction of the acids into benzene at pH 1. The acids are back extracted into sodium hydroxide, and then reextracted into methylene chloride under acidic conditions. The acids are subsequently converted to the methyl esters for GLC analysis by reaction with CH_2N_2. The sensitivity of the method is such that 0.3 μg of drug/ml plasma can be analyzed with an FID; with an ECD ([63]Ni), as little as 2.5 ng of compound/ml can be quantitated. Quantitative determination of the hydroxylated metabolite was made following derivatization of the methyl ester of the metabolite with BSA. A typical ECD-GLC tracing showing the detector response for the internal standard (I.S.), MK-196 and the metabolite is presented in Figure 26. Matin and Rowland [235] devised an ECD-GLC method for the simultaneous determination of tolbutamide and its metabolites in biological fluids. The method involves a pH-dependent solvent extraction system to separate the drug from its two known metabolites. The separated compounds are then converted quantitatively into N-butyl-2,4-dinitroaniline and analyzed by ECD-GLC. The method provides several advantages (increased sensitivity and specificity, and metabolite quantitation) over other published methods. An ECD-GLC approach was also employed by de Silva et al. [31] for the determination of flurazepam and its major metabolites present in blood. The sensitivity of the method is such that 4 to 10 ng of each compound can be detected/ml of plasma using a [63]Ni ECD. The authors discuss the advantages (better sensitivity, amenability to automation, and specificity) of their method over spectrofluorimetric procedures. The overall recoveries of flurazepam, hydroxyethylflurazepam, N-desalkylflurazepam, and the N-desalkyl-3-hydroxy metabolite were 76 ± 6%, 96 ± 8%, 94 ± 6%, and 42 ± 9%, respectively.

Flame ionization detection methods have been reported for many drugs and their metabolites. Karlén et al. [236] reported on the analysis of the major (4-hydroxylated) metabolites of diphenylhydantoin in human urine. Diphenylhydantoin, which is widely used in the treatment of various epileptic disorders, is extensively metabolized before elimination from the body.

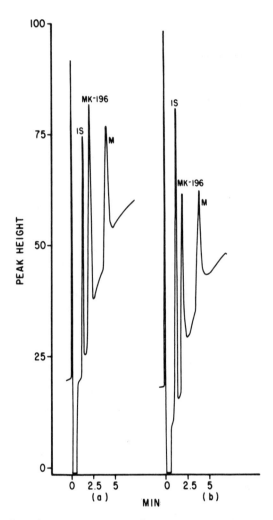

FIG. 26. Gas chromatogram resulting from the analysis of (a) MK-196,
I. S., and metabolite added to control urine in a 2/2/1 ratio and carried
through an ECD method and (b) chimpanzee urine (1-2 h) extract. Five out
of 100 μl were injected and analyzed with a ^{63}Ni detector. (Reprinted from
Ref. 184 by courtesy of the American Pharmaceutical Association.)

Less than 4% of the dose is recovered as unchanged drug in the urine; 50
to 76% of the dose is present in the urine as the conjugated and unconjugated
4-hydroxymetabolite. The recently identified dihydrodiol metabolite [237]
might interfere in the previously published GLC methods (trimethylsilylation

[238], flash methylation [239], methylation with TMAH [51]) since it has
been demonstrated [237] that upon acid hydrolysis the dihydrodiol is de-
hydrated to form the 3- and 4-hydroxy metabolites. The method described
permitted the determination of the excreted conjugated and unconjugated
4-hydroxy metabolite. Mottale and Stewart [240] reported on the ECD-GLC
determination of β-phenethylbiguanide and its p-hydroxy metabolite in serum
and urine. The limit of detection was 0.2 μg of drug and 0.5 μg of metabolite per ml of serum or urine. Other 1974 articles were published by
De Leenheer [23] on phenothiazine drugs, Selly et al. [241] for tolmetin
and its metabolites, Hucker and Stauffer [242] on amitriptyline, Midha et
al. [54] for phenylbutazone and its metabolite oxyphenbutazone, Chan et
al. [243] for the determination of pethidine and its metabolites, and Gallo
et al. [244] for the determination of the urinary metabolite of diftalone,
a new anti-inflammatory drug.

VII. CONCLUSION

GLC is an extremely powerful technique for the separation, identification,
and quantification of a wide variety of drugs and their metabolites present
in biological specimens. GLC methods are often both more specific and
more sensitive than colorimetric, spectrophotometric, and spectrofluorometric assays. The large number of papers in the recent literature attest
to the general acceptance of this technique for the analysis of drugs and
their metabolites.

The technique of microscale derivatization as applied to GLC analyses
should not be underestimated, for without conversion to less polar derivatives many compounds would not be amenable to GLC analysis. The derivatization approach can markedly improve separation patterns, minimize
tailing, and allow the introduction of halogen-containing moieties to permit
sensitive and selective detection of the compounds by electron capture processes. In reality, it is the wide array of highly useful detectors (e.g.,
the flame ionization, electron capture, element selective, and mass spectrometric) which complement the separation aspects of GLC and make it
admirably suited for drug analysis. The development of thin-film thermo-
stable packings, high resolution capillary columns, and sophisticated
detector systems allow assay methods not dreamed of a decade ago.

We have discussed a number of approaches employed by various investigators in the analysis of drugs. Although a single method cannot be recommended because of the diversity of drugs and problems to be resolved, a
few general statements are applicable. The analysis of drugs and their
metab olites by GLC techniques requires the following steps: (1) The drug
(and/or metabolites) must be isolated from the biological specimen; this

usually entails solvent partitioning methods at selected pH values, frequently followed by a wet chromatographic method. (2) An appropriate volatile derivative must be prepared for those compounds not suitable for direct GLC analysis. The resulting derivative may also provide enhanced sensitivity (EC detection methods) and minimize sample adsorption problems. (3) A proper choice of GLC operating conditions (i. e., column temperature, stationary phase, and detector) must be determined. (4) Recognition (e.g., by GLRC if the drug is radiolabeled) and identification of the compound of interest. The judicious choice of an internal standard with properties similar to those of the drug is essential. Addition of the internal standard at the initial step in isolation compensates for losses during sample workup and provides a reliable technique for the quantification aspects. (5) Data acquisition and quantification.

REFERENCES

1. E. C. Horning and M. G. Horning, Metabolic Profiles: Chromatographic Methods for Isolation and Characterization of a Variety of Metabolites in Man, in Methods in Medical Research, Vol. 12 (R. E. Olson, ed.), Year Book Medical Publishers, Chicago, 1970; Clin. Chem., 17, 802 (1971).

2. A. Zlatkis, W. Butsch, H. A. Lichtenstein, A. Tishbee, F. Shumbo, H. M. Liebich, A. M. Coscia, and N. Fleischer, Anal. Chem., 45, 763 (1973).

3. E. C. Horning, W. J. A. VandenHeuvel, and B. G. Creech, Separation and Determination of Steroids by Gas Chromatography, in Methods of Biochemical Analysis, Vol. 11 (D. Glick, ed.), Wiley (Interscience), New York, 1963.

4. E. C. Horning and W. J. A. VandenHeuvel, Qualitative and Quantitative Aspects of the Separation of Steroids, in Advances in Chromatography, Vol. 1 (J. C. Giddings and R. A. Keller, eds.), Dekker, New York, 1965.

5. W. J. A. VandenHeuvel and A. G. Zacchei, Gas-Liquid Chromatography in Drug Analysis, in Advances in Chromatography, Vol. 14 (E. Grushka, ed.), Dekker, New York, 1976.

6. D. Sohn, J. Simon, M. Hanna, and G. Ghali, J. Chromatogr. Sci., 10, 294 (1972).

7. J. Vessman, S. Stromberg, and G. Freij, J. Chromatogr., 94, 239 (1974).

8. L. Helleberg, J. Chromatogr., 117, 167 (1976).

9. L. F. Prescott, K. K. Adjipon-Yamoah, and E. Roberts, J. Pharm. Pharmacol., 25, 205 (1973).

10. D. E. Case, J. Pharm. Pharmacol., 25, 800 (1973).

11. R. J. Flanagan and G. Withers, J. Clin. Pathol., 25, 889 (1972).
12. J. E. O'Brien, W. Zazulak, V. Abbey, and O. Hinsyark, J. Chromatogr. Sci., 10, 336 (1972).
13. N. F. Wood, J. Pharm. Sci., 64, 1048 (1975).
14. J. A. F. de Silva, C. V. Puglisi, and N. Munno, J. Pharm. Sci., 63, 520 (1974).
15. B. Dahlström and L. Paalzow, J. Pharm. Pharmacol., 27, 127 (1975).
16. J. A. F. de Silva, I. Bekersky, M. A. Brooks, R. W. Weinfeld, W. Glover, and C. V. Puglisi, J. Pharm. Sci., 63, 1440 (1974).
17. M. L. Mashford, P. L. Ryan, and W. A. Thomson, J. Chromatogr., 89, 11 (1974).
18. C. Rhodes and P. A. Wright, J. Pharm. Pharmacol., 26, 894 (1974).
19. C. Feyerabend, T. Levitt, and M. A. H. Russell, J. Pharm. Pharmacol., 27, 434 (1975).
20. H. K. L. Hundt, E. C. Clark, and F. O. Müller, J. Pharm. Sci., 64, 1041 (1975).
21. L. C. Bailey and A. P. Shroff, J. Pharm. Sci., 62, 1274 (1973).
22. R. G. Moore, E. J. Triggs, C. A. Shanks, and J. Thomas, Eur. J. Clin. Pharmacol., 8, 353 (1975).
23. A. P. De Leenheer, J. Pharm. Sci., 63, 389 (1974).
24. W. van der Pol, E. van der Kleijn, and M. Lauw, J. Pharmcokin. Biopharm., 3, 99 (1975).
25. T. Walle, J. Pharm. Sci., 63, 1885 (1974).
26. D. G. Kaiser and R. S. Martin, J. Pharm. Sci., 63, 1579 (1974).
27. D. E. Fenimore, R. R. Freeman, and P. R. Loy, Anal. Chem., 45, 2331 (1973).
28. N. Larsen and J. Naestoft, J. Chromatogr., 109, 259 (1975).
29. S. Higuchi, H. Sasaki, and T. Sado, J. Chromatogr., 110, 301 (1975).
30. B. Scales and P. B. Copsey, J. Pharm. Pharmacol., 27, 430 (1975).
31. J. A. F. de Silva, C. V. Puglisi, M. A. Brooks, and M. R. Hackman, J. Chromatogr., 99, 461 (1974).
32. M. G. Horning, P. Gregory, J. Nowlin, M. Stafford, K. Lertratanangkoon, C. Butler, W. G. Stillwell, and R. M. Hill, Clin. Chem., 20, 282 (1974).
33. N. Weissman, M. L. Lowe, J. M. Bithe, and Q. Demetriore, Clin. Chem., 17, 875 (1971).
34. J. R. Shipe and J. Savory, Ann. Clin. Lab. Sci., 5, 57 (1975).
35. J. L. Leeling, B. M. Phillips, R. N. Schut, and O. E. Fancher, J. Pharm. Sci., 54, 1736 (1965).
36. W. Sadee, J. Staroscik, C. Finn, and J. Cohen, J. Pharm. Sci., 64, 998 (1975).
37. K. K. Midha, I. J. McGilveray, and J. K. Cooper, J. Pharm. Sci., 63, 1725 (1974).

38. H. A. Lloyd, H. M. Fales, P. F. Highet, W. J. A. VandenHeuvel, and W. C. Wildman, J. Amer. Chem. Soc., 82, 3791 (1960).
39. A. C. Moffat, J. Chromatogr., 113, 69 (1975).
40. E. A. Fiereck and N. W. Tietz, Clin. Chem., 17, 1024 (1971).
41. D. L. Simmons, R. J. Ranz, and P. Picotte, J. Chromatogr., 71, 421 (1972).
42. L. F. Prescott and D. R. Redman, J. Pharm. Pharmacol., 24, 713 (1972).
43. A. G. Zacchei and L. Weidner, J. Pharm. Sci., 62, 1972 (1973).
44. W. D. Conway and S. Melethil, J. Pharm. Sci., 63, 1551 (1974).
45. D. G. Kaiser and G. J. Vangiessen, J. Pharm. Sci., 63, 219 (1974).
46. D. G. Kaiser and E. M. Glenn, J. Pharm. Sci., 63, 784 (1974).
47. G. P. Tosolini, A. Forgione, E. Moro, and V. Mandelli, J. Chromatogr., 92, 61 (1974).
48. R. M. Thompson, N. Gerber, R. A. Seibert, and D. M. Desiderio, Drug Metab. Disp., 1, 489 (1973).
49. E. Brochmann-Hanssen and T. O. Oke, J. Pharm. Sci., 58, 370 (1969).
50. J. MacGee, Anal. Chem., 42, 421 (1970).
51. A. Estas and P. A. Dumont, J. Chromatogr., 82, 307 (1973).
52. J. MacGee, Clin. Chem., 17, 587 (1971).
53. P. Friel and A. S. Troupin, Clin. Chem., 21, 751 (1975).
54. K. K. Midha, I. J. McGilveray, and C. Charette, J. Pharm. Sci., 63, 1234 (1974).
55. R. H. Hammer, B. J. Wilder, R. R. Streiff, and A. Mayersdorf, J. Pharm. Sci., 60, 327 (1971).
56. R. H. Hammer, J. L. Templeton, and H. L. Panzik, J. Pharm. Sci., 63, 1963 (1974).
57. K. K. Midha and C. Charette, J. Pharm. Sci., 63, 1244 (1974).
58. K. K. Midha, I. J. McGilveray, and C. Charette, J. Pharm. Sci., 63, 1741 (1974).
59. R. Osiewicz, V. Aggarwal, R. M. Young, and I. Sunshine, J. Chromatogr., 88, 157 (1974).
60. H. L. Davis, K. L. Falk, and D. G. Bailey, J. Chromatogr., 107, 61 (1975).
61. W. J. A. VandenHeuvel, V. F. Gruber, R. W. Walker, and F. J. Wolf, J. Pharm. Sci., 64, 1309 (1975).
62. P. W. Feit, K. Roholt, and H. Sorensen, J. Pharm. Sci., 62, 375 (1973).
63. V. Aggarwal and I. Sunshine, Clin. Chem., 20, 200 (1974).
64. E. B. Solow, J. M. Metaxes, and T. R. Summers, J. Chromatogr. Sci., 12, 256 (1974).
65. J. MacGee, The Chemistry and Technique of Flash Alkylation in Gas Chromatography, in Methods of Analysis of Antiepileptic Drugs

(J. W. A. Meijer, H. Meinardi, C. Gardner-Thorpe, and E. Van der Kleijn, eds.), Excerpta Medica, Amsterdam, 1973.
66. W. D. Hooper, D. K. Dubetz, M. J. Eadie, and J. H. Tyer, J. Chromatogr., 110, 206 (1975).
67. R. H. Greeley, J. Chromatogr., 88, 229 (1974).
68. C. J. Least, Jr., G. F. Johnson, and H. M. Solomon, Clin. Chim. Acta, 60, 285 (1975).
69. M. Ervik and K. Gustavii, Anal. Chem., 46, 39 (1974).
70. H. Ehrsson and A. Tilly, Anal. Lett., 6, 197 (1973).
71. H. Ehrsson, Anal. Chem., 46, 922 (1974).
72. B. Lindström and M. Molander, J. Chromatogr., 101, 219 (1974).
73. A. E. Pierce, "Silylation of Organic Compounds," Pierce Chemical Co., Rockford, Illinois, 1968.
74. S. Ahuja, J. Pharm. Sci., 65, 163 (1976).
75. J. F. Nash, R. J. Bopp, and A. Rubin, J. Pharm. Sci., 60, 1062 (1971).
76. D. G. Kaiser and S. R. Shaw, J. Pharm. Sci., 63, 1994 (1974).
77. W. J. A. VandenHeuvel, V. B. Gruber, and R. W. Walker, J. Chromatogr., 87, 341 (1973).
78. W. J. A. VandenHeuvel, R. P. Buhs, J. R. Carlin, T. A. Jacob, F. R. Koniuszy, J. L. Smith, N. R. Trenner, R. W. Walker, D. E. Wolf, and F. J. Wolf, Anal. Chem., 44, 14 (1972).
79. A. G. Zacchei, L. Weidner, G. H. Besselaar, and E. B. Raftery, Drug Metab. Disp., 4, 387 (1976).
80. A. Frigerio, R. M. Baker, and G. Belvedere, Anal. Chem., 45, 1846 (1973).
81. C. P. Talley, N. R. Trenner, G. V. Downing, Jr., and W. J. A. VandenHeuvel, Anal. Chem., 43, 1379 (1971).
82. W. J. A. VandenHeuvel, Applications of Mass Spectrometry in Drug Metabolism and Related Fields, in Applications of the Newer Techniques of Analysis (I. L. Simmons and G. W. Ewing, eds.), Plenum Press, New York, 1973.
83. W. J. A. VandenHeuvel, J. L. Smith, G. Albers-Schönberg, B. Plazonnet, and P. Belanger, Derivatization and Gas Chromatography in the Mass Spectrometry of Steroids, in Modern Methods of Steroid Analysis (E. Heftmann, ed.), Academic Press, New York, 1973.
84. M. W. Anders, personal communication.
85. G. D. Paulson and C. E. Portnoy, J. Agr. Food Chem., 18, 180 (1970).
86. E. C. Horning, M. G. Horning, N. Ikekawa, E. M. Chambaz, P. I. Jaakonmaki, and C. J. W. Brooks, J. Gas Chromatogr., 5, 283 (1967).
87. W. J. A. VandenHeuvel, J. Chromatogr., 28, 406 (1967).
88. S. Billets, P. S. Lietman, and C. Fenselau, J. Med. Chem., 16, 30 (1973).

89. J. B. Knaak, J. M. Eldridge, and L. J. Sullivan, J. Agr. Food Chem., 15, 605 (1967).
90. G. D. Paulson, R. G. Zaylskie, and M. M. Dockter, Anal. Chem., 45, 21 (1973).
91. H. Ehrsson, T. Walle, and S. Wikstrom, J. Chromatogr., 101, 206 (1974).
92. J. E. Mrochek and W. T. Rainey, Jr., Anal. Biochem., 57, 173 (1974).
93. N. Gerber, R. A. Seibert, and R. M. Thompson, Res. Commun. Chem. Pathol. Pharmacol., 6, 499 (1973).
94. D. J. Tocco, R. P. Buhs, H. D. Brown, R. Matzuk, H. E. Mertel, R. E. Harman, and N. R. Trenner, J. Med. Chem., 7, 399 (1964).
95. F. Marcucci, R. Bianchi, L. Airoldi, M. Salmona, R. Fanelli, C. Chiabrando, A. Frigerio, E. Mussini, and S. Garattini, J. Chromtaogr., 107, 285 (1975).
96. R. J. Daun, J. Assoc. Offic. Anal. Chem., 54, 1277 (1971).
97. H. M. Fales and T. Luukkainen, Anal. Chem., 37, 955 (1965).
98. W. L. Gardiner and E. C. Horning, Biochim. Biophys. Acta, 115, 524 (1966).
99. P. G. Devaux, M. G. Horning, R. M. Hill, and E. C. Horning, Anal. Biochem., 41, 70 (1971).
100. C. E. Cook, T. J. Odiorne, M. C. Dickey, M. E. Twine, E. D. Pellizzari, M. E. Wall, and R. Bressler, Life Sci., 15, 1621 (1974).
101. F. Vane and M. G. Horning, Anal. Lett., 2, 357 (1969).
102. B. Samuelsson, M. Hamberg, and C. C. Sweeley, Anal. Biochem., 38, 301 (1970).
103. M. Hamberg, Biochem. Biophys. Res. Commun., 49, 720 (1972).
104. J. W. Horodniak, M. Julius, J. E. Zarembo, and A. D. Bender, Biochem. Biophys. Res. Commun., 57, 539 (1974).
105. R. W. Kelly, Anal. Chem., 45, 2079 (1973).
106. C. J. W. Brooks and I. MacLean, J. Chromatogr. Sci., 9, 18 (1971).
107. M. P. Rabinowitz, P. Reisberg, and J. I. Bodin, J. Pharm. Sci., 63, 1601 (1974).
108. A. J. F. Wickramasinghe, W. Morozowich, W. E. Hamlin, and S. R. Shaw, J. Pharm. Sci., 62, 1428 (1973); A. J. F. Wickramasinghe and R. S. Shaw, Biochem. J., 141, 179 (1974).
109. D. G. Kaiser, S. R. Shaw, and G. J. Vangiessen, J. Pharm. Sci., 63, 567 (1974).
110. J.-P. Thenot, E. C. Horning, M. Stafford, and M. G. Horning, Anal. Lett., 5, 217 (1972).
111. J.-P. Thenot and E. C. Horning, Anal. Lett., 5, 519 (1972).
112. V. S. Venturella, V. M. Gualario, and R. E. Long, J. Pharm. Sci., 62, 662 (1973).

113. W. J. A. VandenHeuvel and V. F. Gruber, J. Chromatogr., 112, 513 (1975).
114. O. Gyllenhaal and H. Ehrsson, J. Chromatogr., 107, 327 (1975).
115. R. J. Perchalski and B. J. Wilder, Clin. Chem., 20, 492 (1974).
116. H. E. Weinberg, U. S. Patent 3,121,084 to E. I. DuPont de Nemours and Co., February 11, 1964.
117. J. A. F. de Silva, M. A. Schwartz, V. Stefanovic, J. Kaplan, and L. D'Arconte, Anal. Chem., 36, 2099 (1964).
118. R. Huffman, J. W. Blake, R. Ray, J. Noonan, and P. W. Murdick, J. Chromatogr. Sci., 12, 382 (1974).
119. J. W. Blake, R. Huffman, J. Noonan, and R. Ray, Amer. Lab., 5, 63 (1973).
120. T. A. Montzka, J. T. Matiskella, and R. A. Partyka, Tetrahedron Lett., 14, 1325 (1974).
121. P. Hartvig and J. Vessman, Acta Pharm. Suecica, 11, 115 (1974).
122. P. Hartvig and J. Vessman, Anal. Lett., 7, 223 (1974).
123. P. Hartvig and J. Vessman, J. Chromatogr. Sci., 12, 722 (1974).
124. R. L. Ellsworth and W. J. A. VandenHeuvel, unpublished results, 1974.
125. T. Walle, J. Chromatogr., 111, 133 (1975).
126. H. P. Burchfield, E. E. Storrs, R. J. Wheeler, V. K. Bhat, and L. L. Green, Anal. Chem., 45, 916 (1973).
127. H. E. Hamilton, J. E. Wallace, and K. Blum, Anal. Chem., 47, 1139 (1975).
128. R. W. Souter, J. Chromatogr., 108, 265 (1975).
129. C. J. W. Brooks and J. D. Gilbert, J. Chromatogr., 99, 541 (1974).
130. G. J. Vangiessen and D. G. Kaiser, J. Pharm. Sci., 64, 798 (1975).
131. G. P. Tosolini, E. Moro, A. Forgione, M. Fanghiere, and V. Mandelli, J. Pharm. Sci., 63, 1072 (1974).
132. S. H. Curry, Anal. Chem., 40, 1251 (1968).
133. G. P. Beharrell, D. M. Hailey, and M. K. McLaurin, J. Chromatogr., 70, 45 (1972).
134. D. M. Hailey, J. Chromatogr., 98, 527 (1974).
135. J. A. F. de Silva, N. Munno, and R. E. Weinfeld, J. Pharm. Sci., 62, 449 (1973).
136. J. A. F. de Silva and I. Bekersky, J. Chromatogr., 99, 447 (1974).
137. E. D. Pellizzari, J. Chromatogr., 98, 323 (1974).
138. J. A. F. de Silva, in Drug Fate and Metabolism: Methods and Techniques (E. R. Garrett and J. L. Hirtz, eds.), Dekker, New York (vol. in preparation).
139. P. Erdtmansky and J. Goehl, Anal. Chem., 47, 750 (1975).
140. J. A. F. de Silva, I. Bekersky, and C. V. Puglisi, J. Chromatogr. Sci., 11, 547 (1973).

141. J. A. Knowles, W. H. Comer, and H. W. Ruelius, Arzneim.
      Forsch., 21, 1055 (1971).
142. K. Nagasawa, A. Ogamo, and T. Shinozuka, J. Chromatogr., 111,
      51 (1975).
143. C. F. Poole, E. D. Morgan, and P. M. Bebbington, J. Chromatogr.,
      104, 172 (1975).
144. J. P. Desager and C. Harvengt, J. Pharm. Pharmacol., 27, 53
      (1975).
145. L. Strömberg and A. C. Machly, J. Chromatogr., 109, 67 (1975).
146. A. G. Zacchei and L. Weidner, J. Pharm. Sci., 64, 814 (1975).
147. R. J. Perchalski, B. J. Wilder, and R. H. Hammer, J. Pharm.
      Sci., 63, 1489 (1974).
148. A. Karmen, J. Assoc. Offic. Agr. Chem., 47, 15 (1964).
149. A. Karmen, Combined Gas-Liquid Chromatography and Radioassay
      of ^{14}C- and ^{3}H-Labeled Compounds, in Methods in Enzymology,
      Vol. 14 (J. M. Lowenstein, ed.), Academic Press, New York,
      1969.
150. W. J. A. VandenHeuvel and G. W. Kuron, Biochemical and Bio-
      medical Applications of Preparative Gas Chromatography, in
      Preparative Gas Chromatography (A. Zlatkis and V. Pretorius,
      eds.), Wiley, New York, 1971.
151. R. C. Pfeger, C. Piantadosi, and F. Snyder, Biochim. Biophys.
      Acta, 144, 633 (1967).
152. N. R. Trenner, O. C. Speth, V. B. Gruber, and W. J. A. Vanden-
      Heuvel, J. Chromatogr., 71, 415 (1972).
153. W. J. A. VandenHeuvel, N. R. Trenner, D. E. Wolf, R. P. Buhs,
      R. W. Walker, J. R. Carlin, F. R. Koniuszy, M. L. Green,
      E. Sestokas, N. Allen, R. L. Ellsworth, T. A. Jacob, and
      F. J. Wolf, unpublished results.
154. D. E. Wolf, W. J. A. VandenHeuvel, F. R. Koniuszy, T. R. Tyler,
      T. A. Jacob, and F. J. Wolf, J. Agr. Food Chem., 20, 1252
      (1972).
155. C. C. Porter, B. H. Arison, V. F. Gruber, D. C. Titus, and
      W. J. A. VandenHeuvel, Drug Metab. Disp., 3, 189 (1975).
156. S. Vickers, E. K. Stuart, H. B. Hucker, and W. J. A. Vanden-
      Heuvel, J. Med. Chem., 18, 134 (1975).
157. F. F. Sun, Biochim. Biophys. Acta, 348, 249 (1974).
158. F. F. Sun and J. E. Stafford, Biochim. Biophys. Acta, 369, 95
      (1974).
159. H. W. Seyberth, B. J. Sweetman, J. C. Frolich, and J. A. Oates,
      Prostaglandins, 11, 381 (1976).
160. M. Hamberg and B. Samuelsson, J. Biol. Chem., 246, 6713
      (1971).
161. W. J. A. VandenHeuvel, V. F. Gruber, K. Hooke, and F. J. Wolf,
      unpublished results, 1975.

162. M. Hamberg and B. Samuelsson, J. Amer. Chem. Soc., 91, 2177 (1969).

163. W. A. Aue, J. Chromatogr. Sci., 13, 329 (1975).

164. D. F. S. Natusch and T. M. Thorpe, Anal. Chem., 45, No. 14, 1184A (1973).

165. H. Maier-Bode and M. Riedman, Gas Chromatographic Determination of Nitrogen Containing Pesticides Using the Nitrogen Flame Ionization Detector, in Residue Reviews (F. A. and J. D. Gunther, eds.), Springer-Verlag, New York, 1975.

166. H. A. McLeod, A. G. Butterfield, D. Lewis, W. E. J. Phillips, and D. E. Coffin, Anal. Chem., 47, 674 (1975).

167. D. M. Hailey, A. G. Howard, and G. Nicklees, J. Chromatogr., 100, 49 (1974).

168. N. K. McCallum, J. Chromatogr. Sci., 11, 509 (1973).

169. C. Jackson, Jr. and P. J. Reynolds, J. Agr. Food Chem., 20, 972 (1972).

170. R. E. Schirmer and R. J. Pierson, J. Pharm. Sci., 62, 2052 (1973).

171. W. M. Lamkin, N. S. Jones, T. Pan, and D. N. Ward, Anal. Biochem., 58, 549 (1974).

172. J. F. Palframan, J. MacNob, and N. T. Crosby, J. Chromatogr., 76, 307 (1973).

173. A. M. J. A. Duchateau, F. W. H. M. Merkus, and F. Schobben, J. Chromatogr., 109, 432 (1975).

174. J. D. Cameron, Clin. Chim. Acta, 56, 307 (1974).

175. L. A. Gifford, P. Turner, and C. M. B. Pane, J. Chromatogr., 105, 107 (1975).

176. A. Jorgensen, Acta. Pharmacol. Toxicol., 36, 79 (1975).

177. P. A. Toseland, M. Albani, and F. D. Gauchel, Clin. Chem., 21, 98 (1975).

178. B. U. Dvorchik, J. Chromatogr., 105, 49 (1975).

179. D. A. Smith and W. J. Cole, J. Chromatogr., 105, 377 (1975).

180. H. B. Hucker and S. C. Stauffer, J. Pharm. Sci., 65, 926 (1976).

181. M. L. Mashford, D. L. Ryan, and W. A. Thomson, J. Chromatogr., 89, 11 (1974).

182. B. Plazonnet and A. Cerdeno, Proceedings of the International Symposium on Chromatography and Electrophoresis, Brussels, May, 1975.

183. P. C. Cala, N. R. Trenner, R. P. Buhs, G. V. Downing, Jr., J. L. Smith, and W. J. A. VandenHeuvel, J. Agr. Food Chem., 20, 337 (1972).

184. A. G. Zacchei and T. I. Wishousky, J. Pharm. Sci., 65, 1770 (1976).

185. W. J. Cole, R. G. Mitchell, and R. F. Salamonsen, J. Pharm. Pharmacol., 27, 167 (1975).

186. C.-G. Hammar, B. Holmstedt, and R. Ryhage, Anal. Biochem.,
     25, 532 (1968).
187. T. E. Gaffney, C.-G. Hammar, B. Holmstedt, and R. E.
     McMahon, Anal. Chem., 43, 307 (1971).
188. R. L. Wolen, E. A. Ziege, and C. M. Gruber, Jr., Clin.
     Pharmacol. Ther., 17, 15 (1975).
189. M. G. Horning, J. Nowlin, M. Stafford, K. Lertratanangkoon,
     K. R. Sommer, R. M. Hill, and R. N. Stillwell, J. Chromatogr.,
     112, 605 (1975).
190. J. T. Biggs, W. H. Holland, S. Chang, P. P. Hipps, and
     W. E. Sherman, J. Pharm. Sci., 65, 261 (1976).
191. H. W. Seyberth, G. V. Segre, J. L. Morgan, B. J. Sweetman,
     J. T. Potts, Jr., and J. A. Oates, New Engl. J. Med., 293,
     1278 (1975).
192. J. Kaplan, L. R. Mandel, R. Stillman, R. W. Walker, W. J. A.
     VandenHeuvel, J. C. Gillin, and R. J. Wyatt, Psychopharmacologia,
     38, 239 (1974).
193. R. W. Walker, H.-S. Ahn, G. Albers-Schönberg, L. R. Mandel,
     and W. J. A. VandenHeuvel, Biochem. Med., 8, 105 (1973).
194. M. Riedmann, J. Chromatogr., 88, 376 (1974).
195. M. Riedmann, Xenobiotica, 3, 411 (1973).
196. J. F. Johnson, Guide to Modern Methods of Instrumental Analysis,
     Wiley (Interscience), New York, 1972.
197. H. M. McNair and E. J. Bonelli, Basic Gas Chromatography,
     5th ed., Varian Aerograph, Walnut Creek, California, 1969.
198. E. Kovats, Helv. Chim. Acta, 41, 1915 (1958).
199. G. Schomburg, Advan. Chromatogr., 6, 211 (1968).
200. W. J. A. VandenHeuvel, W. L. Gardiner, and E. C. Horning,
     Anal. Chem., 36, 1550 (1964).
201. I. A. Zingales, J. Chromatogr., 61, 237 (1971).
202. D. J. Tocco, A. E. W. Duncan, F. A. deLuna, H. B. Hucker,
     and W. J. A. VandenHeuvel, Drug Metab. Disp., 3, 361 (1975).
203. S. Vickers, E. K. Stuart, H. B. Hucker, M. E. Jaffe, R. E.
     Rhodes, W. J. A. VandenHeuvel, and J. R. Bianchine, Drug
     Metab. Disp., 2, 9 (1974).
204. T. R. Tyler, J. K. Lee, H. Flynn, and W. J. A. VandenHeuvel,
     Drug Metab. Disp., 4, 177 (1976).
205. E. C. Horning, R. N. Stillwell, W. G. Stillwell, J. F. Nowlin, and
     M. G. Horning, in Drug Fate and Metabolism: Methods and Tech-
     niques (E. R. Garrett and J. L. Hirtz, eds.), Dekker, New York
     (vol. in preparation).
206. H. B. Hucker, B. M. Michniewicz, and R. E. Rhodes, Biochem.
     Pharmacol., 20, 2123 (1971).
207. J. W. Gorrod, D. J. Temple, and A. H. Beckett, Xenobiotica,
     5, 453 (1975).

208. A. H. Beckett, R. T. Coutts, and F. A. Ogunbona, J. Pharm. Pharmacol., 25, 190 (1973).
209. H. M. Berman and M. A. Spirtes, Biochem. Pharmacol., 20, 2275 (1971).
210. C.-Y. Wang, C.-W. Chin, B. Kaiman, and G. T. Bryan, Biochem. Pharmacol., 24, 291 (1975).
211. H. B. Hucker, L. T. Grady, B. M. Michniewicz, S. C. Stauffer, S. E. White, G. E. Maha, and F. G. McMahon, J. Pharmacol. Exp. Ther., 179, 359 (1971).
212. A. De Leenheer and A. Heyndrickx, J. Pharm. Sci., 62, 31 (1973).
213. A. De Leenheer and A. Heyndrickx, J. Pharm. Sci., 61, 914 (1972).
214. S. D. Nelson, G. D. Breck, and W. F. Trager, J. Med. Chem., 16, 1106 (1973).
215. A. H. Beckett, J. M. Van Dyke, H. H. Chissick, and J. W. Gorrod, J. Pharm. Pharmacol., 23, 812 (1971).
216. W. J. A. VandenHeuvel, Separation Sci., 3, 151 (1968).
217. D. B. Peakall, Phthalate Esters: Occurrence and Biological Effects, in Residue Reviews (F. A. Gunther and J. D. Gunther, eds.), Springer-Verlag, New York, 1975.
218. R. A. De Zeeuw, J. H. G. Jonkman, and F. J. W. Van Mansvelt, Anal. Biochem., 67, 339 (1975).
219. P. W. Albro, R. Thomas, and L. Fishbein, J. Chromatogr., 76, 321 (1973).
220. H. A. H. Oelschläger, D. J. Temple, and C. F. Temple, Xenobiotica, 5, 309 (1975).
221. K. C. Liebman and E. Ortiz, Drug Metab. and Disp., 1, 543 (1973).
222. A. G. Zacchei and T. Wishousky, 23rd Annual Conference on Mass Spectrometry and Applied Topics, Houston, Texas, May 25-30, 1975.
223. W. G. Stillwell, E. C. Horning, M. G. Horning, R. N. Stillwell, and A. Zlatkis, J. Steroid Biochem., 3, 699 (1972).
224. A. Frigerio, N. Sossi, G. Belvedere, C. Pantaratto, and S. Garattini, J. Pharm. Sci., 63, 1536 (1974).
225. E. C. Dinovo, L. A. Gottschalk, E. P. Noble, and R. Biener, Res. Commun. Chem. Pathol. Pharmacol., 7, 489 (1974).
226. L. D. Gruenke, J. C. Craig, E. C. Dinovo, L. A. Gottschalk, E. P. Noble, and R. Biener, Res. Commun. Chem. Pathol. Pharmacol., 10, 221 (1975).
227. J. D. Fitzgerald and S. R. O'Donnell, Brit. J. Pharmacol., 43, 222 (1971).
228. D. A. Saelens, T. Walle, P. J. Privitera, D. R. Knapp, and T. E. Gaffney, J. Pharmacol. Exp. Ther., 188, 86 (1974).

229. A. R. Hansen and L. J. Fischer, Clin. Chem., 20, 236 (1974).

230. L. J. Fischer and J. J. Ambre, J. Chromatogr., 87, 379 (1973).

231. B. Dubinsky, M. C. Crew, M. D. Melgar, J. K. Karpowicz, and
      F. J. Di Carlo, Biochem. Pharmacol., 24, 277 (1975).

232. H. B. Hucker, S. C. Stauffer, S. D. White, R. E. Rhodes,
      B. H. Arison, E. R. Umbenhauer, R. J. Bower, and F. G. McMahon,
      Drug Metab. Disp., 1, 721 (1973).

233. J. F. Nash, I. F. Bennett, R. J. Bopp, M. K. Brunson, and
      H. R. Sullivan, J. Pharm. Sci., 64, 429 (1975).

234. V. D. Reif, J. E. Sinsheimer, J. C. Ward, and D. E. Schteingart,
      J. Pharm. Sci., 63, 1731 (1974).

235. S. B. Matin and M. Rowland, Anal. Lett., 6, 865 (1973).

236. B. Karlén, M. Garle, A. Rane, M. Gutova, and B. Lindborg,
      Eur. J. Clin. Pharmacol., 8, 359 (1975).

237. T. Chang, A. Savory, and A. J. Glazko, Biochem. Biophys. Res.
      Commun., 38, 444 (1970).

238. A. J. Glazko, T. Chang, J. Baukema, W. A. Dill, J. R. Goulet,
      and R. A. Buchanan, Clin. Pharmacol. Ther., 10, 498 (1969).

239. A. J. Atkinson, J. MacGee, J. Strong, D. Garteiz, and
      T. E. Gaffney, Biochem. Pharmacol., 19, 2483 (1970).

240. M. Mottale and C. J. Stewart, J. Chromatogr., 106, 263 (1975).

241. M. L. Selly, J. Thomas, and E. J. Triggs, J. Chromatogr., 89,
      169 (1974).

242. H. B. Hucker and S. C. Stauffer, J. Pharm. Sci., 63, 296 (1974).

243. K. Chan, M. J. Kendall, and M. Mitchard, J. Chromatogr., 89,
      169 (1974).

244. G. G. Gallo, N. Rimorini, L. F. Zerilli, and P. Radaelli,
      J. Chromatogr., 101, 163 (1974).

Chapter 3

STEREOCHEMICAL METHODOLOGY

Bernard Testa

School of Pharmacy
University of Lausanne
Lausanne, Switzerland

and

Peter Jenner

University Department of Neurology
The Institute of Psychiatry and
King's College Hospital Medical School
London, England

143

"The world is chiral and clinal; enjoy symmetry wherever you find it."
(Prelog, cited by Ginsburg [1].)

I. INTRODUCTION

Stereoisomers are molecules that have the same atoms with the same link-
ages among them but are not superimposable in three-dimensional space.
Two stereoisomers can show either an enantiomeric or a diastereoisomeric
relationship; these relationships are mutually exclusive. Thus, any chiral
object (i.e., not superimposable on its mirror image) will share an enantiomeric relationship with its mirror image.

    If two stereoisomeric compounds are not mirror images, they are dia-
stereoisomers. Epimers are a particular type of diastereoisomers:
stereoisomers with two or more centers of chirality that differ in the configuration of one and only one of these centers.

    While the limit between enantiomerism and diastereoisomerism is a
very sharp one, this is not the case for the distinction between configuration
and conformation. The best criterion available is that of energy levels.
Configurational isomers are interconverted through high energy transition
(e.g., covalent bond cleavage), whereas conformers are interconverted
through a low energy transition state (e.g., rotation around a single bond).

    The distinction between enantiomers and diastereoisomers is essential
in discussing both stereochemical factors in drug metabolism and the methods used for their assessment. The distinction between configuration and
conformation, on the other hand, will be much less helpful. Indeed, there
are few studies on conformational factors in drug metabolism as opposed
to studies on configurational factors.

    Enzymes are the chiral "tools" of the chiral biosphere [2] in metabolic
reactions and show stereochemical preferences in their catalyses. Stereospecificity denotes an apparently absolute preference. Stereoselectivity
denotes a partial predominance of one stereoisomer over the other(s) in
metabolic processes [3,4]. Unfortunately, the literature frequently does
not delineate the stereoisomeric-discriminating efficiency of the analytical
methods used, and thus quantitative decisions on the degree of stereoselectivity or a decision as to apparent stereospecificity cannot be made.

Recognition by the enzyme of elements of stereoisomerism in the substrates will result in substrate stereoselectivity, where stereoisomers are metabolized at different rates by the same enzyme. This is due to the fact that the transition states are diastereoisomeric and therefore have different energy levels [4, 5].

Product stereoselectivity designates the preferential generation of stereoisomers from a given substrate in a metabolic process due to competitive reactions catalyzed by the same enzyme. Obviously, not all substrates can be metabolized to stereoisomeric products. A necessary condition for product stereoselectivity is the presence of characteristic structural features at the target site of the substrate. This structural feature is most frequently represented by an element of prostereoisomerism [6]. Such target sites can be enantiotopic or diastereotopic [7] so that stereoselective metabolic attack can occur as in the hydroxylation of a prochiral methylene carbon. Alternatively, product stereoselectivity can occur when the target site has an unresolvable center of chirality so that metabolic attack blocks it in one configuration by the substitution of one ligand as in N-oxidation of some tertiary amines. Substrate-product stereoselectivity encompasses those cases when an additional element of stereoisomerism is introduced into an already stereoisomeric substrate. Product stereoselectivity may be different for stereoisomeric substrates, in which case substrate and product stereoselectivity show some degree of interdependence and cannot be considered separately [4].

There are three main groups of techniques in stereochemical methodology: (1) discrimination of stereoisomers by physical separation of stereoisomers or their generated spectroscopic signals; (2) synthesis of stereoisomers involving stereoisomers as reagents and/or as products, e. g., asymmetric synthesis, coupling of two chiral moieties; and (3) structure determination with assessments of absolute three-dimensional configurations and concomitant thermodynamic factors. Naturally, these groups of techniques overlap. Synthetic procedures are used in the separation of enantiomers by the synthesis of diastereoisomeric salts or derivatives with subsequent crystallization or chromatographic separation. The configurations of diastereoisomers are correlated with those physicochemical properties effective in discrimination methods such as chromatographic separation and spectroscopic identification. Structures can be assigned by unambiguous synthetic routes. Discrimination of diastereoisomeric derivatives of enantiomers can permit structural correlations.

This chapter will be restricted to the discrimination of stereoisomers suitable to drug metabolism studies where the minute amounts of metabolites obtained require high selectivity and sensitivity. Stereochemical synthesis and structure determination will only be considered in this regard.

This review is based on the fundamental differences between diastereoisomers and enantiomers. Diastereoisomers differ in their physicochem-

ical properties and can be discriminated without derivatization by chromatographic, spectroscopic, and other techniques. Enantiomers can be discriminated solely by recourse to a dissymmetric handle (e.g., enzymes,
dissymmetric reagents or solvents, enantiomeric circularly polarized
components of plane polarized light). The diastereoisomeric interaction
thus generated results in feasible discrimination by physicochemical
means [8].

II. STEREOCHEMICAL STUDIES: PROBLEMS IN OBTAINING AND INTERPRETING RESULTS

The proper prelude to studies of stereochemical factors in drug metabolism
is consideration of their design.

A. Metabolic Studies of Separate Stereoisomers

When a drug which exists in enantiomeric forms is investigated for stereoselective metabolism not involving the introduction of further asymmetric
centers (substrate stereoselectivity), it is feasible to administer the separate enantiomers and racemate on different occasions and to obtain stereochemical data by subsequently comparing the resulting recoveries or levels
of drug or metabolite(s) obtained. Such methodology avoids stereochemical
analysis of the drug or its metabolite(s) in biological samples after administration of the racemate and allows the use of simpler more available
nonstereochemical techniques [e.g., UV, gas chromatography (GC), liquid
chromatography (LC), fluorimetry]. A comparison of individual data for
the enantiomers might seem more simplistic in approach by not involving
some costly and complex physicochemical techniques [e.g., circular dichroism (CD), optical rotatory dispersion (ORD), and nuclear magnetic
resonance (NMR)].

It is nevertheless important to know the degree of resolution of the
administered enantiomeric forms. The stereospecificity of benzhexol for
the postganglionic acetylcholine receptors of guinea pig ileum has clearly
demonstrated that one enantiomer has an appreciably higher biological
activity [9]. If only 95% resolution has been effected, the highest possible
stereospecific index or ratio of activity of enantiomers would be 19. An
experimental stereospecific index of 100 would indicate a minimum degree
of resolution of 99%. A stereospecific index of 1,000 was obtained [9] and
indicated a minimum of 99.9% resolution (Fig. 1). Metabolism of high
stereoselectivity should also serve as the basis for the estimation of minimum degrees of resolution of administered enantiomers or of the stereoisomeric ratios of administered mixtures.

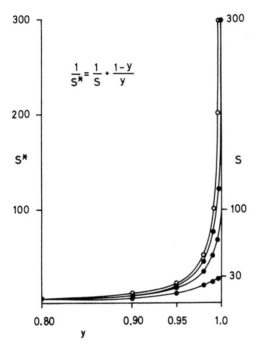

FIG. 1. The effect of the degree of resolution on the stereospecific index. The stereospecific index observed (S*) is plotted against the degree of resolution (Y) for particular values [30, 100, 300, and ∞ (open circles)] of the true stereospecific index (S). (Reproduced from Ref. 9 by courtesy of the Journal of Pharmacy and Pharmacology.)

Proper <u>statistical analysis</u> of the extent of stereoselective metabolism in vivo is necessary since intersubject and temporal variations can obscure significances. The number of observations required depends more on intersubject variations than intrasubject variations [10-12] and the degree of metabolic stereoselectivity. Ideally, the enantiomer metabolism should be compared in each individual animal or subject at a discrete time interval. Intersubject stereoselective metabolic variations can be assessed from the enantiomers (Table 1). Five individuals provided adequate evidence for probable enantiomeric stereoselectivity in many cases.

B. Experimental and Biological Factors Influencing
   Stereochemical Studies

Stereochemical studies of drug metabolism can be carried out either in vitro or in vivo. The former method is preferable since less processes

TABLE 1

Comparison of Intersubject Variation in the Extent of Stereoselective
Metabolism of Propranolol[a], Hexobarbital[b], and Warfarin[c]

Compound administered	Individual plasma $t_{1/2}$ (h)					$\bar{x}$	S.D. $\%$ of $\bar{x}$
	1	2	3	4	5		
(+)-Propranolol	2.1	2.4	1.7	1.3	2.6	2.02	26
(-)-Propranolol	3.6	3.5	3.4	2.8	2.7	3.20	13
ratio (+)/(-)	0.58	0.69	0.50	0.46	0.96	0.64	31
(+)-Hexobarbital	6.3	4.7	4.0	3.5	4.3	4.56	23
(-)-Hexobarbital	1.6	1.6	1.3	1.4	1.3	1.44	10
ratio (+)/(-)	3.94	2.94	3.08	2.50	3.31	3.15	17
(+)-Warfarin	64.2	34.9	45.0	37.5	--	45.4	29
(-)-Warfarin	51.6	28.8	26.0	23.5	--	32.5	40
ratio (+)/(-)	1.24	1.21	1.73	1.60	--	1.44	18

[a] From [12].

[b] From [13].

[c] From [14].

of biotransformation and disposition are involved, some of which may display stereoselectivity and affect the pharmacokinetic profile of the enantiomers. However, the drug will be used in the in vivo situation, and such studies must therefore be complementary. Whichever approach is adopted, a number of fundamental problems of protocol must be surmounted.

Drug metabolism studies demand the establishment of an index of stereoselectivity. It is tempting to assume that both stereoisomers will be metabolized by the same route and that the enantiomorphic content of the unchanged substrate is indicative of the metabolic stereoselectivity of that pathway. However, the metabolic pathways may differ for stereoisomers. The metabolism of N-substituted amphetamines [Structure (1)] is stereochemically governed in vivo and in vitro [15, 16], but the activation energies of α-carbon oxidation and N-oxidation of enantiomeric amphetamines [17] by rat liver microsomes suggested different mechanisms to be involved. α-Carbon-oxidation seemed to be the rate-limiting step in dealkylation and deamination of the (+)-enantiomers of secondary amphetamines, while the (-)-isomers were apparently N-oxidized. The N-dealkylation of tertiary amphetamines apparently proceeded by N-oxidation regardless of stereochemistry [17], although the route showed marked

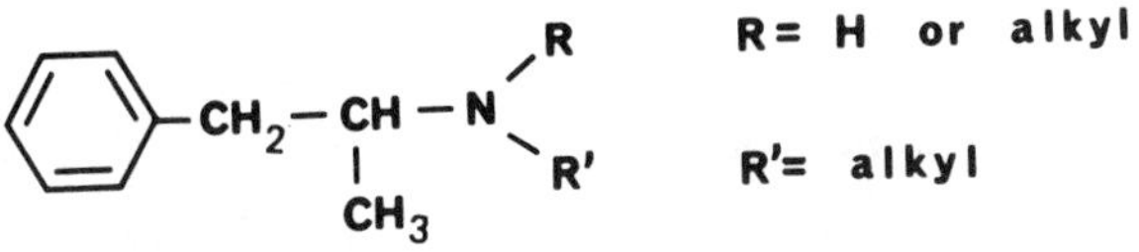

(1)

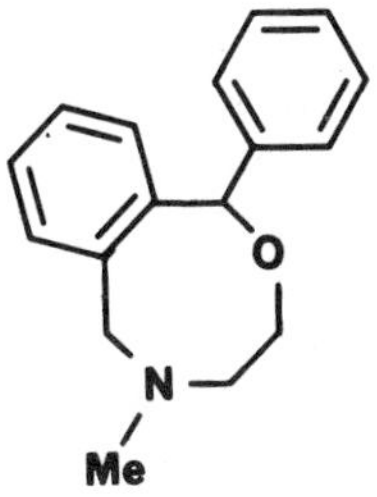

(2)

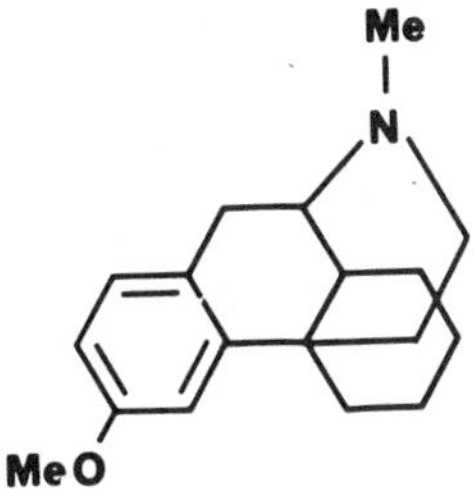

(3)

stereoselectivity [4]. Kinetic studies can show if two enantiomers are substrates for the same enzyme, such as with nefopam (2) and methorphan (3). In both cases, the same enzyme dealkylated the enantiomers [18, 19]. Measurement of one metabolic route alone may give rise to a false value for stereoselectivity. If one enantiomer is metabolized preferentially by one route of metabolism and the other enantiomer by an alternate route, the amount of substrate available for metabolism by the alternate route will be small. Measurement of either route alone would suggest apparent but false stereoselectivity for one route. The same situation may arise when the amount of enantiomeric substrate available for a nonstereoselective route is governed by the stereoselectivity of a competing route. For example, after administration of the enantiomers of dimethylamphetamine [(1), R = R' = Me] to man under conditions of acidic urinary pH, more methylamphetamine was excreted from (+)-dimethylamphetamine, while the (-)-enantiomer gave rise to larger quantities of the N-oxide [4]. According to the authors of the study the apparent stereoselectivity of N-oxidation is probably due to the faster demethylation of the (+)-enantiomer leaving an excess of (-)-substrate for N-oxidation.

Misleading answers are possible if the further metabolism of the primary metabolite of enantiomers occurs stereoselectively. After separate administration of fenfluramine (4) enantiomers to man, greater recoveries of R-(-)- than S-(+)-fenfluramine were found [15], as with other β-phenylethylamine derivatives. However, recoveries of the dealkylation product norfenfluramine were similar, suggesting that either the stereoselectivity of fenfluramine metabolism was due to an alternate route of metabolism

$$CF_3$$
(benzene ring)—CH_2—$\underset{\underset{CH_3}{|}}{CH}$—$NHC_2H_5$

(**4**)

(benzene ring)—$\underset{\underset{OH}{|}}{CH}$—$\underset{\underset{CH_3}{|}}{CH}$—$NHCH_3$

(**5**)

and not to dealkylation, or that further stereoselective metabolism of nor-fenfluramine occurred. Recent stereochemical analytical studies with racemic fenfluramine and norfenfluramine conclusively demonstrated the stereoselectivity of fenfluramine dealkylation and the further metabolism of norfenfluramine [4].

The choice of the moiety to measure is important. Formaldehyde production was monitored in the in vitro metabolism of ephedrine (5) stereo-isomers [20,21]. Small differences in the demethylation of the stereo-isomers were observed, and the isomers of (2S) configuration were more rapidly metabolized. These isomers subsequently underwent deamination, a metabolic route more highly stereoselective and not necessarily preceded by dealkylation. Therefore, formaldehyde production alone did not permit the observation of the specificity of deamination which would have been demonstrated by monitoring substrate disappearance. Only by the subsequent measurement of benzoic acid production was the stereoselectivity of deamination conclusively shown. One wonders whether specific investigations of the mechanism of deamination might have revealed even further selectivity.

It follows that the routes and mechanisms of enantiomer metabolism should be delineated before embarking upon studies of stereochemical metabolism unless the only interest is in the overall stereoselectivity of total metabolism. Analytical procedures need development for unchanged drug and as many metabolites as possible in order to assess the true stereoselectivity of the specific metabolic processes.

The manner of comparison of the drug enantiomers and their products is also of significance. Monitoring of total urinary recovery of unchanged drug after the separate administration of enantiomers is a frequent index of stereoselective metabolism but may be misleading as to the extent of stereoselectivity. A study published several years ago showed that the urinary recovery of unchanged R-(-)-amphetamine under conditions of acidic urinary pH was only slightly greater than that of the S-(+)-isomer [22]. However, a sensitive GC method (see Section IV) later showed that approximately equal amounts of both isomers were in the pooled urine containing 75% of the drug renally excreted during the first 12 h after the administration of racemic amphetamine. In the terminal stage of excretion, the enantiomeric ratio changed markedly in the urine aliquots analyzed at various times [23]. This explains why only slight enantiomeric differences are apparent when analyzing bulked urine samples. If single point measurements are to be made, a truer indication of stereoselectivity will be obtained from samples collected during the later stages of drug elimination when differences between the enantiomers will be maximal. However, for exact measurements of stereoselectivity it is necessary to establish the time course of drug elimination and the variation with time of the enantiomeric ratio.

Metabolic interactions between enantiomers may result in discrepancies in the observed rates and ratios when the administration of racemates and of the separate enantiomers are compared. Comparison of the stereoselectivity of the in vitro metabolism of the analgesics methadone (6) and phenadoxone (7) showed (+)/(-) metabolic ratios of 1.14 to 1.45 for the separate enantiomers. This ratio decreased to 1.07 to 1.17 when the racemates were studied [24] due to the apparent inhibition of their S-(+)-isomer metabolism by the R-(-)-enantiomers [4]. These findings were confirmed in vivo in man where $25.5 \pm 1.5\%$ of administered S-(+)-methadone was recovered in urine compared to $32.3 \pm 1.7\%$ after administration of the racemate [24]. Similarly, the separately studied enantiomers of isomethadone (8) with guinea pig microsomes showed faster demethylation of S-(-)-isomethadone, whereas racemic isomethadone had preferential metabolism of the R-(+)-enantiomer [25,26]. It is suggested that the R-(+)-isomer in the racemic mixture acts as a competitive inhibitor of the metabolism of the S-(-) form. Similarly, in vivo inhibition of levomethorphan metabolism in mice by its enantiomer dextromethorphan resulted in increased and prolonged analgesic activity of the former compound [19].

The route of drug administration may also influence the degree of stereoselectivity. The metabolic clearance of the (-)-enantiomer of hexobarbital (9) in man is at least three times greater than that of (+)-hexo-

$$R = \quad CH_2 - \underset{\underset{CH_3}{|}}{CH} - N(CH_3)_2 \qquad (6)$$

$$R = \quad CH_2 - \underset{\underset{CH_3}{|}}{CH} - N \bigcirc O \qquad (7)$$

$$R = \quad \underset{\underset{CH_3}{|}}{CH} - CH_2 - N(CH_3)_2 \qquad (8)$$

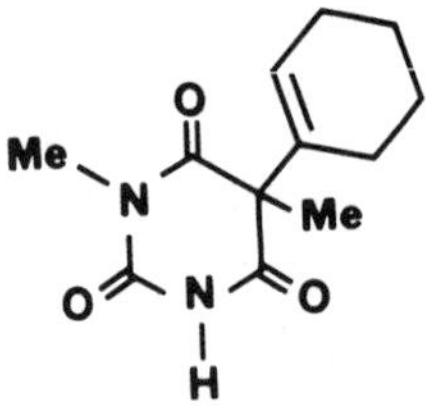

(9)

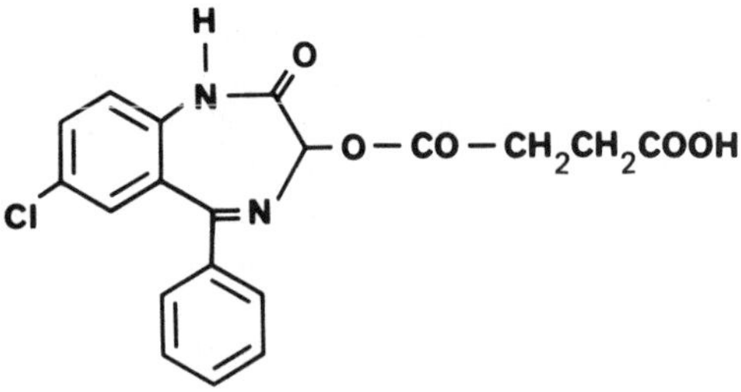

(10)

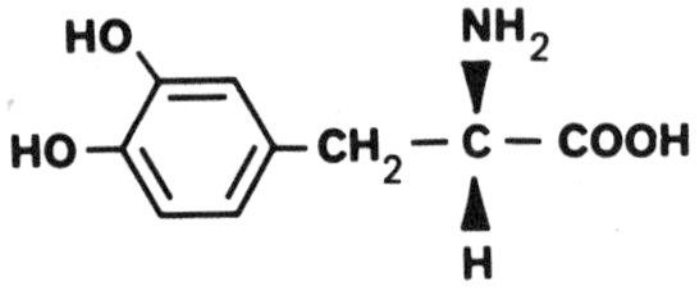

(11)

barbital. A substantial relative first pass phenomenon for the former compound is very probable after oral administration [13] and would increase the relative stereoselectivity of its metabolism compared to the (+)-isomer relative to intravenous administration. On the contrary, the stereoselective metabolism of enantiomeric oxazepam succinate half-esters (10) observed on i.v. administration to rats was not observed on oral administration [27]. Similarly, the tissue uptake of intravenously administered L-dopa (11) was significantly higher than D-dopa [28], but oral administration diminished tissue uptake of L-dopa which exceeded the D-isomer in only a few tissues. D-dopa generally showed higher accumulation and a longer retention on oral administration. Significant metabolism of L-dopa to dopamine occurred in gastric and intestinal mucosa and in liver, while untransformed D-dopa was absorbed and accumulated in tissues.

Dose-related effects also influence the observed stereoselectivity. Saturable or autoinhibition phenomena are best studied under in vitro conditions. The stereoselective demethylation of the (+)-enantiomer of nefopam (2) by a 9,000g supernatant fraction of rabbit liver was more rapid than that of the (-)-isomer at low substrate concentrations. At higher concentrations, however, there was little difference between the routes of demethylation of the two isomers. The demethylation of racemic nefopam was inhibited to a greater extent than the demethylation of either isomer alone [18], indicating complex phenomena.

Other factors governing the pharmacokinetic profile influence apparent metabolic stereoselectivity of enantiomers in vivo. For example, the absorption of the amino acids dopa and α-methyldopa is stereochemically governed. The D-forms are poorly absorbed relative to the natural enantiomers [28-31]. Similarly, plasma and brain levels of hexobarbital (9) [32] and fenfluramine (4) [33] suggested stereoselective uptake into brain tissue. The enantiomeric ratio of drug levels in the brain showed an accumulation of the more extensively metabolized form relative to plasma.

All the above examples outline some of the more important problems that investigators may encounter in stereochemical studies of drug metabolism. Other indirect approaches in this field may lead to similar difficulties. For example, studies of enantiomeric drug binding to cytochrome P-450 have failed to show a correlation between the enantiomer-cytochrome interaction and the known stereoselectivity of metabolism [34,35].

III. DISCRIMINATION OF DIASTEREOISOMERS

A. Chromatographic Techniques

Effective chromatographic separation of diastereoisomeric molecules depends on proper utilization of structure-related properties such as electronic distribution, volatility, solubilities (highly significant in partition chromatography), and steric hindrance (particularly significant in adsorption chromatography). Systematized chromatographic separations of diastereoisomers are rare (e.g., [36]), especially for compounds related to drug metabolism. This section will consider relevant examples illustrative of functional groups that generate diastereoisomerism. Alicyclic molecules with their restricted conformational freedoms and reduced numbers of diastereoisomeric conformers are better model compounds than their open-chain analogs and will be stressed. Combined diastereoisomeric and enantiomeric discrimination will be discussed in Section V.

Paper chromatography is more time-consuming and in general gives smaller resolution than TLC, but has utility. The nicotine-1'-N-oxide (12) product of the metabolic N-oxidation of nicotine exists as two diastereoisomers, the cis form (R,S and/or S,R) and the trans form (R,R and/or S,S). Separation by paper chromatography (see Table 2) permitted elution for structure elucidation and quantification [37,38]. The cis and trans diastereoisomers of 3-aminocyclohexanol [(13) and (14), respectively] and of 4-aminocyclohexanol [(15) and (16)] are metabolites of cyclohexylamine, in turn a metabolite of the sweetening agent cyclamate. Separation of the stereoisomers gave insight into the stereochemical aspects of cyclohexylamine hydroxylation [39].

Metabolic hydroxylation of 17β-estradiol by rat liver microsomes generated the epimeric 6α-hydroxyestradiol (17) and 6β-hydroxyestradiol

TABLE 2

Paper Chromatographic Separation of Some Diastereoisomeric Metabolites

Compound	Form	R_f	Paper	Mobile phase	Reference
Nicotine-1'-N-oxide	cis	0.41	Whatman 3MM	n–Butanol/n–propanol/ammonia 2 M (2:1:1, by volume)	[37]
	trans	0.52			
3–Aminocyclohexanol	cis (13)	0.59	Whatman No. 1	n–Butanol/acetic acid/water (4:1:2, by volume)	[39]
	trans (14)	0.43			
4–Aminocyclohexanol	cis (15)	0.40			
	trans (16)	0.49			
3–Aminocyclohexanol	cis	0.55		n–Butanol/isopropanol/water/acetic acid (8:4:2:1, by volume)	
	trans	0.43			
4–Aminocyclohexanol	cis	0.42			
	trans	0.50			
6α–17β–Hydroxyestradiol (17)		a	Schleicher and Schüll 2043b Mgl formamide	CHCl$_3$/ethyl acetate (5:1, by volume)	[40]
6β–17β–Hydroxyestradiol (18)					

aR_f not reported, save that the 6α–epimer migrates faster than the 6β–epimer.

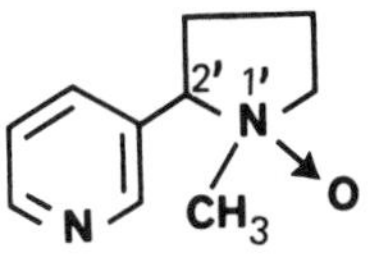

(12) 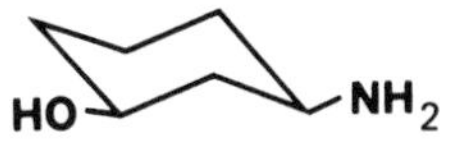   (13) 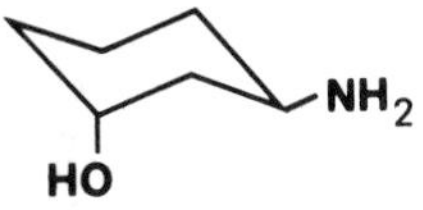   (14)

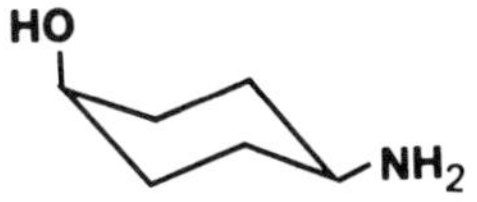

(15) 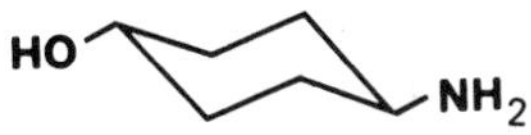   (16)

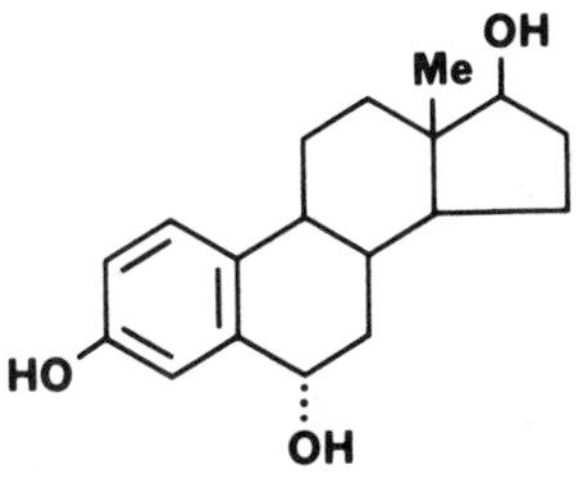

(17) 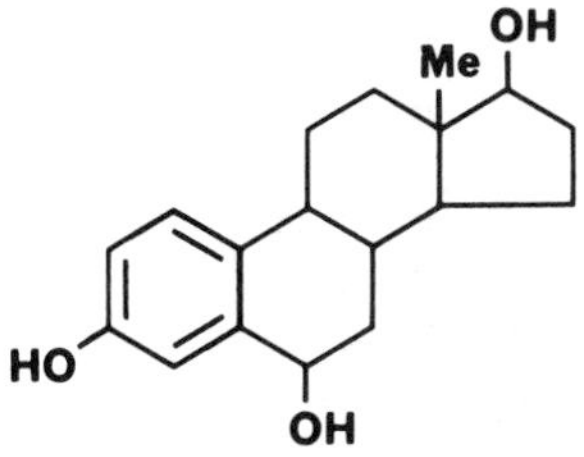   (18)

(18) and these were successfully separated by paper chromatography (Table 2) [40].

TLC is a fast and convenient method for diastereoisomeric separations. The expectedly difficult separations of alicyclic diastereoisomers such as the metabolites of bromhexine [(19), (20), and (21)] and of cyproheptadine [(22) and (23)] were reported (Table 3). An interesting example of compounds exhibiting open-chain elements of diastereoisomerism is that of the reduced metabolites of warfarin, the alcohols (24); the conditions for their separation are reported in Table 3.

GC, and more specifically gas-liquid chromatography, has long been recognized as a method of immense value for the separation of stereoisomers. More space will be devoted to this method in Section IV. B (e.g., assessment of peak resolution) while the following paragraphs are limited to the consideration of a few selected examples.

Diastereoisomers separated by GC may vary in their conformational freedom. Rigid structures are exemplified by the metabolites of D-camphor

TABLE 3

Thin-layer Chromatographic Separation of Some Diastereoisomeric Metabolites (Stationary Phase: Silica Gel)

Compound	Form	R_f	Mobile phase	Reference
N-(3-Hydroxycyclohexyl)-N-methyl-(2-amino-3,5-dibromobenzyl)amine (19)	cis	0.58	Ethyl acetate	[41]
	trans	0.66		
N-(3-Hydroxycyclohexyl)-(2-amino-3,5-dibromobenzyl)amine (20)	cis	0.35		
	trans	0.42		
6,8-Dibromo-3-(3-hydroxycyclohexyl)-1,2,3,4-tetrahydroquinazoline (21)	cis	0.16		
	trans	0.22		
10,11-Dihydroxycyproheptadine (22)	cis	0.41	Acetone/ammonia (100:1)	[42]
	trans	0.31		
10,11-Dihydroxydesmethylcyproheptadine (23)	cis	0.09		
	trans	0.07		
(22)	cis	0.22	Benzene/dioxane/ammonia (60:35:5), upper phase	
	trans	0.09		
(23)	cis	0.07		
	trans	0.03		

Compound	Isomer	R_f	Solvent system	Ref
(22)	cis	0.53	CHCl$_3$/methanol/acetic acid (47.5:47.5:5)	
	trans	0.45		
(23)	cis	0.48		
	trans	0.40		
(22)	cis	0.60	CHCl$_3$ sat. with ammonia/ methanol (19:1)	
	trans	0.48		
(23)	cis	0.20		
	trans	0.06		
	cis	0.52	Benzene/dioxane/ammonia (10:80:10)	
	trans	0.30		
(22)	cis	0.30	CHCl$_3$ sat. with ammonia	
	trans	0.07		
	cis	0.49	n–Butanol/acetic acid/water (65:15:20)	
	trans	0.43		
3-[α-(2-Hydroxypropyl)benzyl]-4-hydroxycoumarin (24)	RS + SR	0.46	Toluene/ethyl formate/ formic acid (10:5:1)	[43]
	RR + SS	0.21		

that result from either keto reduction [borneol and isoborneol, (25) and (26), respectively] or 5-hydroxylation [(27) and (28)]. The diol metabolites of cyproheptadine [(22) and (23)], discriminated by TLC (see above), were also resolved by GC (Table 4), although poorly for the desmethyl analogs. TMS-derivatization in each case presumably yielded the mono- and di-derivatives. The presumed mono-derivatives of longer retention time were better resolved than the unreacted compounds [42].

The stereoisomeric metabolites of cyclohexylamine (see above) were resolvable by GC (Table 4). Another example was the diastereoisomeric 4-hydroxylated metabolites (29) of propylhexedrine; configurational assignment of the two separated forms was, however, not made [45].

As representative of compounds containing a cyclic diastereoisomeric moiety, we report the GC resolution of 1,2-dihydroxy-1-phenylpropane (31),

TABLE 4

Gas Chromatographic Separation of Some Diastereoisomeric Metabolites

Compound	Form		Retention time (min)	Column	Oven temp. (°C)	Reference
2-Hydroxybornane	2-endo	(25)	2.3	20% Carbowax 20M on Chromosorb W, 6 ft	195	[44]
	2-exo	(26)	2.15			
5-Hydroxycamphor	5-endo	(27)	6.6		225	
	5-exo	(28)	5.4			
10,11-Dihydroxycyproheptadine (22)	cis		8.3 $(4.3 + 5.8)^a$	1.5% OV-17 on Gas-Chrom Q, 6 ft	238	[42]
	trans		8.7 $(5.4 + 4.3)^a$			
10,11-Dihydroxydesmethylcyproheptadine (23)	cis		10.4 $(5.1 + 7.0)^a$		233	
	trans		10.3 $(6.5 + 5.2)^a$			
3-Aminocyclohexanol	cis	(13)	19	3% E-301 on Chromosorb G, 5 ft	100	[39]
	trans	(14)	15			
4-Aminocyclohexanol	cis	(15)	21			
	trans	(16)	25			

TABLE 4 (Continued)

Compound	Form	Retention time (min)	Column	Oven temp. (°C)	Reference
4-Hydroxypropyl-hexedrine (29)	b	12.0 15.2	5% Carbowax 20M + 5% KOH on Chromo-sorb G, 2 m	c	[45]
	b	18.7 23.9	7% Carbowax 20M on Chromosorb W, 2 m	145	
1,2-Dihydroxy-1-phenylpropane (31)	erythro threo	7.9 7.2	7.5% Carbowax 20M on Chromosorb W, 1 m	165	[46]
Norephedrine (30)	erythro threo	4.1 3.9			

aTrimethylsilyl (TMS) derivatives; two peaks were observed in each case, the major one being listed first [42].
bConfigurations not reported.
cNot reported due to a printing error.

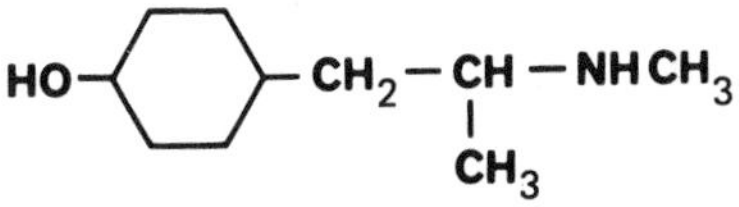

(29)

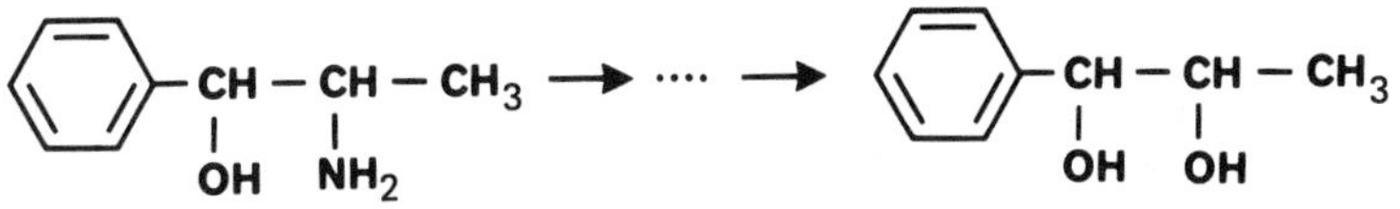

(30)   (31)

a metabolite of norephedrine resulting from oxidative deamination and subsequent keto reduction, in Table 4. For comparison, the separation of the diastereoisomeric forms of the parent compound (30) are also given. Further examples of GC and TLC separation of norephedrine and analogs can be found in Section V.

B. Proton Magnetic Resonance Spectroscopy

Protons in diastereoisomeric environments experience nonequivalent electromagnetic influence due to different spatial relationships among atoms and to the magnetic anisotropic shielding effects of many functional groups, resulting in differences in their proton magnetic resonance (PMR) signals. The theoretical and experimental aspects of PMR spectroscopy are well presented in the outstanding book by Casy [47] which considers detailed applications of PMR spectroscopy in medicinal and biological chemistry.

A limiting factor in drug metabolism studies is the quantity of material available, and this is particularly true for PMR. Although it varies with the number of protons in the molecule, approximately 30 mg is needed for a good spectrum with a continuous wave instrument without a signal averager system for spectrum accumulation, provided that solubility is adequate. Microtubes may permit the use of one-tenth of this amount. Fourier-transform (FT) NMR may further decrease the amount needed by 10 to 50 times. FT-PMR thus permits studies on fractions of a milligram and is of great promise in drug metabolism studies.

An interesting illustration of epimeric discrimination with these spectroscopic techniques was with the narcotic antagonist naltrexone (32) which underwent a metabolic keto reduction to the 6β-OH metabolite [(33), iso-

(<u>32</u>)   (<u>33</u>)   (<u>34</u>)

morphine configuration] in man, and to the 6α-OH epimer (<u>34</u>) in the
chicken with an apparently high degree of stereoselectivity [48]. TLC
could not discriminate the two epimers. The determination of the PMR
spectrum of the isolated 0.5 mg of pure human urinary metabolite (<u>33</u>)
was possible by a FT instrument. The 6α-H was found to resonate at
δ = 3.38 to 3.68 ppm (CDCl$_3$, TMS), whereas the 6β-H of the chicken
metabolite (<u>34</u>) resonated at δ = 4.16 to 4.40 ppm. The 5β-H resonates
at δ = 4.52 and 4.66 ppm, respectively. The configurational assignments
were rendered possible by the excellent PMR discrimination of the epimers,
and were achieved by comparison with the spectra of codeine and isocodeine
derivatives [48].

PMR spectroscopy also discriminates diastereotopic protons, as in
enantiomeric compounds of the type W−CH$_2$−CXYZ. Chemical shift differences typically in the range of 0.02 to 0.10 ppm may be observed, and
they are of potential interest in drug metabolism studies.

IV. DISCRIMINATION OF ENANTIOMERS

The discrimination of enantiomers can only be achieved by diastereoisomeric interaction. A dissymmetric "handle" is thus necessary. Three
methods of utility and promise are based on optical activity, and on interaction with optically active compounds allowing discrimination by GC or
NMR.

A. Optical Activity

Plane-polarized light is the vectorial resultant of two in-phase beams of
right and left circularly polarized light, ϵ_R and ϵ_L. These vectors trace
a right-handed and a left-handed helix, respectively, which provide the
required dissymmetric handles.

In a solution of a dissymmetric compound the diastereoisomeric interaction results in different refractive indices of the two beams ($n_R \neq n_L$) and in different molar extinction coefficients ($\epsilon_R \neq \epsilon_L$).

The difference in refractive indices n_R and n_L is known as circular birefringence. Rotation of the plane of polarization permits the detection of optical rotation. The angle of rotation (α) in degrees per centimeter is

$$\alpha = \frac{180}{\lambda} \, (n_L - n_R) \tag{1}$$

The magnitude of α for a given solute depend on wavelength (λ), solvent, temperature, and the number of molecules in the path of light, assuming no interaction between these molecules (see page 165).

Optical rotation can be expressed as specific rotation [α] or as molecular rotation [ϕ] at a given wavelength and temperature:

$$[\alpha]_\lambda^T = \frac{\alpha_\lambda^T \times 100}{Lc} \tag{2}$$

$$[\phi]_\lambda^T = \frac{MW \times [\alpha]_\lambda^T}{100} \tag{3}$$

where α is in degrees, L is in dm, and c is in g/100 ml. In a mixture of enantiomers, the optical purity is:

$$\% \text{ optical purity} = \frac{[\alpha]}{[\alpha_0]} \times 100 \tag{4}$$

where [α] is the specific rotation of the enantiomeric mixture and [α_0] is the specific rotation of one pure enantiomer. Optical purity is equal to the enantiomeric purity:

$$\% \text{ enantiomeric purity} = \frac{(R - S)}{(R + S)} \times 100 \quad \text{(for R > S)} \tag{5}$$

where R and S are the concentrations of the two enantiomers [8]. The enantiomeric percentages (or enantiomeric compositions) are derived from:

$$\% \text{ R-enantiomer} = \frac{R}{R + S} \times 100 \tag{6}$$

$$\% \text{ S-enantiomer} = \frac{S}{R + S} \times 100 \tag{7}$$

which are calculated from the enantiomeric purity, e. g. :

$$100 \times \frac{(R - S)}{(R + S)} + \frac{100 - 100 \times \frac{(R - S)}{(R + S)}}{2} = 100 \times \frac{R}{(R + S)} \qquad (8)$$

Frequent use is made in drug metabolism studies of the equivalence of optical and enantiomeric purity. The steps in the determination of the enantiomeric percentages are:

1. Isolation and purification of the metabolite (i. e., mixture of enantiomers) by any suitable method: TLC, column chromatography, preparative GC, etc.

2. Preparation of a solution of known concentration in an adequate solvent. The concentration of the solution can either be obtained by weighing the sample and/or by subsequent determination (UV, GC, etc.).

3. Measurement of the optical rotation in a micropolarimeter (sensitivity in the range of 1 millidegree). Measurements are usually carried out at the wavelength of the sodium D-line (589 nm) or at any other suitable and accessible wavelength.

4. Determination of optical purity from the specific rotation of pure individual enantiomers under the same experimental conditions. If an authentic sample of a pure enantiomer is not available, its specific rotation can be calculated indirectly from the specific rotation and enantiomeric composition of an incompletely resolved sample determined by various techniques such as GC, NMR, and kinetic resolution [49].

Interesting applications of optical rotation are in the metabolic studies of ethylbenzene (35) and indane (38) [50-53]. The two achiral compounds were oxidized to chiral hydroxylated metabolites [1-phenylethanol (36) and indanol (39), respectively]. The absolute configurations and specific rotations of their pure enantiomers were known. These underwent dehydrogenation to yield achiral ketones [acetophenone (37) and indanone (40), respectively]. The product and substrate stereoselectivities of the various reactions were determined after isolation, purification, and measurement of the specific activity of (36) and (39) either produced metabolically or as re-

(35)   (36)   (37)

(38)   (39)   (40)

(41)   (42)

mainders of metabolism of the racemates, and this permitted comparison of
in vitro and in vivo situations, the influence of inducers, etc.

Conditions necessary to calculate enantiomeric percentages from the
known specific rotation of one pure enantiomer are not always available.
Nevertheless, measurements of the specific activity of an isolated metabolite may be of value in recognition of a stereoselective reaction. To illustrate, the in vitro metabolic studies of acetophenone oxime (41) showed the
corresponding hydroxylamine (42) generated by a reductive pathway to be
optically active [54]. It was the first time that product stereoselectivity
was detected in metabolic C=N reduction, a phenomenon already observed
in C=C reduction.

The equivalence of optical purity and enantiomeric purity is valid only
in the absence of enantiomeric interactions in solution. Horeau has shown
that such interactions may occur [55, 56]. The specific rotations of chloroform solutions of 2-methyl-2-ethylsuccinic acid with known enantiomeric
percentages showed wide discrepancies between the calculated enantiomeric
purities and the measured optical purities which were functions of concentration and disappeared at greater dilutions. Although this may not be a
frequent occurrence at the low concentrations generally used, e.g., 1%,
in metabolic studies, there is a potential difficulty.

Some micropolarimeters allow measurements at wavelengths other than
the sodium D-line, such as the mercury lines of 578, 546, 435, and 365 nm.
Spectropolarimeters can use the spectral regions scanned by UV and visible
spectrophotometers. The optical rotatory dispersion (ORD) curves generated
by spectropolarimeters are proportional at a given wavelength to the difference between n_R and n_L. Molecular rotation increases regularly with
decreasing wavelength when no absorption maximum is observed. If the

compound does give rise to a peak of absorption (presence of a chromophore), the resultant <u>Cotton effect</u> has two aspects:

1. The sign and/or amplitude of the difference $n_L - n_R$ varies, and the Cotton effect perturbs the normal ORD curve to yield an anomalous curve.

2. Differences in molar extinction coefficients ($\epsilon_L - \epsilon_R = \Delta\epsilon \neq 0$) are known as <u>circular dichroism</u> (CD) and can be measured on dichrographs or spectropolarimeters with CD attachments by the molecular ellipticity

$$[\Theta]_\lambda^T = 3,300 \, (\Delta\epsilon) \tag{9}$$

The fundamental aspects and general applications of ORD and CD are well detailed [8, 57-66]. The following brief discussion presents applications to drug metabolism studies.

Rotatory power usually increases rapidly with decreasing wavelength, thus sensitivity is enhanced. ORD curves should be recorded and the wavelength region of maximum rotary power selected. In addition to increased sensitivity there is an accompanying gain in specificity, since peaks in molecular rotations often result from Cotton effects characteristic of chromophores in molecular structures.

CD curves are "pure" representations of Cotton effects, and their specificity for a given optically active compound is even greater than that of an ORD curve. One reason for the limited use of molecular ellipticities in determinations of enantiomeric percentages is a generally decreased sensitivity as compared to molecular rotations.

A wider application of the ORD technique than in the determination of enantiomeric percentages is exemplified by metabolic studies of pentobarbital (43) in dogs [67, 68]. This drug was metabolized by (ω - 1) hydroxylation to 3'-hydroxypentobarbital (44). R-(+)-Pentobarbital yielded approximately 33% of hydroxylated metabolites, with the (1'R;3'R)- and

(<u>43</u>)   (<u>44</u>)

(1'R;3'S)-diastereoisomers in a 1:1 ratio. S-(-)-Pentobarbital yielded approximately 38% of hydroxylated metabolites, with the (1'S;3'S)- and (1'S;3'R)-diastereoisomers in a 1:5 ratio. The ORD curves of the four isolated metabolites were obtained and, with other spectroscopic techniques, permitted elucidation of their configurations, particularly which metabolites were enantiomers and had mirror image curves, and which were diastereo-isomers. Specific rotations of the four metabolites alone would not have provided conclusive evidence for such interrelationships. Administration of racemic pentobarbital resulted in the excretion of two hydroxylated metabolites, the (R;S + S;R)- and (R;R + S;S)-diastereoisomers, which were optically active due to the substrate-product stereoselectivity of the metabolic reaction. The signs and amplitudes of the optical rotations of these two metabolites agreed with the predictions based on studies with the separate enantiomers.

The chiroptical techniques (ORD and CD) are also extremely powerful tools for delineating fundamental enzymic mechanisms. An interesting application of CD simultaneously elucidated substrate stereoselectivity and reaction rates of asparaginase [69] and may be applicable to genuine drug metabolism studies. Racemic mixtures that yielded either optically inac-tive or optically active metabolites were substrates for asparaginase. Diaminosuccinic acid monoamide (45) was incubated as a racemic mixture of the (2R;3S)- and (2S;3R)-enantiomers, and each had a CD maximum of 222 nm. The molecular ellipticity showed increasing negative values on continuous CD monitoring of the incubation mixture at this wavelength due to the regular enrichment of the medium with the unhydrolyzed (2S;3R)-isomer; the (2R;3S)-meso product of hydrolysis (46) was optically inactive and per-mitted kinetic analysis. This method is directly applicable only if the enzymic reaction has substrate stereospecificity. The generation of opti-cally active products of hydrolysis from racemic mixtures was also studied. In these cases regular spectral scanning was necessary to monitor the enzymic reaction, since the observed curve resulted from the contributions of both unhydrolyzed substrate and product.

Magneto-ORD (MORD) and magnetic CD (MCD) techniques based on the optical activity of achiral compounds in a strong magnetic field (Faraday effect) are useful in the study of microsomal cytochromes. MCD was used

COOH
|
2 CH NH$_2$
|
3 CH NH$_2$
|
CONH$_2$

(45)

→

COOH
|
CH NH$_2$
|
CH NH$_2$
|
COOH

(46)

for the quantitative determination of cytochromes P-450 and b_5, and possibly also P-420, in microsomal suspensions with a single measurement. It may find application in investigating structural changes of cytochrome P-450 induced by binding of substrates [70] to give insight into fundamental aspects of drug metabolism.

B. Gas Chromatography

Thin-layer and paper chromatographic methods, currently used in diastereoisomer discrimination (see Section III), have limited application in enantiomer discrimination, whereas GC has proven extremely useful [71].

GC resolution demands separate signals for the two enantiomers, with the possibility of physical separation by preparative GC. Gaussian peaks can be readily resolved by triangulation. In the theoretical chromatogram of Figure 2, the inflection tangents AB, CB, MN, and ON define the two triangles ABC and MNO. The <u>resolution factor</u> R can be defined from these triangles [72] by

$$R = 2 \frac{\overline{DP}}{\overline{AC} + \overline{MO}} = 2 \frac{t - t'}{a + b} \tag{10}$$

where t and t' are the retention times in min of the two peaks and a and b are $\overline{AC}$ and $\overline{MO}$ expressed in min.

Optimally, the two triangles ABC and MNO do not overlap, and the resolution is complete (R > 1). The internal triangles BDC and NPM can

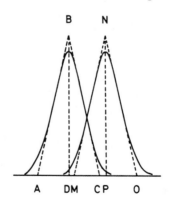

FIG. 2. Idealized representation of a two-compound chromatogram. (Reproduced from Ref. 82 by courtesy of the Journal of Pharmacy and Pharmacology.)

overlap moderately (0.5 < R < 1) or drastically so that the internal triangles BDC and NPM overlap on the external triangles BDA and NPO
(R < 0.5).

When R > 1 and when 0.5 < R < 1, quantitative assessment of enantiomeric composition is possible from appropriate calibration curves. When
R < 0.5 or if the peaks are markedly asymmetric or tailing, enantiomeric
composition can be approximated as by the peak height ratio method [73]
where the contributions of the overlapping peaks are subtracted to estimate
the true peak height.

Dissymmetric "handles" to resolve signals can be an optically active
stationary phase or derivatization of enantiomers with an optically active
reagent prior to separation on an ordinary stationary phase.

A few years ago, the use of optically active stationary phases raised
great hopes. These stationary phases often necessitate capillary columns
in order to achieve resolution, and are severely limited by the temperature
factor. Indeed, these phases are far from having the temperature stability
of ordinary phases, and may racemize and decompose readily above working temperature. They are thus suitable only for compounds of sufficient
volatility, or for highly volatile derivatives such as N-TFA- and particularly
N-PFP-derivatives of amines. Selected examples of optically active stationary phases, experimental conditions, and completely resolved compounds
are given in Table 5. Typical retention times were in the range of 1/2 to
2 h. Unfortunately, the separated compounds had relatively low molecular
weights and were not proper drugs, nor was this technique applied to drug
analysis and metabolism. Expertise and experience is also needed with
capillary columns and may partially explain this lack of interest.

Optically active reagents yield diastereoisomeric derivatives which can
be separated on ordinary stationary phases. Acceptable discrimination
requires optically pure chiral reagents, no racemization in the generated
diastereoisomers, and no stereoselectivity in the reaction (kinetic resolution) [49]. The optically active reagent must generate diastereoisomers
that have sufficient differences in physicochemical properties (i.e., adequate spatial disposition of the two chiral centers), chemical and stereochemical stability under GC conditions, and good volatility. Although capillary columns were first used [49], new optically active reagents permit
the use of packed columns.

The most commonly used reagent has been N-trifluoroacetyl-S-prolyl
chloride [TPC (47)]. Newer reagents include: S-(-)-N-pentafluorobenzoyl-
prolyl 1-imidazolidide [PFBPI (48)], (+)-α-methyl-α-methoxypentafluoro-
phenylacetyl 1-imidazolidide (49), and the terpinoid derivatives drimanoyl
chloride (50) and chrysanthemoyl chloride (51). These reagents are
acylating agents, and discriminate enantiomeric amines and alcohols.
They react smoothly within minutes at room temperature or upon mild

TESTA and JENNER

TABLE 5

A Few Selected Examples of Optically Active GC Stationary Phases Used in Capillary Columns
for the Separation of Enantiomers

Stationary phase[a]	Column temp. (°C)	Coating[b] (%)	Column length	Enantiomers studied	Reference
Ureide of L-valine isopropyl ester	100–120	5–40	40 m	N-TFA-, N-PFP-, and N-HFB-derivatives of simple alkyl- and cycloalkylamines	[74]
N-TFA-L-phenylalanyl-L-leucine cyclohexyl ester	110–140	10	100–400 ft	TFA amides–isopropyl esters and PFP amides–isopropyl	[75] [76]
N-TFA-L-valyl-L-valine cyclo-hexyl ester	max. 110			esters of amino acids	[76]

[a] TFA, trifluoroacetyl; PFP, pentafluoropropionyl; HFB, heptafluorobutyryl.
[b] w/v Concentration of the coating solution.

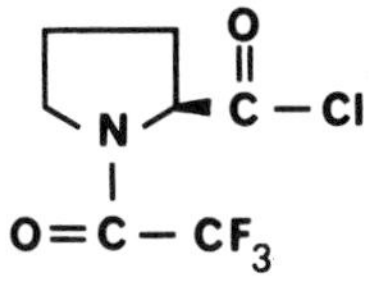

(47) 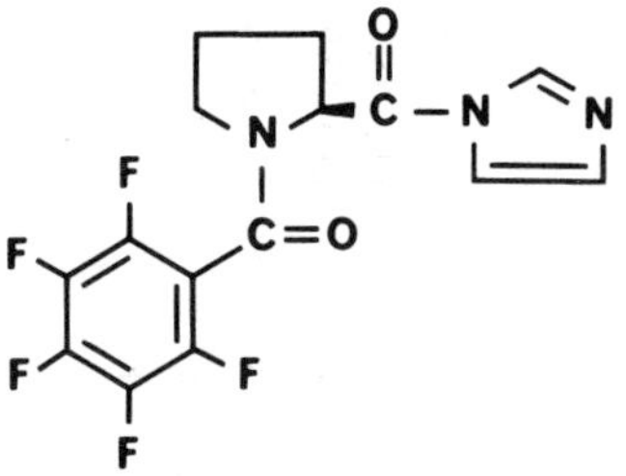 (48) 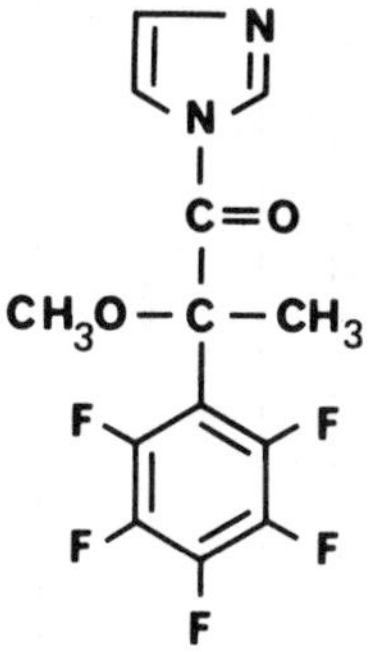 (49)

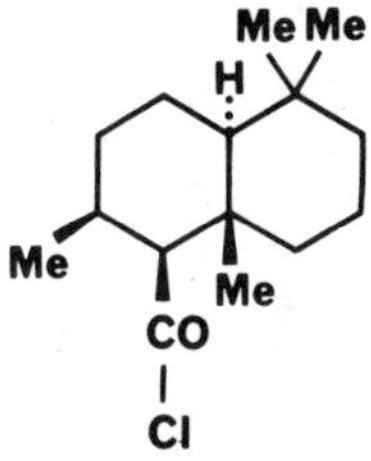

(50) 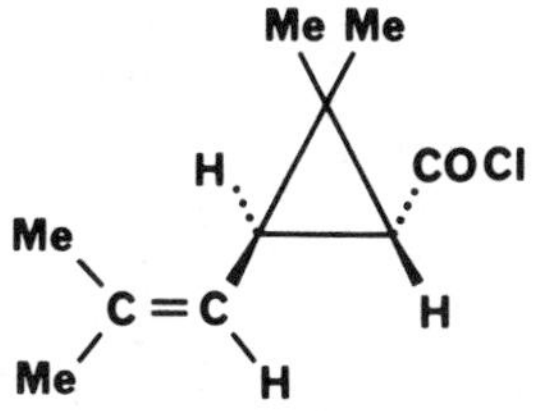 (51)

warming in dry solvents such as benzene, toluene, tetrahydrofuran, and chloroform. The reaction can be achieved on the microliter scale and followed directly by injection into the gas chromatograph.

Selected applications and important experimental conditions are listed in Tables 6 and 7. Due to the unique importance of amino functional groupings in drug molecules, the major efforts have been directed toward the resolution of amines, as apparent in these tables.

The achieved discriminations are exemplified in the chromatograms of Figures 3a-c which were obtained under uniform conditions after TPC derivatization of amphetamine [($\underline{1}$), R = R' = H] and N-n-alkyl-substituted amphetamines (Fig. 3a), of ring-substituted amphetamines, (Fig. 3b) and of β-hydroxyamphetamines (ephedrines, Fig. 3c).

The minute amounts of material needed have allowed these techniques to be applied to several metabolic studies. Recent examples include the use of PFBPI ($\underline{48}$) in studying the stereochemistry of α-methyldopamine formed metabolically from α-methyldopa and in proving the large if not complete retention of configuration of the metabolic reaction [84]. The same reagent established the overall substrate stereoselectivity of the in vivo metabolism of 1-(2,5-dimethoxy-4-methylphenyl)-2-aminopropane [87].

TABLE 6

Some Applications of N-TFA-S-Prolyl chloride[a] in the Resolution of Enantiomeric Drugs and Other Molecules

Enantiomers studied	Typical retention times (min)	Column	Column temp. (°C)	Reference
Amino acids methyl esters	5-15 5-30	5% SE-30 on Chromosorb W, 5 ft 0.5% EGA on Chromosorb W, 5 ft	176 185	[77]
Amino acids n-butyl esters	3-12	5% OV-1 on Supelcoport, 5.5 ft 2% Carbowax adipate on Supelcoport, 4 ft	210 220	[78]
Aminoalkanes	35-80 12-25 10-20	0.75% DEGS + 0.25% EG SS-X on Chromosorb W, 15 ft 5% SE-30 on Chromosorb W, 5 ft	110-130 140-185 140-185	[77]
Phenylalkyl-, (substituted phenyl)alkyl-, diphenylalkyl-, and naphthyl-amines	8-85	3% SE-30 on Chromosorb W, 3 m 2% QF-1 on Chromosorb W, 2 m 2% DEGS on Chromosorb W, 1 m	160-200	[79]
Heterocyclic amines and phenylethylamines	3-20	5% DC LSX-3-0295 on Chromosorb W, 5 ft	210	[77]
Amphetamine	12.5 + 15	1% Carbowax 20M on Gas Chrom Q, 2 m	185	[80]
N-Alkylamphetamines	30-100	3% SE-30 on Chromosorb G, 2 m	170	[81]
Ring-substituted amphetamines	25-65			
Ephedrines	60-120			[82]

TABLE 7

Applications of Some Recent Chiral Reagents in the GC Resolution of Enantiomeric Molecules

Reagent[a]	Enantiomers studied	Typical retention times (min)	Column	Column temp. (°C)	Reference
(48)[b]	Amphetamine	11.25 + 12	3% OV-17 on Chromosorb W, 6 ft	250	[83]
	Di- and trimethoxy ring-substituted amphetamines	12-18		250, 270	
	O-Methylated α-methyl-dopamine	28.5 + 33.4	3% SE-30 on Chromosorb W, 6 ft	190	[84]
(49)[b]	Amphetamine	12.0 + 12.5	3% SE-30 on Varaport 30, 5 ft	170	[85]
	2,5-Dimethoxy-4-methyl-, 3,4,5-trimethoxy-, and 2,3,5-trimethoxy-amphetamine	15-30		190	
(50), (51)	Amphetamine	45-60	1% SE-30 on Gas Chrom Q, 5 m	100, 160	[86]
	Terpenic alcohols	30-50		143, 190	
	Methyl esters of hydroxy fatty acids	30-50			

[a]Reagents: S-(−)-N-pentafluorobenzoylpropyl 1-imidazolidide (48); (+)-α-methyl-α-methoxypentafluorophenylacetyl 1-imidazolidide (49); drimanoyl chloride (50); chrysanthemoyl chloride (51).

[b]Reagent with good electron capture properties.

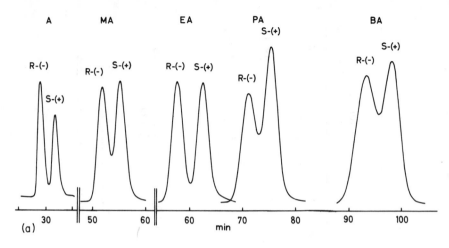

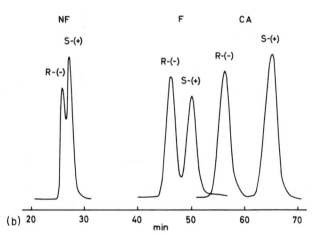

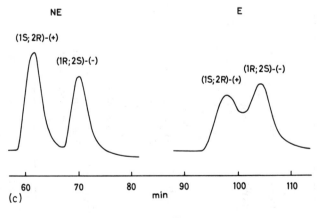

FIG. 3

174

A promising approach [88] may permit the neglected GC separation of enantiomeric carboxylic acids. The enantiomers of the anti-inflammatory agent α-[4-(1-oxo-2-isoindolinyl)phenyl]propionic acid (52) were separated after the formation of the acid chloride, which was reacted with (-)-α-methylbenzylamine, and GC analysis (conditions: 1% OV-17 on Chromosorb W, column temperature 280°C). The retention times of the derivatives of (+)- and (-)- (52) were 24.9 and 28.2 min, respectively, with a resolution factor better than 1. The plasma levels of both enantiomers after administration of the racemic compound could be monitored. This should be a generally applicable procedure.

(52)

C. Proton Magnetic Resonance Spectroscopy

Protons in enantiomeric environments are chemically and magnetically equivalent. A diastereoisomeric relationship is necessary to permit discrimination which can be achieved either by derivatization with optically active reagents and/or by intermolecular interactions [89, 90]. The diastereoisomeric products of such interactions must show differences between chemical shifts sufficient for separate integration of diastereoisomeric signals.

Optically active reagents are used to synthesize derivatives which must be isolated and purified before the recording of NMR spectra, in contrast to GC where isolation and purification of the derivatives is often unnecessary. Derivatization (see Section IV.B) must occur without racemization or kinetic resolution. Favorable structural features of the reagent include (1) the presence of a highly magnetically anisotropic group (e.g., a phenyl

FIG. 3. GC separation of TPC derivatives. Conditions: 3% SE-30 on Chromosorb G; 2 m column; oven temperature 170°C; N_2 flow rate 25 ml/ min. (a) A, amphetamine [(1), R = R' = H]; MA, N-methylamphetamine; EA, N-ethylamphetamine; PA, N-n-propylamphetamine; BA, N-n-butyl-amphetamine. (b) NF, norflenfluramine (meta-trifluoromethylamphetamine); F, fenfluramine (4); CA, para-chloroamphetamine. (c) NE, norephedrine [β-hydroxyamphetamine, (30)]; E, ephedrine (5). (Reproduced from Refs. 81 and 82 by courtesy of Elsevier Publishing Co. and the Journal of Pharmacy and Pharmacology, respectively.)

ring) to increase the probability of chemical shift nonequivalence, and (2) the presence of groups that generate singlet resonance signals; suitable signals from either component of the diastereoisomers may permit discrimination [90].

Salt formation can permit discrimination, but the usual procedure is by covalent bond formation with acylating reagents. An effective reagent is α-methoxy-α-trifluoromethylphenylacetic acid [MTPA (54)] [91], which is available in either enantiomeric form. Differences in the chemical shifts of diastereoisomeric derivatives are usually in the range of 0.01 to 0.15 ppm.

Some optically active reagents have proven useful in both GC and PMR studies. Diastereoisomeric derivatives of α-methoxy-α-methylpentafluoro-phenylacetyl 1-imidazolidide (49) showed chemical shift differences in the range of 0.06 to 0.18 ppm [85]. Both reagents (49) and (54) improve on O-methylmandelyl chloride (53), which gave racemization in some cases [90]. Derivatives of (+)-10-camphosulfonic acid (55) with enantiomeric arylalkyl amines were separated by GC and showed differences as great as 0.55 ppm in the chemical shifts of either methylene proton and methyl group of the camphor moiety [92].

The alternative method in PMR discrimination of enantiomers involves diastereoisomeric intermolecular interactions. Optically active solvents give rise to small differences in chemical shifts (less than 0.1 ppm). A typical example is 2,2,2-trifluoro-1-phenylethanol (56), with amines, esters, and sulfur compounds [90,93].

Chiral lanthanide shift reagents are a tool of great interest in stereochemical studies. A lanthanide shift reagent (LSR) consists of a six-

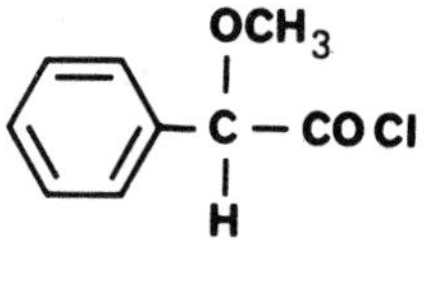

(53)

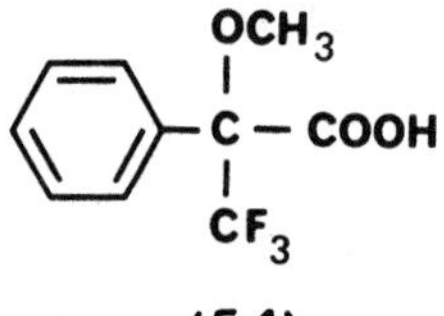

(54)

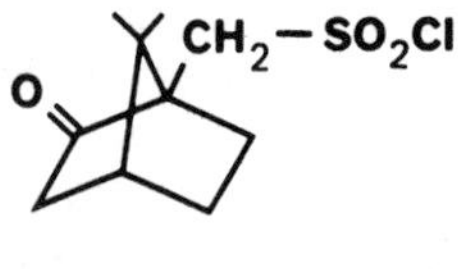

(55)

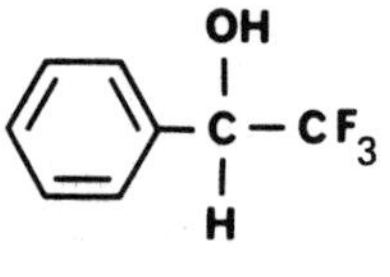

(56)

coordinate metal complex which, by expanding its coordination, accepts further ligands. Heteroatoms exhibiting some degree of Lewis basicity provide the required ligands, and are a necessary requirement for a substrate to form a complex with a LSR. As a result of such paramagnetic lanthanide complexes, large pseudocontact shifts (designated $\Delta\delta$) are induced in nuclei close to the heteroatoms. A wide variety of compounds has been shown to exhibit lanthanide-induced shifts; they include alcohols, phenols, oximes, ketones and aldehydes, esters and lactones, amides and lactams, ethers and peroxides, amines, aza heterocyclic compounds, nitriles, sulfoxides and sulfones, N-oxides, and nitrones.

The equilibrium constant of the complex is induced by the magnitudes of the Lewis basicity and steric hindrance about the heteroatoms. LSR with increased acidity bind more strongly to a given substrate and extend the range to weaker substrates; LSR thus often contain fluorine atoms to increase the acidity of the metal ion.

LSR must be used in solvents not capable of coordinating with them, e.g., CCl_4, C_6D_6, and CS_2. Successive amounts of the LSR are added to the solution of the compound, and the changes in chemical shifts that occur with varying LSR/substrate ratios are followed by recorded spectra. The solubility of the reagent may be a limiting factor. Two outstanding reviews [94, 95] and a recent book [96] give the theory and applications of lanthanide-induced shifts.

Achiral LSR have been applied to stereochemical studies for increased resolution and assignment of signs from diastereoisomeric and diastereotopic protons. On the other hand, chiral LSR raise considerable interest in the discrimination of enantiomers. Useful reagents include Tris[3-(tert-butylhydroxymethylene)-d-camporato]europium(III) [(57), Ln = Eu], Tris-(3-trifluoroacetyl-d-camphorato)europium(III) (or Eu(facam)₃) and its praseodymium analog Pr(facam)₃ [(58), Ln = Eu and Pr, respectively], and Tris(3-heptafluorobutyryl-d-camphorato)europium(III) (or Eu(hfbc)₃) and Pr(hfbc)₃ [(59), Ln = Eu and Pr, respectively] [94, 97, 98].

In the presence of such reagents, corresponding protons in enantiomeric molecules experience differences in the pseudocontact shifts ($\Delta\Delta\delta$) which are usually in the range of 0.00 to 0.20 ppm, but are not infrequently much larger.

$$R = C(CH_3)_3 \quad (\underline{57})$$

$$R = CF_3 \quad (\underline{58})$$

$$R = n\text{-}C_3F_7 \quad (\underline{59})$$

Optimal ranges of molar ratios of LSR/substrate with a proper reagent can be found which maximally separate enantiomeric signals and quantitatively discriminate two enantiomers. Amusingly, this technique has been coined "polarimetry by NMR." Table 8 illustrates the separations obtained for the model compounds 1-phenylethylamine and 1-phenylethanol, where phenylethanol, the weaker Lewis base, demands stronger Lewis acid reagents to permit resolution.

The relative signal shifts of the R/S enantiomers are not predictable, thus chiral LSR are at present unsuitable for the determination of absolute configuration.

Chiral LSR, chiral solvents, and the derivatization with chiral reagents are methods of potential utility in drug metabolism studies, especially in the discrimination of enantiomers. Relevant examples in this field are still rare but may be anticipated within the next years.

TABLE 8

Enantiomeric Shift Differences ($\Delta \Delta \delta$ in ppm)[a]

Substrate	Signal	LSR		
		Eu-(57)[b]	Eu-(58)[b]	Eu-(59)[c]
1-Phenylethylamine	CH_3	0.21	0.50	0.08
	CH	0.55	--[d]	0.00
	ortho-H	0.13	0.05	0.06
1-Phenylethanol	CH_3	0.00	0.00	0.05
	CH	0.00	0.40	0.07
	ortho-H	0.00	0.00	--[d]

[a]From [98, 99].

[b]Concentrations of LSR and substrate: 0.3 ± 0.1 M; solvents: phenylethylamine $CDCl_3$, phenylethanol CCl_4 [99].

[c]Molar ratio LSR/substrate > 0.6; solvent CCl_4 [98].

[d]Data not available.

V. COMPLEX CASES

Sections III and IV separately considered diastereoisomeric and enantiomeric molecules. Metabolic studies frequently are made with compounds
that possess two or more elements of stereoisomerism and exist as chiral
diastereoisomers. The following are examples which need combinations of
the techniques described in the previous sections.

Nortriptyline [NT (60)] is metabolized by hydroxylation at the 10-position
(benzylic hydroxylation) to yield 10-hydroxynortriptyline (10-OH-NT). This
major human metabolite exists as two π-diastereoisomers, the Z- and E-
isomer (or cis- and trans-isomer), each of which is chiral and exists as
two enantiomers. The two racemic diastereoisomers were available as
authentic compounds, but since their configurations were unknown they were
designated as I and II [100]. The separation of I and II from human urine
was achieved by TLC (silica gel; cyclohexane/chloroform/diethylamine,
70:20:10, v/v; five developments; retention factor (R_f) values 0.39 and
0.33, respectively). Repeated chromatography resulted in complete separation, and the eluted spots were analyzed by GC. The two isolated metabolites were optically active and the stereoselectivity of the hydroxylation
reactions was investigated. The CD curves were almost mirror images of
each other (I: negative maximum at 251 nm, positive maximum at 233 nm;
II: positive maximum at 250 nm, negative maximum at 228 nm) and indicated that I and II had opposite configurations at their asymmetric carbon
(10R and 10S). This suggested that the two predominant stereoisomers of
10-OH-NT were either (S)-(Z) and (R)-(E), or (R)-(Z) and (S)-(E), where
the R- and S-isomers would have the hydroxyl group on the same side of
the tricyclic plane when the side-chain is fixed in one position.

The configuration of the two diastereoisomers of 10-OH-NT were later
determined [101]. Comparison of TLC data suggests that I and II are the
E- and Z-isomers, respectively. The absolute configuration of the enantiomers is not known at present.

$$(R)\text{-}(E) \quad (S)\text{-}(Z)$$
$$(S)\text{-}(E) \quad\quad (R)\text{-}(Z)$$

$$\text{H} \quad \text{CH}_2\text{CH}_2\text{NHCH}_3$$

(60)

Dieldrin (61), a polychlorinated insecticide, has an epoxide group, and
its metabolic fate was elucidated only recently [102]. The first identified
metabolite was the trans-dihydrodiol derivative, trans-dihydroaldrindiol
[TAD (63)]; cis-dihydroaldrindiol [CAD (62)] was detected later under in
vitro conditions. These two epimeric metabolites were separated by two-
dimensional TLC (silica gel; mobile phase 1: hexane/acetone, 1:1; mobile
phase 2: ether/hexane, 9:1) and quantified by liquid scintillation counting.
The main metabolic pathway involved hydrolysis of the exo-epoxide group-
ing to the cis-dihydrodiol derivative and microsomal epimerase converted
this metabolite to TAD. The cis-(exo-exo) compound CAD, a meso stereoisomer, is achiral; TAD on the other hand is chiral and showed negative
rotation when generated as a metabolite of dieldrin. The enantiomeric composition of this metabolite was determined by chiral LSR, Eu(hfbc)$_3$ (59).
Four mg of TAD were isolated from a series of incubations after TLC purification. The NMR spectra recorded in the FT mode in the presence of the
shift reagent showed that TAD contained approximately 64% of one enantiomer (which must be the levorotatory enantiomer, see above) and 36% of the
other [103]. The epimerization reaction thus occurs with a moderate degree
of stereoselectivity. The absolute configuration of the predominant enantiomer remains to be determined.

The anorectic drug diethylpropion (64) is rapidly and extensively metabolized in humans. The two major pathways are N-dealkylation and keto
reduction [104]. Diethylpropion and its amino-ketone metabolites, (65) and
(66), are chiral, whereas the amino-alcohols N-diethylnorephedrine [DENE
(67)] N-ethylnorephedrine [ENE (68)], and norephedrine [NE (69)] each
exist as four stereoisomers. A complex procedure has been developed to
determine the ratios of the four stereoisomers of each amino-alcohol
excreted in man after the administration of diethylpropion [105]. All the

stereoisomers separated and quantified in this study were available as
authentic compounds, and their absolute configuration was known: (1S;2R)-
(+)-erythro, (1R;2S)-(-)-erythro, (1S;2S)-(+)-threo, (1R;2R)-(-)-threo.
Only analytical methods were needed to study diethylpropion metabolism.

The diastereoisomeric ratios of the three amino-alcohols were determined by GC (oven temperature 180°C; column: 5% KOH + 5% Carbowax
20M on Chromosorb G, 2 m) and resulted in complete separation of the
threo- and erythro-isomers of DENE (retention times 13.0 and 16.5 min,
respectively) and of threo- and erythro-NE (18.7 and 20.0 min), but not
of the isomers of ENE (threo and erythro, 14.5 min). Calibration curves
allowed simple determination of the threo/erythro ratios of DENE and NE.

The threo and erythro forms of ENE could not be separated on a variety
of columns without their peaks interfering with those of the other metabolites.
Thus, advantage was taken of the differences in the rates of oxazolidine
formation of the two forms. Under carefully standardized conditions, threo-
ENE reacted with acetone and gave the oxazolidine much faster than did
erythro-ENE. GC measurements of the percent of reacted ENE determined
the diastereoisomeric ratios with a calibration curve (percentages of reaction: threo-ENE, 80%; erythro-ENE, 20%).

The enantiomeric ratios of the individual diastereoisomers were determined after their separation from each other and from the other metabolites by TLC (silica gel; acetone/methanol 88:12; R_f values of threo- and erythro-isomers, respectively; DENE 0.53 and 0.32, ENE 0.13 and 0.20, NE 0.70 and 0.61). The elution of the spots corresponding to threo- and erythro-DENE showed complete diastereoisomeric separation, but the eluates were contaminated with ENE and NE. Purification was achieved by acetylating the impurities and removing the resultant nonbasic amides. The purified solutions of threo- and erythro-DENE were then analyzed by optical rotation at 222 nm (using a spectropolarimeter) to yield the concentrations of optically active compounds from the known rotations of the pure enantiomers, and by GC for total concentration. Enantiomeric ratios or percentages were easily derived from these two concentrations. The method required at least 100 µg of optically active erythro-DENE, and at least 50 µg of optically active threo-DENE.

The two diastereoisomers of ENE were insufficiently separated by TLC. They were thus eluted together to yield an eluate containing the four stereoisomers of ENE [(+)- and (-)-erythro, whose concentrations are designated a, b, c, and d, respectively]. The eluate was found to be free from all other metabolites. Four determinations are necessary in order to calculate a, b, c, and d. These determinations are

a. Total concentration M (determined by GC):

$$M = a + b + c + d \tag{11}$$

b. Fraction L of erythro form (determined by GC as described above):

$$L = \frac{a + b}{a + b + c + d} \tag{12}$$

c. Optical rotation at 222 nm (m and n being calibration factors):

$$K = m(a - b) + n(c - d) \tag{13}$$

d. Enantiomeric determination by GC, using TPC-derivatization and conditions described in Table 6 [82]; the derivatives of (+)-erythro- plus (-)-threo-ENE produce one peak (114 min) fairly well separated from a second peak (120 min) corresponding to (-)-erythro plus (+)-threo-ENE. Therefore

$$N = \frac{a + d}{a + b + c + d} \tag{14}$$

Equations (11) to (14) can be solved for a, b, c, and d to yield the $(+)/(-)$ ratio of erythro-ENE and the $(+)/(-)$ ratio of threo-ENE. The same amounts of material as for DENE were required.

The eluates from the two spots corresponding to threo- and erythro-NE showed that only a partial separation has been obtained. The concentrations of the four stereoisomers in the two eluates were designated a_1, b_1, c_1, and d_1, and a_2, b_2, c_2, and d_2, respectively. Determination of the diastereoisomeric fractions R of the two eluates by GC (see above) yielded

$$R_1 = \frac{c_1 + d_1}{a_1 + b_1 + c_1 + d_1} \tag{15}$$

$$R_2 = \frac{c_2 + d_2}{a_2 + b_2 + c_2 + d_2} \tag{16}$$

Enantiomeric determination by GC analysis of TPC-derivatives, carried out separately for the two eluates, again differentiated two peaks, the first (63 min) corresponding to $(+)$-erythro- plus $(-)$-threo-NE, the second peak (70 min) to $(-)$-erythro- plus $(+)$-threo-NE, yielding the fractions

$$P_1 = \frac{a_1 + d_1}{a_1 + b_1 + c_1 + d_1} \tag{17}$$

$$P_2 = \frac{b_2 + c_2}{a_2 + b_2 + c_2 + d_2} \tag{18}$$

Since

$$s = \frac{a_1}{b_1} = \frac{a_2}{b_2} \tag{19}$$

and

$$t = \frac{c_1}{d_1} = \frac{c_2}{d_2} \tag{20}$$

where s and t are the $(+)/(-)$ ratios of erythro- and threo-NE, respectively, s and t can be expressed in terms of P_1, P_2, R_1, and R_2 to give the required answer.

The reader is referred to the original publication [105] for full details on this unusually lengthy procedure and for its validation using solutions containing known diastereoisomeric and enantiomeric ratios of the aminoalcohols. Extensive studies on the stereochemical aspects of diethylpropion metabolism in man were then possible [104, 106, 107].

VI. MECHANISTIC STUDIES WITH STEREOSPECIFICALLY LABELED COMPOUNDS

Stereospecifically labeled substrates have permitted fundamental insight into the steric and mechanistic aspects of enzymic reactions and have been well reviewed [108-111].

The difference between their use and that of the methods previously described lies in the actual stereochemical stage of the method. With stereospecifically labeled compounds this stage must occur during the synthesis of the substrate (as in Section II.A) and may or may not also occur during analysis of metabolites. Stereospecific synthesis is outside the scope of this review and discussion is restricted to selected examples which illustrate applications and potentialities.

The high degree of stereoselectivity in the enzymic hydroxylation of prochiral benzylic carbons was confirmed by the use of stereospecifically labeled substrates. Configuration was retained with front side displacement of a hydrogen atom. Ethylbenzene (35) metabolism was studied with (S)-(+)-[1-^{2}H$_1$]-ethylbenzene (70) as a substrate for rat liver mono-oxygenases. The metabolite (R)-(+)-[1-^{2}H$_1$]-1-phenylethanol (71) retained 86% of the deuterium present in the substrate and had an optical activity corresponding to 92% of the (R)-(+)-enantiomer [112]. These two values clearly show the mechanism of front side displacement.

The stereochemical course of hydroxylation by dopamine-β-hydroxylase was investigated with several substrates. (1S;2S)-[2-^{3}H$_1$]Amphetamine (72) was β-hydroxylated to (1S;2R)-[2-^{3}H$_1$]norephedrine (73), with a high

(70)   (71)

(72)   (73)

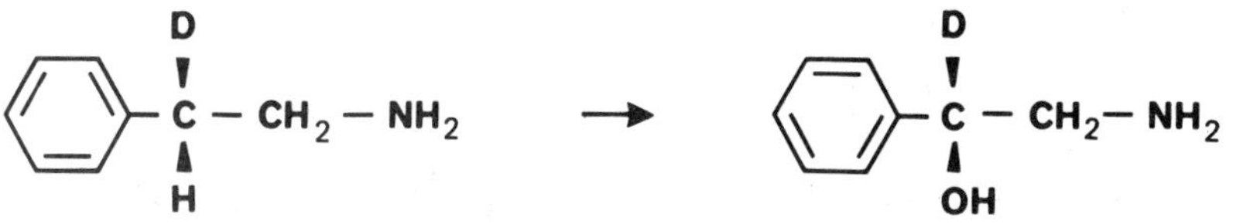

Ph–C(D)(H)–CH$_2$–NH$_2$ → Ph–C(D)(OH)–CH$_2$–NH$_2$

(74) (75)

Ph–C(H)(D)–CH$_2$–NH$_2$ → Ph–C(H)(OH)–CH$_2$–NH$_2$

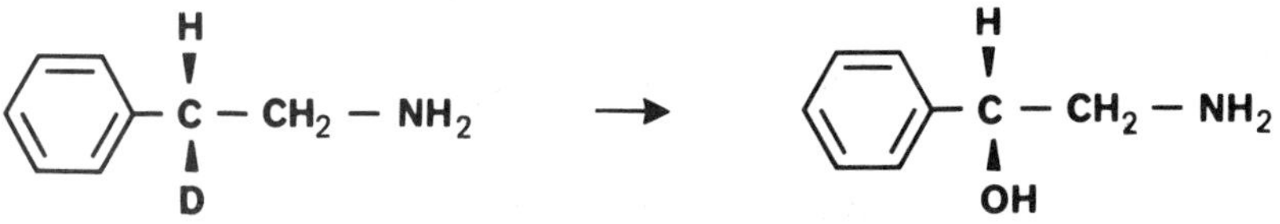

(76) (77)

retention of configuration and radioactivity [113]. Similarly, (2S)-[2-^{2}H$_1$]-phenylethylamine (74) and (2S)-[2-^{3}H$_1$]dopamine were hydroxylated to (2R)-[2-^{2}H$_1$]-2-hydroxyphenylethylamine (75) and to (2R)-[2-^{3}H$_1$]noradrenaline, respectively, with practically complete retention of deuterium or tritium. On the other hand, (2R)-[2-^{2}H$_1$]phenylethylamine (76) and (2R)-[2-^{3}H$_1$]dopamine were hydroxylated to the (2R)-enantiomers [e.g., (77)] with practically complete loss of label [114, 115].

The well known 3-hydroxylation of 1,4-benzodiazepine-2-ones also proceeds at a chiral center. The metabolism of (3R)-[3-^{14}C;3-^{3}H$_1$]demethyl-diazepam (78) and of (3R)-[3-^{14}C;3-^{3}H$_1$]diazepam (80) was studied with mouse hepatic microsomes. The 3-hydroxylated metabolites, oxazepam (79) and methyloxazepam (81), respectively, retained 94% and 80% of the tritium label (as determined by measurements of ^{3}H/^{14}C ratios). Strong evidence supports the absolute configurations shown for (79) and (81). When the (3S)-enantiomers of (78) and (80) were assayed, the retention of tritium was 30% [116]. Again, a mechanism of front side displacement was indicated for hydroxylation of a carbon atom adjacent to a carbonyl group. The product stereoselectivity of metabolic generation of oxazepam was previously unknown; this study indicated a strongly predominant (3S) product.

Stereochemical studies also have made use of stereospecifically labeled coenzymes. The best known examples are NADH and NADPH. The dihydro-nicotinamide moiety of these coenzymes has a prochiral center (C-4) carrying a pro-R- (H$_R$) and a pro-S-hydrogen (H$_S$) (82). NADH and NADPH with ^{2}H or ^{3}H either in the (4R) or in the (4S) position were prepared and used as hydride donors for many reductases. Two classes of reductases are

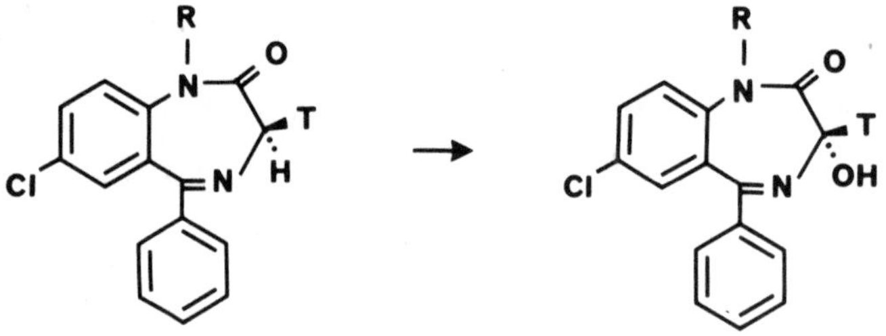

(78)   R = H   (79)

(80)   R = CH₃   (81)

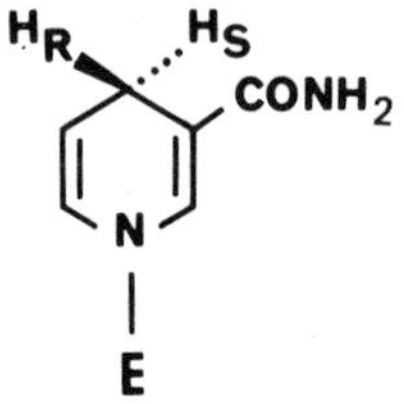

(82)

distinguished, the H_R- and the H_S-stereospecific enzymes [111]. Alcohol dehydrogenase is H_R-stereospecific, and aromatic aldehyde-ketone reductase and steroid alcohol dehydrogenase are H_S-stereospecific [117, 118]. Many drugs undergo stereoselective metabolic reduction (mainly exemplified by carbonyl reduction). The reduction of model compounds with labeled NADH and NADPH [117] could be applied to actual drugs to establish the governing rules of substrate and product stereoselectivity in metabolic reductions.

VII. RECENT DEVELOPMENTS

Since the completion of this manuscript, several relevant publications have appeared which describe new stereochemical techniques and reagents of proven or potential interest in drug metabolism studies.

A method of kinetic resolution allowing calculation of the maximum rotatory power of an enantiomer has been proposed [119] and may prove useful for the determination of optical purity in complementing classical procedures (Section IV. A).

A workable separation of the enantiomers of amphetamine [(1), R = R' = H" and methylamphetamine [(1), R = CH_3, R' = H] has been achieved using thin-layer chromatography [120] by derivatization with TPC (47) or N-benzyloxycarbonyl-L-prolyl chloride. Differences in R_f of up to 11% were obtained, but the method presumably lacks the sensitivity and accuracy of gas-chromatographic techniques (Section IV. B).

Gas-chromatographic discrimination of enantiomers has been actively investigated [121], and a few new optically active stationary phases of improved performance described. For example, good or very good resolution of enantiomeric amino acids (such as N-TFA methyl or isopropyl esters) has been achieved on packed columns (2-4 m) coated with N-docosanoyl-L-valine tert-butylamide or N-lauroyl-L-valine-2-methyl-2-heptadecylamide at temperatures up to 190 and 180°C, respectively [122].

In the field of optically active GC reagents a systematic investigation of structure-resolution relationships has been undertaken. By derivatizing various aralkylamines (e.g., amphetamine) with four different N-acyl amino acid chlorides, the separation was shown to be dependent on substitution at the chiral centers of both amino acid and amine [123]. Modification of the pyrrolidine ring of TPC (47) did not markedly alter the separation of aralkylamines [124]. Such systematic studies are of value in the rational design of better resolution reagents.

Terpinoid derivatives appear to be promising resolving agents. Besides drimanoyl chloride (50) and chrysanthemoyl chloride (51) mentioned in Section IV. B, the bicyclo and tricyclo terpinoid derivatives (+)-isoketopinyl chloride, (-)-dihydroteresantalinyl chloride, and (-)-teresantalinyl chloride led to the resolution of methyl esters of amino acid enantiomers [125]. The utility of such rigid reagents in separating drug and metabolite enantiomers can be predicted with reasonable confidence.

An elegant study has shown that metabolic conjugation of a racemic drug with β-D-glucuronic acid may correspond to derivatization with an optically active reagent. Indeed, the administration to man and dog of (±)-propranolol resulted in the urinary excretion of the diastereoisomeric propranolol-O-glucuronides. These conjugates were separated by GC as the methyl-TFA derivatives on a 1% OV-1 column at 200°C; the retention times were approximately 3.5 and 5 min for the derivatives of the (+)- and (-)-enantiomer, respectively [126].

A new stereochemical methodology involving metabolic studies of pseudo-racemates appears of exceptional interest and promise. Pseudo-racemates are racemic mixtures in which one enantiomer is labeled with deuterium (further suitable stable isotopes will certainly be used in the future). Consider for example a chiral drug D; the pseudo-racemates $[(+)-D/(-)-D-d_n]$ and $[(+)-D-d_n/(-)-D]$ are studied in turn for their in vivo fate or in vitro metabolism. Measurements of $(+)/(-)$ ratios are achieved by a mass-discriminating system (e.g., mass fragmentography). The position of labeling in the molecule is critical in designing this type of metabolic study. By labeling a position sufficiently removed from the center(s) of metabolic attack(s), stereoselectivity in distribution and excretion can be assessed, as well as the stereoselectivity of overall biotransformation and of the generation and transformation of individual metabolites. If on the other hand the label is close to the center of metabolic attack, factors such as the deuterium isotope effect of the metabolic reaction(s) can be investigated. Recent applications of this methodology include studies on the stereoselective disposition of propoxyphene in the dog [127], and on the in vitro metabolism of 1-2, 5-dimethoxy-4-methylphenyl)-2-aminopropane [128].

VIII. CONCLUSION

Drug metabolism utilizes medicinal chemistry and biochemistry where stereochemical factors have long been recognized to be of major importance. A major limitation in the consideration of these factors has been experimental difficulties.

The main purpose of this review was to demonstrate the existence of sensitive and specific stereochemical methods applicable to drug metabolism. The categorization and discussion of the major techniques should provide useful guidelines in the consideration of stereochemical factors in this field.

REFERENCES

1.   D. Ginsburg, Acc. Chem. Res., 7, 286 (1974).
2.   J. L. Abernethy, J. Chem. Educ., 49, 455 (1972).
3.   P. S. Portoghese, Ann. Rev. Pharmacol., 10, 51 (1970).
4.   P. Jenner and B. Testa, Drug Metab. Rev., 2, 117 (1973).
5.   V. Prelog, Ind. Chim. Belge, 11, 1309 (1962).
6.   H. Hirschmann and K. R. Hanson, J. Org. Chem., 36, 3293 (1971).
7.   K. Mislow and M. Raban, Stereoisomeric Relationships of Groups in Molecules, in Topics in Stereochemistry, Vol. 1 (N. L. Allinger and E. L. Eliel, eds.), Wiley, New York, 1967, pp. 1-38.
8.   K. Mislow, Introduction to Stereochemistry, Benjamin, New York, 1966, pp. 119.

9. R. B. Barlow, F. M. Franks, and J. D. M. Pearson, J. Pharm. Pharmacol., 24, 753 (1972).
10. R. A. Alvarez, Ph. D. Thesis, University of Nijmegen, 1971.
11. D. D. Breimer and J. M. van Rossum, Eur. J. Pharmacol., 26, 321 (1974).
12. C. F. George, T. Fenyvesi, M. E. Conolly, and C. T. Dollery, Eur. J. Clin. Pharmacol., 4, 74 (1972).
13. D. D. Breimer and J. M. van Rossum, J. Pharm. Pharmacol., 25, 762 (1973).
14. D. S. Hewick and J. McEwen, J. Pharm. Pharmacol., 25, 458 (1973).
15. A. H. Beckett and L. G. Brookes, in International Symposium on Amphetamines and Related Compounds (E. Costa and S. Garattini, eds.), Raven Press, New York, 1970, pp. 109-120.
16. A. H. Beckett and E. V. B. Shenoy, J. Pharm. Pharmacol., 25, 793 (1973).
17. P. T. Henderson, T. B. Vree, C. A. M. van Ginneken, and J. M. van Rossum, Xenobiotica, 4, 121 (1974).
18. A. G. Bolt, G. Graham, and P. Wilson, Xenobiotica, 4, 355 (1974).
19. M. J. Cooper and M. W. Anders, Life Sci., 15, 1665 (1974).
20. R. E. Dann, D. R. Feller, and J. F. Snell, Eur. J. Pharmacol., 16, 233 (1971).
21. D. R. Feller, P. Basu, W. Mellon, J. Curott, and L. Malspeis, Arch. Int. Pharmacodyn. Ther., 203, 187 (1973).
22. A. H. Beckett and M. Rowland, J. Pharm. Pharmacol., 17, 628 (1965).
23. L. M. Gunne, Biochem. Pharmacol., 16, 863 (1967).
24. J. F. Taylor, Ph. D. Thesis, University of London, 1968.
25. A. H. Beckett, M. Mitchard, and A. A. Shihab, J. Pharm. Pharmacol., 23, 941 (1971).
26. A. A. Shihab, Ph. D. Thesis, University of London, 1971.
27. E. Mussini, F. Marcucci, R. Fanelli, A. Guaitani, and S. Garattini, Biochem. Pharmacol., 21, 127 (1972).
28. H. Shindo, E. Nakajima, K. Kawai, N. Miyakoshi, and K. Tanaka, Chem. Pharm. Bull. (Tokyo), 21, 817 (1973).
29. W. V. U. Au, L. G. Dring, D. G. Grahame-Smith, P. Isaac, and R. T. Williams, Biochem. J., 129, 1 (1972).
30. C. T. Dollery and M. Harington, Lancet, 759 (1962).
31. B. Duhm, W. Maul, H. Medenwald, K. Patzschke, and L. A. Wegner, Z. Naturforsch. B, 20b, 434 (1965).
32. W. Rummel, U. Brandenberger, and H. Buch, Med. Pharmacol. Exp., 16, 496 (1967).
33. C. D. Morgan, F. Cattabeni, and E. Costa, J. Pharmacol. Exp. Ther., 180, 127 (1972).
34. M. W. Anders, M. J. Cooper, and A. E. Takemori, Drug Metab. Disp., 1, 642 (1973).

35. I. Hoffström and S. Orrenius, FEBS Lett., 31, 205 (1973).
36. L. R. Snyder, Principles of Adsorption Chromatography, Marcel Dekker, New York, 1968, pp. 295-334.
37. A. H. Beckett, P. Jenner, and J. W. Gorrod, Xenobiotica, 3, 557 (1973).
38. P. Jenner, J. W. Gorrod, and A. H. Beckett, Xenobiotica, 3, 573 (1973).
39. A. G. Renwick and R. T. Williams, Biochem. J., 129, 857 (1972).
40. H. Breuer, R. Knuppen, and G. Pangels, Biochim. Biophys. Acta, 65, 1 (1962).
41. E. Schraven, F. W. Koss, J. Keck, and G. Beisenherz, Eur. J. Pharmacol., 1, 445 (1967).
42. H. B. Hucker, A. J. Balletto, S. C. Stauffer, A. G. Zacchei, and B. H. Arison, Drug Metab. Disp., 2, 406 (1974).
43. K. K. Chan, R. J. Lewis, and W. F. Trager, J. Med. Chem., 15, 1265 (1972).
44. K. C. Leibman and E. Ortiz, Drug Metab. Disp., 1, 543 (1973).
45. K. K. Midha, A. H. Beckett, and A. Saunders, Xenobiotica, 4, 627 (1974).
46. A. H. Beckett, G. R. Jones, and S. Al-Sarraj, J. Pharm. Pharmacol. 26, 945 (1974).
47. A. F. Casy, PMR Spectroscopy in Medicinal and Biological Chemistry, Academic Press, New York, 1971, pp. 86-134.
48. N. Chatterjie, J. M. Fujimoto, C. E. Inturrisi, S. Roerig, R. I. H. Wang, D. V. Bowen, F. H. Field, and D. D. Clarke, Drug Metab. Disp., 2, 401 (1974).
49. M. Raban and K. Mislow, Modern Methods for the Determination of Optical Purity, in Topics in Stereochemistry, Vol. 2 (N. L. Allinger and E. L. Eliel, eds.), Wiley, New York, 1967, pp. 199-230.
50. R. E. McMahon and H. R. Sullivan, Life Sci., 5, 921 (1966).
51. R. E. McMahon and H. R. Sullivan, in Microsomes and Drug Oxidations (J. R. Gillette, A. H. Conney, G. J. Cosmides, R. W. Estabrook, J. R. Fouts, and G. J. Mannering, eds.), Academic Press, New York, 1969, pp. 239-247.
52. R. E. Billings, H. R. Sullivan, and R. E. McMahon, Biochem., 9, 1256 (1970).
53. G. A. Maylin, M. J. Cooper, and M. W. Anders, J. Med. Chem., 16, 606 (1973).
54. J. Hes and L. A. Sternson, Drug Metab. Disp., 2, 345 (1974).
55. A. Horeau, Tetrahedron Lett., 3121 (1969).
56. A. Horeau and J. P. Guetté, Tetrahedron, 30, 1923 (1974).
57. P. Crabbé, Recent Applications of ORD and OCD in Organic Chemistry, in Topics in Stereochemistry, Vol. 1 (N. L. Allinger and E. L. Eliel, eds.), Wiley, New York, 1967, pp. 94-198.

58. G. Snatzke, Angew. Chem. Int. Ed., 7, 14 (1968).
59. H. Eyring, H.-C. Liu, and D. Caldwell, Chem. Rev., 68, 525 (1968).
60. L. Velluz and M. Legrand, Bull. Soc. Chim. Fr., 1785 (1970).
61. P. Crabbé, ORD and CD in Organic Chemistry, Holden Day, San Francisco, 1965.
62. L. Velluz, M. Legrand, and M. Grosjean, Optical Circular Dichroism, Academic Press, New York, 1965.
63. G. Snatzke, ed., ORD and CD in Organic Chemistry, Heyden, London, 1967.
64. W. Klyne and P. M. Scopes, Farmaco Ed. Sci., 24, 760, 847 (1969).
65. L. A. Mitscher and G. W. Clark, Lloydia, 35, 311 (1972).
66. F. Ciardelli and P. Salvadori, eds., Fundamental Aspects and Recent Developments in ORD and CD, Heyden, London, 1973.
67. K. H. Palmer, M. S. Fowler, M. E. Wall, L. S. Rhodes, W. J. Waddell, and B. Baggett, J. Pharmacol. Exp. Ther., 170, 355 (1969).
68. K. H. Palmer, M. S. Fowler, and M. E. Wall, J. Pharmacol. Exp. Ther., 175, 38 (1970).
69. J. E. Coleman and R. E. Handschumacher, J. Biol. Chem., 248, 1741 (1973).
70. P. M. Dolinger, M. Kielczewski, J. R. Trudell, G. Barth, R. E. Linder, E. Bunnenberg, and C. Djerassi, Proc. Nat. Acad. Sci. U.S., 71, 399 (1974).
71. S. Wilen, Resolving Agents and Resolutions in Organic Chemistry, in Topics in Stereochemistry, Vol. 6 (N. L. Allinger and E. L. Eliel, eds.), Wiley, New York, 1971, pp. 107-176.
72. J. B. Pattison, A Programmed Introduction to Gas-liquid Chromatography, Heyden, London, 1969, p. 55.
73. Y. Mori, J. Chromatogr., 66, 9 (1972).
74. J. A. Corbin and L. B. Rogers, Anal. Chem., 42, 974 (1970).
75. W. A. Koenig, W. Parr, H. A. Lichtenstein, E. Bayer, and J. Oró, J. Chromatogr. Sci., 8, 183 (1970).
76. W. Parr, J. Pleterski, C. Yang, and E. Bayer, J. Chromatogr. Sci., 9, 141 (1971).
77. J. W. Westley and B. Halpern, in Gas Chromatography 1968 (C. L. A. Harbourn, ed.), The Institute of Petroleum, London, 1969, pp. 119-128.
78. H. Iwase, Chem. Pharm. Bull. (Tokyo), 22, 2075 (1974).
79. A. Murano, Agr. Biol. Chem. (Tokyo), 37, 981 (1973).
80. C. E. Wells, J. Ass. Offic. Anal. Chem., 53, 113 (1970).
81. A. H. Beckett and B. Testa, J. Chromatogr., 69, 285 (1972).
82. A. H. Beckett and B. Testa, J. Pharm. Pharmacol., 25, 382 (1973).

83.   S. B. Matin, M. Rowland, and N. Castagnoli, Jr., J. Pharm. Sci.,
      62, 821 (1973).
84.   K. S. Marshall and N. Castagnoli, Jr., J. Med. Chem., 16, 266
      (1973).
85.   L. R. Pohl and W. F. Trager, J. Med. Chem., 16, 475 (1973).
86.   C. J. W. Brooks, M. T. Gilbert, and J. D. Gilbert, Anal. Chem.,
      45, 896 (1973).
87.   S. B. Matin, P. S. Callery, J. S. Zweig, A. O'Brien, R. Rapoport,
      and N. Castagnoli, Jr., J. Med. Chem., 17, 877 (1974).
88.   G. P. Tosolini, E. Moro, A. Forgione, M. Ranghieri, and V.
      Mandelli, J. Pharm. Sci., 63, 1072 (1974).
89.   Perkin-Elmer NMR Quarterly, No. 7, 2 (1973).
90.   A. F. Casy, PMR Spectroscopy in Medicinal and Biological Chem-
      istry, Academic Press, New York, 1971, pp. 170-187.
91.   J. A. Dale, D. L. Dull, and H. S. Mosher, J. Org. Chem., 34,
      2543 (1969).
92.   G. A. Hoyer, D. Rosenberg, C. Rufer, and A. Seeger, Tetrahedron
      Lett., 985 (1972).
93.   W. H. Pirkle and S. D. Beare, J. Amer. Chem. Soc., 91, 5150
      (1969).
94.   B. C. Mayo, Chem. Soc. Rev., 2, 49 (1973).
95.   A. F. Cockerill, G. L. O. Davies, R. C. Harden, and D. M.
      Rackham, Chem. Rev., 73, 553 (1973).
96.   R. E. Sievers, ed., Nuclear Magnetic Resonance Shift Reagents,
      Academic Press, New York, 1973.
97.   H. L. Goering, J. N. Eikenberry, G. S. Koermer, and C. J.
      Lattimer, J. Amer. Chem. Soc., 96, 1493 (1974).
98.   C. Kutal, cited in [96], pp. 87-98.
99.   M. D. McCreary, D. W. Lewis, D. L. Wernick, and G. M.
      Whitesides, J. Amer. Chem. Soc., 96, 1038 (1974).
100. L. Bertilsson and B. Alexanderson, Eur. J. Clin. Pharmacol.,
      4, 201 (1972).
101. D. C. Remy, W. A. Van Saun, Jr., E. L. Engelhardt, and B. H.
      Arison, J. Org. Chem., 38, 700 (1973).
102. H. B. Matthews and J. D. McKinney, Drug Metab. Disp., 2, 333
      (1974).
103. J. D. McKinney, H. B. Matthews, and N. K. Wilson, Tetrahedron
      Lett., 1895 (1973).
104. B. Testa and A. H. Beckett, J. Pharm. Pharmacol., 25, 119
      (1973).
105. B. Testa and A. H. Beckett, J. Chromatogr., 71, 39 (1972).
106. B. Testa, Acta Pharm. Suec., 10, 441 (1973).
107. A. H. Beckett and D. Mihailova, Biochem. Pharmacol., 23, 3347
      (1974).
108. H. R. Levy, P. Taladay, and B. Vennesland, The Steric Course

of Enzymatic Reactions at meso Carbon Atoms: Application of Hydrogen Isotopes, in Progress in Stereochemistry, Vol. 3 (P. B. D. de la Mare and W. Klyne, eds.), Butterworths, London, 1962, pp. 299-349.

109. D. Arigoni and E. L. Elial, Chirality due to the Presence of Hydrogen Isotopes at Non-cyclic Positions, in Topics in Stereochemistry, Vol. 4 (E. L. Eliel and N. L. Allinger, eds.), Wiley, New York, 1969, pp. 127-243.

110. J. W. Cornforth, Tetrahedron, 30, 1515 (1974).

111. W. L. Alworth, Stereochemistry and its Application in Biochemistry, Wiley, New York, 1972.

112. R. E. McMahon, H. R. Sullivan, J. C. Craig, and W. E. Pereira, Jr., Arch. Biochem. Biophys., 132, 575 (1969).

113. K. B. Taylor, J. Biol. Chem., 249, 454 (1974).

114. L. Bachan, C. B. Storm, J. W. Wheeler, and S. Kaufman, J. Amer. Chem. Soc., 96, 6799 (1974).

115. A. R. Battersby, P. W. Sheldrake, J. Staunton, and D. C. Williams, J. Chem. Soc. Chem. Commun., 566 (1974).

116. A. Corbella, P. Gariboldi, G. Jommi, A. Forgione, F. Marcucci, P. Martelli, E. Mussini, and F. Mauri, J. Chem. Soc. Chem. Commun., 721 (1973).

117. H. W. Culp and R. E. McMahon, J. Biol. Chem., 243, 848 (1968).

118. J. M. George, J. C. Orr, A. G. C. Renwick, P. Carter, and L. L. Engel, Bioorganic Chem., 2, 140 (1973).

119. A. Horeau, Tetrahedron, 31, 1307 (1975).

120. D. Eskes, J. Chromatogr., 117, 442 (1976).

121. E. Gil-Av and D. Nurok, in Advances in Chromatography, Vol. 10 (J. C. Giddings and R. A. Keller, eds.), Dekker, New York, 1974, pp. 99-172.

122. R. Charles, U. Beitler, B. Feibush, and E. Gil-Av, J. Chromatogr., 112, 121 (1975).

123. R. W. Souter, J. Chromatogr., 108, 265 (1975).

124. R. W. Souter, J. Chromatogr., 114, 307 (1975).

125. T. Nambara, J. Goto, K. Taguchi, and T. Iwata, J. Chromatogr., 100, 180 (1974).

126. H. Ehrsson, J. Pharm. Pharmacol., 27, 971 (1975).

127. R. E. McMahon and H. R. Sullivan, Res. Comm. Chem. Pathol. Pharmacol., 14, 631 (1976).

128. R. J. Weinkam, J. Gal, P. Callery, and N. Castagnoli, Jr., Anal. Chem., 48, 203 (1976).

Chapter 4

FLUORESCENCE SPECTROSCOPY

Stephen G. Schulman

Department of Pharmaceutical Chemistry
College of Pharmacy
University of Florida
Gainesville, Florida

and

Datta V. Naik

Department of Chemistry
Manhattanville College
Purchase, New York

I. INTRODUCTION

The emission of light by molecules which are electronically excited as a result of the absorption of visible or UV radiation forms the basis of fluorescence spectroscopy. Due to its relatively low cost and high analytical sensitivity (concentrations of fluorescing analytes $\leq 1 \times 10^{-9}$ mol liter^{-1} are routinely determined), this technique is widely employed in the quantitative analysis of drugs and metabolites and, to a lesser extent, in the evaluation of the interactions of these substances with biological macromolecules. These applications are derived from the relationship between analyte concentrations and fluorescence intensity and are therefore similar in concept to most other physicochemical methods of analysis. However, other features of fluorescence spectral bands, such as position in the electromagnetic spectrum (wavelength or frequency), bandform, emission lifetime, and excitation spectrum, as well as fluorescence intensity, are related to molecular structure and environment and therefore have broad analytical value. Moreover, because fluorescence originates from the lowest excited singlet state, certain aspects of the chemistry of that excited electronic state occasionally cause interferences in fluorometric analysis. In some cases they even form the basis for optimization of analysis.

The great sensitivity and selectivity of fluorescence spectroscopy and the strong dependence of the fluorescence spectrum upon molecular structure, molecular environment, and singlet state photochemistry are well known. These features permit the analyst to carry out qualitative identification of metabolites at concentrations far lower than possible with other techniques for organic structure determination (e.g., NMR and IR spectroscopy). Moreover, although the fluorescence methods lack the generality of NMR and IR spectroscopy, they compensate by allowing studies of interactions of fluorescing metabolites with biological or model biological systems in aqueous media where the other spectroscopic methods are drastically reduced in applicability. This chapter will consider the origin, nature and measurement of molecular fluorescence and the dependence of fluorescence upon molecular structure, reactivity, and interactions with the environment. Rather than being an exhaustive reference work, it is intended to provide the investigator with sufficient appreciation of the physical and instrumental principles to be able to intelligently devise fluorometric analyses and to understand the interferences that frequently limit and occasionally obviate fluorescence spectroscopy as a practical method of analysis. In addition, the related field of phosphorescence spectroscopy will also be considered here. However, because the practice of phosphorimetry usually requires low temperatures and some cumbersome equipment it is not, at present, as widely employed for analytical purposes as fluorometry. Accordingly, the treatment of phosphorimetry here will be brief. For a deeper view into phosphorescence and its analytical applications, the reader is referred to the excellent references by Winefordner and coworkers [1-3].

II. THE PHYSICOCHEMICAL BASIS OF FLUORESCENCE SPECTROSCOPY

A. The Origin and Nature of Molecular Fluorescence [3-7]

Fluorescence consists of the emission of light accompanying the transition of an electronically excited molecule to its ground electronic state. In order to best appreciate the nature of fluorescence and its dependence upon chemical and physical factors it is appropriate to begin by considering how the fluorescing molecule came to be electronically excited and what events transpire between excitation and emission.

The electronic excitation of molecules occurs as the result of the absorption of near UV or visible light. The absorption or excitation process consists of the interaction of the electric field vector, associated with the exciting light, with the π or nonbonded electrons of the absorbing molecule. This interaction causes the electronic distribution of the absorbing molecule to be distorted and energy to be absorbed from the light-wave, a process that occurs in $\sim 10^{-15}$ sec. The intensity of light absorbed (I_a) is expressed macroscopically by the Lambert-Beer law:

$$I_a = I_0 - I_t = I_0 (1 - 10^{-\epsilon c \ell}) \tag{1}$$

where I_0 and I_t are, respectively, the incident and transmitted light intensities, ϵ is the molar absorptivity, c is the concentration of absorber
species and ℓ is the path-length of light through the sample. The energy
of the light absorbed is equal to the difference in energy between the ground
and excited state of the absorbing molecule and given by the Planck frequency relation

$$E = Nh\nu = Nhc/\lambda \tag{2}$$

where E is the energy associated with light of frequency ν or wavelength λ,
c is the velocity of light, and N is Avogadro's number. The absorption
spectrum of a molecular species consists of a graphic representation of
the intensity of absorption as a function of the wavelength of the exciting
light.

It should be noted that most molecules of interest to the pharmaceutical
scientist, which will absorb near UV or visible light, are derived from
benzene or naphthalene and exhibit two or three absorption bands corresponding to excitation from the ground electronic state to two or three
excited states.

Subsequent to excitation to an electronically excited singlet state, in
which the molecule of interest may be vibrationally excited as well, the
process of return to the ground electronic state begins. The loss of excess
vibrational energy, known as vibrational or thermal relaxation, takes place
in a stepwise fashion, each step taking about 10^{-14} sec, and proceeds, in
solution, by inelastic collisions with solvent molecules. Because of the
overlap between higher and lower electronically excited states, there is
also an efficient vibrational pathway for the demotion of the excited molecule from higher to lower electronically excited singlet states. The latter
process is called internal conversion and is not directly observable spectroscopically. In aliphatic molecules with a high degree of vibrational
freedom, vibrational relaxation and internal conversion may return the
excited molecule to the ground electronic state. Under this circumstance
fluorescence does not occur. However, in aromatic and a few other highly
conjugated molecules, the degree of vibrational freedom is restricted,
resulting in a very inefficient thermal mechanism of return to the ground
state. In this case, the molecule of interest may, as the result of direct
excitation or internal conversion and vibrational relaxation, rapidly arrive
in the lowest vibrational level of the lowest electronically excited singlet
state. After the relatively long period of 10^{-11} to 10^{-7} sec, it may then
return to the ground electronic state, radiating away the difference in
energy between the ground and lowest excited singlet states in the form of
near UV or visible fluorescence. The frequency or wavelength of the

fluorescent light is related to its energy by Equation (2). However, because of vibrational relaxation in the excited state (Fig. 1) subsequent to absorption and, in the ground state, subsequent to emission, the energy of fluorescence is generally lower (and the wavelength of fluorescence therefore longer) than that of absorption to the lowest excited singlet state, even though the same electronic states are involved in both transitions. Moreover, if the spacing between vibrational sublevels in ground and lowest excited singlet states is equal in a given molecular species, the longest wavelength absorption band and the fluorescence band will appear as mirror images of one another when plotted on an abcissa linear in frequency or energy (Fig. 2).

It is important from the analytical point of view to keep in mind that fluorescence almost invariably occurs from the lowest excited singlet state. This means that only one fluorescence band may be observed from any given molecular species, even though it will generally have several absorption bands. Therefore, the observation of several fluorescence bands in a solution of a supposedly pure sample suggests either the occurrence of a chemical reaction or the presence of impurities.

If all molecules arriving in the lowest excited singlet state emitted fluorescence, the observed intensity of fluorescence would be given by I_a in Equation (1). However, because of the relatively long lifetime of the potentially fluorescent excited state, several processes may compete with fluorescence for deactivation of the lowest excited singlet state. Consequently, the intensity of fluorescence I_f is obtained by multiplying I_a by the fraction of molecules ϕ_f, which are deactivated by fluorescence. Hence,

$$I_f = \phi_f I_a \tag{3}$$

ϕ_f is called the quantum yield of fluorescence or the fluorescence efficiency, is always one or a fraction, and is related to the rates of fluorescence (k_f) and competitive deactivating processes (k_d) by

$$\phi_f = \frac{k_f}{k_f + \Sigma k_d} \tag{4}$$

Thus, the greater the numbers or rates of processes competing with fluorescence for deactivation of the lowest excited singlet state, the lower the value of ϕ_f and, hence, the intensity of fluorescence. On most commercial instrumentation ϕ_f must be greater than 1×10^{-4}, for fluorescence to be observable. From Equations (1) and (3) it follows that

$$I_f = \phi_f I_0 (1 - 10^{-\epsilon c \ell}) \tag{5}$$

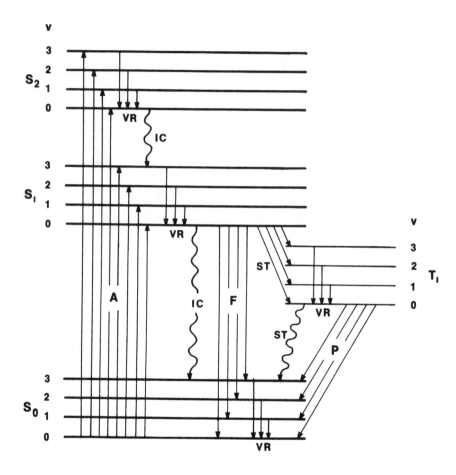

FIG. 1. Photophysical processes of conjugated molecules. Electronic
absorption (A) from the lowest vibrational level (v = 0) of the ground state
(S$_0$) to the various vibrational levels (v = 0, 1, 2, 3) of the excited singlet
states (S$_1$ and S$_2$) is followed by rapid, radiationless internal conversion
(IC) and vibrational relaxation (VR) to the lowest vibrational level (v = 0)
of S$_1$. Competing for deactivation of the lowest excited singlet state S$_1$
are the radiationless internal conversion and singlet-triplet intersystem
crossing (ST) as well as fluorescence (F). Fluorescence is followed by
vibrational relaxation (VR) in the ground state. Intersystem crossing (ST)
is followed by vibrational relaxation (VR) in the triplet state (T$_1$). Phosphorescence (P) and nonradiative triplet-singlet intersystem crossing (ST)
return the molecule from the triplet state (T$_1$) to the ground state (S$_0$).
Vibrational relaxation in S$_0$ then thermalizes the "hot" ground state molecule.

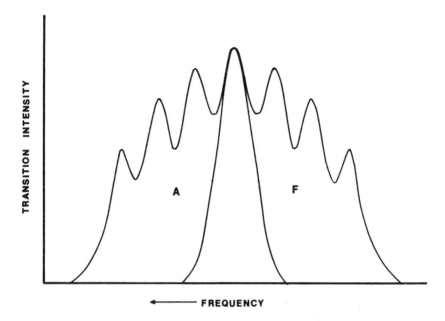

FIG. 2. The mirror-image relationship between absorption (A) and fluorescence (F), extant when the vibrational spacings are identical in ground and electronically excited states.

indicating that fluorescence intensity is not linear but rather exponential in its variation with absorber concentration. However, Equation (5) may be expanded, in series, to

$$\phi_f I_0 (I - 10^{-\epsilon c \ell}) = (2.3\epsilon c \ell - \frac{(2.3\epsilon c \ell)^2}{2!} + \frac{(2.3\epsilon c \ell)^3}{3!} - \cdots) \phi_f I_0 \qquad (6)$$

For values of $\epsilon c \ell < 0.02$, the higher terms in Equation (7) may be neglected (to within 2.3% error) by comparison with the first, so that

$$I_f = 2.3 \phi_f I_0 \epsilon c \ell \qquad (7)$$

Thus, at very low absorbance I_f is linear with analyte concentration, and under constant experimental conditions Equation (8) may be employed analytically in the relative form

$$\frac{I_{f_u}}{I_{f_s}} = \frac{C_u}{C_s} \qquad (8)$$

where the subscripts u and s refer to unknown and standard solutions, respectively. However, it must be borne in mind that at higher absorbances Equation (7) breaks down and correction for higher terms in Equation (6) or the preparation of a calibration curve must be employed for analytical purposes.

Another important property of fluorescing molecules is the lifetime of the lowest excited singlet state (τ). If the mean rate of fluorescence is the number of fluorescence events per unit time, the mean lifetime of the excited state is the reciprocal rate, or the mean time per deactivation event. The greater the number and the faster the processes that compete with fluorescence for deactivation of the lowest excited singlet state, the shorter will be τ. It will later be shown that fluorescence lifetime measurement is a valuable technique in the measurement of macromolecules and micelles and in the analysis of multicomponent samples containing analytes with overlapping fluorescence bands.

Among the processes which compete with fluorescence for deactivation of the lowest excited singlet state is intersystem crossing from the lowest excited singlet state to the lowest excited triplet state. Intersystem crossing is a radiationless process which results in a change in the spin angular momentum of the excited molecule. Although it diminishes the quantum yield of fluorescence, it results in population of the lowest triplet state. The return of molecules from the lowest triplet state to the ground state may be accompanied by a long-duration light emission known as phosphorescence.

Phosphorescence, as fluorescence, is most often observed in molecules having rigid molecular skeletons and large energy separations between the lowest excited triplet state and the ground singlet state (i.e., aromatic molecules). Because triplet states are so long-lived, chemical and physical processes in solution compete effectively with phosphorescence for deactivation of the lowest excited triplet state. This is the primary reason for the importance of the triplet state in photochemistry. Except for the shortest-lived phosphorescences, collisional deactivation by solvent molecules, quenching by paramagnetic species (e.g., oxygen), photochemical reactions, and certain other processes preclude the observation of phosphorescence in fluid media. Rather, phosphorescence is normally studied in glasses, at liquid nitrogen temperature, or in solution in very viscous liquids where collisional processes cannot completely deactivate the triplet state.

Because fluorescence normally originates only from the lowest excited singlet state and phosphorescence only from the lowest triplet state, only one fluorescence band and one phosphorescence band may be observed from any given molecular species. Since phosphorescence is precluded in fluid solutions, only a single emission band, that due to fluorescence, may be observed from a single molecular species. However, at low temperatures, in rigid matrices both fluorescence and phosphorescence may appear in the emission spectrum if both types of emission are comparable in intensity, so that one does not completely mask the other. In this case the band occurring at longer wavelength will be the phosphorescence band because the lowest triplet state always lies lower in energy than the lowest excited singlet state. In low temperature luminescence spectroscopic measurements, phosphorescence is usually distinguished from fluorescence by taking advantage of the differences in the mean lifetimes of the two processes. For very long-lived phosphorescences (> 0.1 sec) mechanical chopping of the exciting light eliminates the fluorescence signal while the long-lived phosphorescence persists as an afterglow. For short lived phosphorescences (< 0.1 sec), electronic chopping devices are employed to distinguish between fluorescence and phosphorescence.

Phosphorescence is analytically useful in much the same way as fluorescence. This is especially so in the study of metabolites that phosphoresce but do not fluoresce. For example, p-nitrophenol, one of the metabolites of parathion, does not fluoresce. Yet it can be detected and determined by its intense phosphorescence at concentrations down to about 10^{-10} M [8]. However, where both luminescences can be employed analytically, fluorescence would generally be the method of choice, because it is not restricted to rigid media.

B. Chemical Structural Effects upon Fluorescence
    Spectra [9-13]

Most fluorescence spectra of analytical interest arise from electronic transitions in functionally substituted aromatic molecules. Consequently, the metabolites of interest in this chapter are those derived from drugs possessing aromatic rings such as benzene, naphthalene or anthracene, or their heteromatic analogs pyridine, quinoline, acridine, etc. The fluorescence spectra of these substances may often be understood in terms of the electronic interactions between the simple aromatic structures and their substituents. The understanding of the spectra-structure relationships can be extremely valuable in assessing the feasibility of a fluorometric method for a given compound, in qualitative analysis, and in the evaluation of interactions of drugs and metabolites with biological structures and with their environment in general. The influence of exocyclic and heterocyclic substituents, in aromatic rings, upon the intensities and positions of the fluorescence spectra of aromatic molecules will be considered in this section.

1. Chemical Structure and Fluorescence Intensity

The intensity of fluorescence observable from a given molecular species depends upon the molar absorptivity of the transition excited and the quantum yield of fluorescence. The molar absorptivity determines the number of molecules ultimately arriving in the lowest excited singlet state. For most aromatic molecules, the π, π^* absorption bands lying in the near UV and visible regions of the spectrum have molar absorptivities of $1,000$ to $10,000$, so that the proper choice of the transition to excite can affect the intensity of fluorescence by about one order of magnitude.

Far more important is the quantum yield of fluorescence, which may affect the intensity of fluorescence over about four orders of magnitude and may, in fact, determine whether or not fluorescence is observable at all. The quantum yield of fluorescence is dependent upon the rates of processes competing with fluorescence for the deactivation of the lowest excited singlet state.

The current state of spectroscopic theory does not permit the quantitative prediction of how efficiently nonradiative deactivation processes compete with fluorescence from molecule to molecule. However, some qualitative generalizations are possible.

Aromatic molecules, containing lengthy aliphatic side chains, generally tend to fluoresce less intensely than those without the side chains. This is brought about by the introduction of a large number of vibrational degrees of freedom by the aliphatic moieties. The greater vibrational freedom introduces vibrational coupling between the ground and lowest excited singlet states and thus reduces the quantum yield of fluorescence by providing an efficient pathway for internal conversion. In the unsubstituted aromatic molecules, the rigidity of the aromatic ring results in wide separation of the ground and lowest excited singlet states. In general, molecular rigidity and high quantum yield of fluorescence are closely related to one another.

The fluorescence of aromatic molecules is quenched (diminished in intensity) partially or completely by heavy atom substitutents such as $-As(OH)_2$, Br, and I and by certain other groups such as $-NO_2$, $-CHO$, $-COR$, and nitrogen in six-membered heterocyclic rings (e. g., quinoline). Each of these substituents has the ability to cause mixing of the spin and orbital electronic motions of the aromatic system (spin-orbital coupling). Spin-orbital coupling destroys the concept of molecular spin as a well-defined property of the molecule and thereby enhances the probability or rate of singlet $\rightarrow$ triplet intersystem crossing. This process favors population of the lowest triplet state at the expense of the lowest excited singlet state and thus decreases the fluorescence quantum yield. However, the efficient population of the lowest triplet state favors a high yield of phosphorescence. Consequently, aromatic arsenates, nitro compounds, bromo and iodo derivatives, aldehydes, ketones and N-heterocyclics tend to fluo-

resce very weakly or not at all. However, most of them phosphoresce
quite intensely. In the heavy atom substituted aromatics, spin-orbital
coupling results from the high nuclear charge of the heavy atom substituent
which causes the π-electrons of the aromatic system to spend more time,
on the average, near the heavy nuclei. This situation causes juxtaposition
of the spin and orbital angular momentum vectors at the heavy nucleus and
thereby favors their coupling. In the aldehyde, ketone, and N-heterocyclic
molecules, however, the phenomenon which causes high electron density
at an atomic nucleus and therefore spin-orbital coupling, is somewhat different. In these molecules, the oxygen atoms of the carbonyl groups and
the heterocyclic nitrogen atoms have nonbonded electron pairs in orbitals
which are sp^2 hybridized. The promotion of a nonbonded electron to a
vacant π^* orbital (n $\rightarrow$ π^* transition) usually occurs at lower energy and
with lower molar absorptivity than the lowest energy $\pi \rightarrow \pi^*$ transition.
Hence, in molecules having nonbonded electrons the n, π^* state is the lowest excited singlet state. The low molar absorptivity of the n, π^* state
means that the natural lifetime of the latter is longer than that of the former. Moreover, the greater degree of s character in the sp^2 hybridized
nonbonding orbital than in the pπ orbitals of the aromatic system results
in a higher degree of spin-orbital coupling in molecules having nonbonded
electrons than in those that do not. These factors combine to result in a
high degree of intersystem crossing in molecules having functional groups
with nonbonded electrons. Hence, these molecules tend to fluoresce weakly
and phosphoresce strongly. A rather interesting distinction between the
molecules having heavy atom substituents and those having nonbonded electrons is that, upon going to a highly polar or hydrogen-bonding solvent
from a weakly interacting solvent, the quantum yield of fluorescence of
the latter group of compounds increases and the quantum yield of phosphorescence decreases. This is due to the binding of the nonbonded electrons,
which stabilizes them and causes the lowest π, π^* state to drop below the
n, π^* state, thereby diminishing the role of the n, π^* state in populating the
triplet. Strongly interacting solvents do not have a dramatic effect upon
the fluorescence yields of heavy atom substituted aromatic molecules. The
role of solvents in the fluorescent properties of molecules will be discussed
at length in Section II. C. 1.

2. Chemical Structure and Position of the
    Fluorescence Maximum

The energies of the ground and lowest excited singlet states of fluorescing
molecules are affected by such features of molecular structure as the
presence of substituents and the molecular geometry. This is reflected
in the position (energy) of the fluorescence band maximum. While the
wavelength corresponding to the band maximum is perfectly suitable for
purposes of identification, it is inadequate as a parameter by which structural effects can be compared in a series of molecules. For example, a

100 nm shift from 200 to 300 nm is equivalent to five times the energy difference represented by a 100 nm shift from 500 to 600 nm. It is necessary, therefore, to convert spectral maxima measured in wavelength units to frequency units which are proportional to energy, in order to intelligently consider the effects of substituents on fluorescence spectra. All future references to spectral maxima in this section will present the maxima in μm^{-1} ($cm^{-1} \times 10^{-4}$) and will refer to the maxima in terms of frequency (denoted by $\bar{\nu}_f$).

According to Equation (1), the greater the separation between the ground and lowest excited singlet states, the greater the frequency and the shorter the wavelength of fluorescence. This separation depends upon the energy difference between the highest occupied and lowest unoccupied molecular orbitals and the repulsion energy between the electronic configurations corresponding to the ground and lowest excited singlet states. It can be shown by molecular orbital theory that for aromatic molecules, the greater the extension of the conjugated system, the smaller is the energy separation between the highest occupied (π) and lowest unoccupied (π^*) orbitals. Thus, the frequencies of fluorescence decrease with increasing extension of conjugation in the direction of linear annulation, in the linearly annullated series benzene ($\bar{\nu}_f = 3.82\ \mu m^{-1}$), naphthalene ($\bar{\nu}_f = 3.18\ \mu m^{-1}$), and anthracene ($\bar{\nu}_f = 2.64\ \mu m^{-1}$).

The frequencies of the fluorescence maxima of aromatic compounds with exocyclic substitutents vary from those of the parent hydrocarbons in ways which depend upon the differences between the electronic interactions of the substituents and the aromatic rings in the ground and excited states. Groups such as $-NH_2$, $-OH$, and $-SH$ have unshared electron pairs which can be transferred into vacant π orbitals belonging to the aromatic ring. Such groups are best treated by considering the lone pair, in the ground state of the molecule, as residing in a molecular orbital which is largely localized on the exocyclic group. The energy of this molecular orbital is slightly lower than that of a pure 2p orbital and is considerably greater than that of the highest occupied π orbital of the aromatic ring (Fig. 3). Thus, the energy gap between the highest occupied and lowest unoccupied orbitals of the substituted molecule is considerably less than that between the highest occupied and lowest unoccupied orbitals of the unsubstituted (parent) molecule. For example, 1-naphthylamine fluoresces at $2.69\ \mu m^{-1}$ in hexane while naphthalene fluoresces at $3.18\ \mu m^{-1}$ in the same solvent.

Groups such as $-COOH$, $-CHO$ (in polar solvents), and $-C \equiv N$ have localized, vacant, low energy π orbitals in the ground state of the substituted molecule. This type of substituent introduces a vacant orbital between the highest occupied and lowest unoccupied π orbitals of the unsubstituted molecule (Fig. 3). The energy gap between the highest occupied and lowest unoccupied orbitals of the substituted molecule is therefore smaller than the gap between the highest occupied and lowest unoccupied orbitals

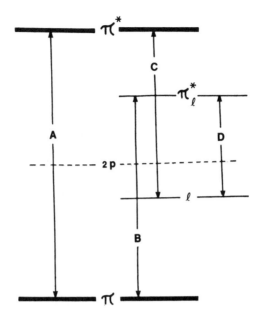

FIG. 3. The effect of exocyclic substituents upon the energies of electronic transitions of aromatic molecules. $\pi, \pi^*, \ell, \pi^*\ell$, and 2p denote the energies of the highest occupied π orbital of the parent hydrocarbon, the lowest unoccupied π orbital of the parent hydrocarbon, a lone-pair orbital derived from a donor substituent, a vacant π orbital derived from an acceptor substituent and the carbon atom 2p orbital, respectively. A, B, C, and D denote the transitions in an aromatic molecule which is A, unsubstituted; B, substituted with an acceptor group; C, substituted with a donor group; D, substituted with both a donor and an acceptor group.

of the unsubstituted molecule. Fluorescence thus appears at lower frequency in the substituted molecule than in the unsubstituted molecule. For example, the fluorescence of 2-naphthoic acid lies at 2.91 μm^{-1} in hexane, 0.27 μm^{-1} lower in frequency than the fluorescence of naphthalene.

Substituent groups such as $-CH_3$ and $-NH_3^+$ neither donate nor accept electrons from the aromatic ring. This type of substituent exerts a polarizing (inductive) effect upon the electronic distributions in the ground and excited states of the aromatic ring. This polarizing effect, however, only slightly affects the position of the fluorescence band. The methyl group has a negatively polarizing influence. The exact nature of the effect of this group is not simple, however, as hyperconjugative interactions may be considered as weak intramolecular charge-transfers. Methyl groups generally produce small shifts to longer wavelengths relative to the fluorescences of the unsubstituted aromatic rings. A positive polarization is produced by ammonium groups. These groups may produce small shifts to longer or shorter wavelengths depending on the site of substitution in the individual aromatic ring.

When an electron-withdrawing and an electron-donating group are attached to the same aromatic ring, fluorescence may be viewed as involving transition between the lone-pair orbital of the donor group and the vacant π orbital of the acceptor group. In this case the energy of the transition is lower, and hence the fluorescence wavelength longer than when either group alone is attached to the ring. This is the well-known auxochromic effect. Depending on one's point of view, either the donor or the acceptor group may be considered to be the chromophore or auxochrome. When two donor groups or two acceptor groups are attached to the aromatic ring, the position of the fluorescence band is usually determined by the donor group with the highest energy lone pair or the acceptor group with the lowest energy vacant orbital.

The presence of a heteroatom in the aromatic ring may be thought of as a special case of a substituent. Two types of heteroatoms may be distinguished. If the heteroatom contributes one π electron to the aromatic system, it will be bonded to the adjacent atoms very much like aromatic carbon. It will exert its effect upon the electronic structure of the molecule by virtue of its possession of nonbonded electron pairs and by its ability, relative to that of aromatic carbon, to attract π electrons. Nitrogen as it occurs in pyridine, quinoline, isoquinoline, acridine, phenanthroline, etc. is the only common member of this class of heteroatoms and will hereafter be referred to as pyridinic nitrogen.

If the heteroatom contributes two electrons to the π-electronic structure of the molecule (e.g., nitrogen in pyrrole or indole, oxygen in furan, sulfur in thiophene) it essentially represents a charge-transfer donor type substituent. Its effect on the electronic structure and spectra will be dominated by this property and to a lesser extent by considerations of electronegativity. Thus the interactions of nitrogen, oxygen, and sulfur in, say, carbazole, dibenzofuran, and dibenzothiophene with their aromatic systems are similar to the interactions of amino, hydroxy, and mercapto exocyclic groups with their aromatic systems. This type of spectroscopic behavior has already been discussed at length.

The pyridinic nitrogen atom is slightly more electronegative than the carbon atoms to which it is bonded. Thus the heteroatom has a slight polarizing effect on the electric distribution of the heterocyclic ring. However, if no charge transfer donor (e.g., $-NH_2$, $-OH$) substitutents are substituted onto the aromatic ring, the effect of the pyridinic nitrogen atom on the ground and π, π^* states of the aromatic ring is so small that the separations between these states in the heterocyclic ring are practically the same as in the corresponding homocyclic molecules. Thus, the fluorescence maximum of the heterocyclic molecule is almost identical with that of the parent homocyclic molecule. However, protonation at the pyridinic nitrogen atom has a substantial effect upon the fluorescence spectrum. This arises from the dramatic increase in electronegativity of the heteroatom resulting from the acquisition of a formal positive charge. The increase in electronegativity of the ring nitrogen upon protonation results in strong stabilization of the excited singlet state dipole with respect to that of the ground state. Thus protonation effects a fluorescence shift to lower frequency.

C. Environmental Effects on Fluorescence Spectra

   1. Solvent Effects [9, 10, 14, 15]

The solvents in which fluorescence spectra are observed play a major role in determining the spectral positions and intensities with which fluorescence bands occur. In some cases the solvent may determine whether or not fluorescence is to be observed at all. The effects of the solvent on the fluorescence spectra are determined by the nature and degree of the interactions of the solvent molecules with the electronic configurations representing the ground and lowest electronically excited singlet state of the fluorescing solute molecules.

Solvent interactions with solute molecules are predominantly electrostatic in nature and may be classified as dipolar or hydrogen bonding. The position of the fluorescence band maximum in one solvent relative to that in another depends upon the relative separations between ground and excited state in either solvent and therefore the relative strengths of ground and excited state solvent stabilization.

The strengths of dipolar interactions depend upon the magnitudes of the dipole moments of the solvent molecules and those of the solute molecules in ground and excited states. If the excited state of a polar molecule has a higher dipole moment than its ground state (most molecules fall into this class), the excited state will be more stabilized by interaction with a polar solvent than the ground state. As a result, upon going from a less polar to a more polar solvent, the fluorescence spectrum will shift to lower frequency. In a few cases, the ground state of a solute is more polar than the excited state, in which case going to a more polar solvent stabilizes the ground state more than the excited state, causing a shift to higher frequency with increasing solvent polarity (dielectric strength). Dipolar interactions decrease with the third power of the distance between interacting molecules. As a result, dilution of a solution of a polar solute, in a polar solvent, with a nonpolar solvent results in an essentially continuous shifting of the fluorescence maximum with increasing mole fraction of unpolar diluent.

Hydrogen bonding solvents having positively polarized hydrogen atoms are said to be hydrogen-bond donor or protic solvents. They interact with the nonbonded and lone electron pairs of solute molecules. Hydrogen bonding solvents having atoms with lone or nonbonded electron pairs are said to be hydrogen-bond acceptor or basic solvents. They interact with positively polarized hydrogen atoms on electronegative atoms belonging to the solute molecules (e.g., in $-COOH$, $-NH_2$, $-OH$, $-SH$).

Hydrogen bonding is a stronger interaction than nonspecific dipole-dipole interaction and is manifested only in the primary solvent cage of the solute. Dilution of a solution of a solute in a hydrogen bonding solvent by an apolar, nonhydrogen bonding solvent will not normally disrupt the hydrogen bonding in the primary solvent cage and thus will cause very small spectral shifts. Because most hydrogen bonding solvents are also polar, hydrogen bonding and nonspecific dipolar interaction are usually both present as modes of solvation of functional molecules. Accordingly, the spectral shifts actually observed upon going from one solvent to another are a composite of dipolar and hydrogen bonding effects which may be constructively or destructively additive.

Due to the involvement of nonbonded and lone electron pairs in n, π^* and intramolecular charge-transfer transitions, hydrogen bonding effects play a major role in the appearances of these spectra. Dipolar effects are most pronounced in π, π^* and intramolecular charge-transfer spectra because of the large dipole moment changes accompanying the associated transitions.

Protic solvents interacting with lone pairs on functional groups which are electron-withdrawing in the excited state (e.g., $\gtrless N$, $>C=O$) enhance charge-transfer by introducing a partial positive charge into the electron acceptor group. This interaction stabilizes the charge-transfer excited state relative to the ground state so that the fluorescence spectra shift to lower frequency with increasing hydrogen-bond donor capacity of the solvent. Increasing hydrogen-bond donor capacity of the solvent produces shifts to higher frequency when interacting with lone pairs on functional groups which are electron donors in the excited state (e.g., $-OH$, $-NH_2$). Hydrogen bond acceptor solvents produce shifts to lower frequency solvating hydrogen atoms on functional groups which are electron donors in the excited state (e.g., $-OH$, $-NH_2$). This is effected by the partial withdrawal of the positively charged proton from the functional group, thereby facilitating transfer of electronic charge away from the functional group. Finally, solvation of hydrogen atoms on functional groups which are charge transfer acceptors in the excited state (e.g., $-COOH$) inhibits charge-transfer by leaving a residual negative charge on the functional group. Thus, the latter interaction results in shifting of the fluorescence spectrum to higher frequency.

Hydrogen bonding in the lowest excited singlet state occasionally results in the diminution or loss of fluorescence intensity in molecules whose lowest excited singlet states are of the intramolecular charge transfer type. This is observed as a decrease in fluorescence quantum yield upon going from hydrocarbon to hydrogen bonding solvents. Many arylamines and phenolic compounds demonstrate this behavior which presently is not predictable. It can be avoided as an analytical interference by making fluorescence measurements in nonhydrogen bonding media.

Molecules having lowest excited singlet states of the n, π^* type rarely fluoresce in hydrocarbon solvents (aprotic, nonpolar) because the n, π^* singlet state is efficiently deactivated by intersystem crossing. However, in polar, hydrogen bonding solvents such as ethanol or water these molecules become fluorescent. This results from the stabilization, relative to the ground state, of the lowest singlet π, π^* state, by dipole-dipole interaction and the destabilization of the lowest singlet n, π^* state by hydrogen bonded interaction. If both of these interactions are sufficiently strong, the π, π^* state drops below the n, π^* state in the strongly solvated molecule, thereby permitting intense fluorescence. Quinoline and 1-naphthaldehyde, for example, do not fluoresce in cyclohexane but do so in water.

Finally, solvent containing atoms of high atomic number (e.g., alkyl iodide) also have a substantial effect on the intensity of fluorescence of solute molecules. However, this effect is not directly related to the polarity or hydrogen bonding properties of the "heavy atom solvent." Atoms of of high atomic number in the solvent cage of the solute molecule enhance spin-orbital coupling in the lowest excited singlet state of the solute. This favors the radiationless population of the lowest triplet state at the expense of the lowest excited singlet state. Thus in heavy atom solvents, all other things being equal, fluorescence is always less intense than in solvents of low molecular weight. In frozen solutions the heavy atom effect favors the enhancement of phosphorescence intensity. Thus in analytical practice, heavy atom solvents are to be avoided in fluorometry and to be desired in phosphorimetry.

2. pH Effects [9, 16-19]

pH effects on fluorescence spectra are primarily derived from the dissociation of acidic functional groups or protonation of basic functional groups associated with the aromatic portions of fluorescing molecules. Since fluorescence spectra are often measured in concentrated acid or base solutions as well as in aqueous solutions containing high concentrations of buffer species, the proton donor and acceptor species in solution are frequently species other than H_3O^+ and OH^- and are not, strictly speaking, represented by the pH scale. Nevertheless, this section will consider the effects of all types of Bronsted acid-base reactions on the appearance of the fluorescence spectra.

Protolytic dissociation may be regarded as an extreme form of interaction with a hydrogen-bond acceptor solvent, while protonation of a heteroatom or basic functional group may be regarded as an extreme case of interaction with a hydrogen-bond donor solvent. Consequently, the spectral shifts observed when basic groups are protonated or when acidic groups are dissociated are greater in magnitude but qualitatively similar in direction to the shifts resulting from interaction of lone or nonbonded electron pairs with hydrogen-bond donor solvents or from interaction of acidic hydrogen atoms with hydrogen-bond acceptor solvents, respectively. Thus, the protonation of electron-withdrawing groups such as carboxyl, carbonyl, and pyridinic nitrogen results in shifts of the fluorescence spectra to longer wavelengths while the protonation of electron donating groups such as the amino group produces spectral shifts to shorter wavelengths. The protolytic dissociation of electron-donating groups such as hydroxyl, sulfhydryl, or pyrrolic nitrogen produces spectral shifts to longer wavelengths, while the dissociation of electron-withdrawing groups, such as carboxyl, produces shifting of the fluorescence spectra to shorter wavelengths.

In some molecules, notably the carbonyl derivatives of benzene, the presence of nonbonded electrons obviates the occurrence of fluorescence even in strongly hydrogen-bonding solvents, such as water. However, protonation of the functional group possessing the nonbonded electron pair, or dissociation of electron donor groups in the molecule, raises the n, π^* lowest excited singlet state above the lowest excited singlet π, π^* state and thereby allows fluorescence to occur. Salicylaldehyde, for example, does not fluoresce as the neutral molecule but does so, moderately intensely, as the cation in concentrated sulfuric acid and as the anion in aqueous sodium hydroxide solutions. Benzophenone, which is obtained as an oxidation product of diphenylhydantoin, fluoresces in its protonated form in concentrated sulfuric acid. However, benzophenone is nonfluorescent in aqueous media.

One of the more interesting aspects of acid-base reactions of fluorescent or potentially fluorescent molecules is derived from the occurrence of protonation and dissociation during the lifetime of the lowest excited singlet state. This phenomenon affects the fluorescence intensity-pH profile in ways which are not anticipated on the basis of ground state acid-base chemistry (pK_a) and occasionally poses a serious threat to the intelligent assessment of the solution conditions under which to carry out fluorometric analysis.

The lifetimes of molecules in the lowest excited singlet state are typically of the order of 10^{-11} to 10^{-7} sec. Typical rates of protolytic reactions are 10^{11} M^{-1} sec^{-1} or lower. Consequently, excited state protolytic reactions may be much slower, much faster, or competitive with radiative deactivation of the excited molecules. Whether or not protonation or dissociation can occur during the lifetime of the excited state depends upon which of the latter three circumstances is extant.

a. Excited state proton-exchange is much slower
than fluorescence

In this case, if the acid form of the analyte is excited, the excited acid will fluoresce before it can convert to the excited conjugate base. The same argument applies to the excitation of the conjugate base species. Thus, which species emits is governed only by which species absorbs. The relative intensities of emission from acid and conjugate base are determined exclusively by the molar absorptivities of acid and conjugate base at the wavelength of excitation and by the thermodynamics (pK_a) of the ground state prototropic reaction. The fluorometric pH titration curve in this case is thus identical with the absorptiometric (ground state) titration curve (Fig. 4a).

b. Excited state proton-exchange is much faster
than fluorescence

If the rates of dissociation of the excited acid and of protonation of the excited conjugate base are much greater than the rate of deactivation of the lowest excited singlet state by fluorescence, prototropic equilibrium in the lowest excited singlet state will be achieved. In this event it is the dissociation constant of the excited state prototropic reaction (pK_a^*) which predominately determines the fluorescence behavior of the analyte. Since the electronic distribution of an electronically excited molecule is generally different from that of its ground state, the pK_a^* of the excited acid is usually very different from the pK_a of the ground state acid. Differences between pK_a^* and pK_a are commonly six or more orders of magnitude and mean that the conversion of acid to conjugate base in the excited state occurs in a pH region different from the corresponding ground state reaction, the inflection point in the fluorometric titration occurring at pH = pK_a^* (Fig. 4a). The unwary analyst may thus find that pH adjustment of the test solution, based upon the ground state acid-base properties of the analyte, may leave the sample in a pH region where the excited state acid-base reaction causes fluorometric interferences. However, the pK_a^* can also be employed to the analyst's benefit as it provides an additional parameter for species identification.

c. Excited state proton transfer and fluorescence
occur at comparable rates

If the rates of proton transfer in the excited state are comparable to the rates of deactivation of acid and conjugate base by fluorescence, the variations of the relative quantum yields of fluorescence of acid and conjugate base with pH will be governed by the kinetics and mechanisms of the excited state prototropic reactions (Fig. 4b). In general, the pH region over which the emissions of both conjugate acid and conjugate base are observed will extend from the general vicinity of pK_a to that of pK_a^*.

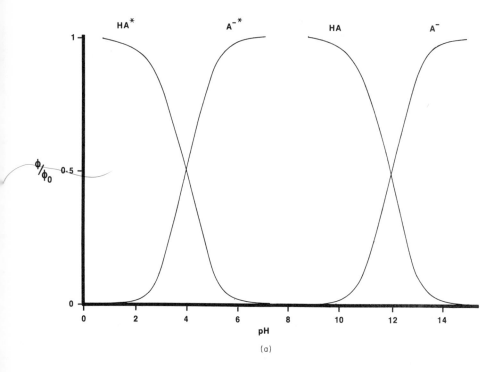

FIG. 4a. pH dependences of the relative quantum yields of fluorescence (ϕ/ϕ_0) of a weak acid HA ($pK_a = 12.0$) and its conjugate base A⁻, in which proton exchange during the lifetime of the lowest excited singlet state is too slow to compete with fluorescence; and of a weak acid HA* ($pK_a = 12.0$) and its conjugate base A⁻*, in which proton exchange during the lifetime of the excited state attains equilibrium ($pK_a^* = 4$) prior to fluorescence of HA*.

Since pK_a and pK_a^* may differ considerably, the probability that excited state proton exchange will be an analytical problem is greatest in the event that it occurs on a time scale comparable to that of fluorescence. In this regard, it is worth noting that buffer ions act as proton donors and acceptors with excited potentially fluorescent molecules. In solutions containing high concentrations of buffer ions the latter may induce excited state proton-transfer in molecules which would not enter into this process in water. Consequently, the intelligent practice of fluorometry in buffered aqueous solutions requires the use of very dilute buffers and therefore a compromise between optimal buffer capacity and optimal fluorometric parameters.

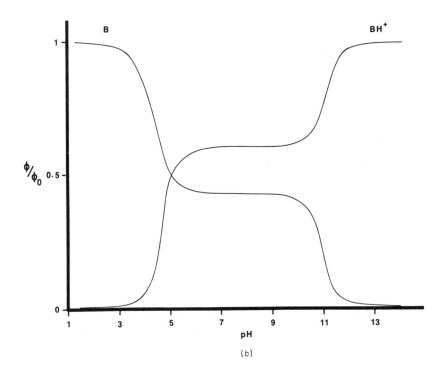

(b)

FIG. 4b. pH dependences of the relative quantum yields of fluorescence (ϕ/ϕ_0) of a base (B) and its conjugate acid (BH$^+$) resulting from B becoming a stronger base in the lowest excited singlet state, ($pK_{BH^+} = 5$, $pK^*_{BH^+} =$ 11.5) but having insufficient time, prior to the fluorescence of B, for complete protonation. Acid base equilibrium is therefore not truly attained during the lifetime of the lowest excited singlet state.

3. Concentration Effects [6, 10, 20, 21]

The discussion of fluorescence has, up to the present, been based upon the properties of dilute solutions in which the analyte molecules were presumed to be isolated from interactions with one another. It has already been established that at high absorbance at the wavelength of excitation, deviations from linearity of the fluorescence intensity vs. concentration relationship may occur because of the actual exponential variation of fluorescence intensity with concentration and, therefore, cause analytical complications. However, over a wide range of solute concentrations, solute-solute interactions may also account for loss of fluorescence intensity with increasing solute concentration.

Several types of excited state solute-solute interaction are common. The aggregation of excited solute molecules with ground state molecules of the same type produces an excited polymer or "excimer" which by virtue of the coupling of the aromatic systems of the excited and unexcited molecules usually luminesces at lower frequency than the monomeric excited molecule. The excimer fluorescence occurs at the expense of monomer fluorescence and if unanticipated, can cause serious errors in fluorometric analysis. Because excimer fluorescence takes place in the excited state, it is demonstrable in the fluorescence spectrum. However, after fluorescence, the deactivated polymer rapidly falls apart. Hence, the absorption spectrum does not reflect the presence of the excited state complexes. Occasionally, excited state complex formation may occur between two different solute molecules. The phenomenon is comparable to excimer formation, however, the term "exciplex" has been coined to describe a heteropolymeric excited state complex. Excimer and exciplex formation are generally observed only in fluid solution because diffusion of the excited species is necessary to form the excited complexes. However, one concentration effect that is observed in molecules in fluid or rigid media is resonance energy transfer. Energy transfer entails the excitation of a molecule which, during the lifetime of the excited state, passes its excitation energy off to a nearby molecule. This process falls off in probability as the inverse sixth power of the distance between donor and acceptor (dipole-dipole interaction) and can occur between molecules which are separated by up to 10 nm. If the energy donor is a different chemical species from the energy acceptor and is of analytical interest, the analytical interference due to loss of fluorescence intensity of this species should be obvious. Because the mean distance between molecules decreases with increasing concentration, energy transfer is favored by increasing concentration of both energy donor and acceptor. For energy transfer to occur between two dissimilar molecules, the fluorescence spectrum of the energy donor must overlap the absorption spectrum of the energy acceptor.

At very high absorber concentrations, ground state aggregation effects may come into play and may ultimately result in the decrease of luminescence intensity with increasing absorber concentration. Moreover, when very highly absorbing solutions are studied, the loss in fluorescence intensity with increasing absorber concentration may also be due to absorption of all of the exciting light before it completely traverses the sample. Fluorescence is then observed from only part of the sample cell. If the absorption spectrum and the fluorescence spectrum of the solute overlap, diminution of fluorescence intensity may result from the reabsorption of part of the emitted radiation. This effect is called trivial reabsorption and is observed as a concentration dependent effect in fluorescence spectroscopy.

Fluorescence may be quenched (diminished in intensity or eliminated) due to the deactivation of the lowest excited singlet state of the analyte by interaction with other species in solution. The mechanisms of quenching are not well understood but appear to employ internal conversion, inter-system crossing, and photodissociation as modes of deactivation of the excited analyte-quencher complexes. Quenching, in most cases, is an interference in fluorometric analysis because it diminishes analytical sensitivity. However, in a few instances analytical methodology based upon the selective quenching of fluorescence has proven extremely useful.

Quenching processes may be divided into two broad categories. In dynamic or diffusional quenching, interaction between the quencher and the potentially fluorescent molecule takes place during the lifetime of the excited state. As a result, the efficiency of dynamic quenching is governed by the lifetime of the excited state of the potential fluorescer and the concentration of the quenching species. Interaction between quencher and excited analyte results in the formation of a transient excited complex which is nonfluorescent and may be deactivated by any of the usual radiationless modes of deactivation of excited singlet states. Because interaction occurs only after excitation of the potentially fluorescing molecule, the presence of the quenching species has no effect on the absorption spectrum of the analyte. Many aromatic molecules, for example, the aminobenzoic and hydroxybenzoic acids and their metabolites, are dynamically quenched by halide ions such as Cl^- and Br^-. Static quenching is characterized by complexation in the ground state between the quenching species and the molecule which, when alone excited, should eventually become a potential fluorescing molecule. The complex is generally not fluorescent and although it may dissociate in the excited state to release the fluorescing species, this phenomenon is, at most, only partially effective in producing fluorescers because radiationless conversion to the ground state may be much faster than photodissociation. As a result, the ground state reaction diminishes the intensity of fluorescence of the potentially fluorescent species. The quenching of the fluorescence of adriamycin by complexation with double helical DNA is an example of static quenching.

It should be noted that in dynamic quenching, the quantum yield of fluorescence is governed by the kinetics of photoreaction. However, in static quenching it is generally governed by the strength of ground state complexation. Thus, conversion of an excited fluorescing acid or base to its non-fluorescent conjugate, by dissociation or protonation, represents static quenching by H_2O, OH^-, or H_3O^+ if the quenching is centered at $pH = pK_a$ and dynamic quenching if it is centered at $pH \neq pK_a$.

The dependence of the relative quantum yield of fluorescence (ϕ/ϕ_0) upon quencher concentration [Q] may be derived from steady-state kinetics and is

$$\frac{\phi}{\phi_0} = \frac{1 - \gamma\alpha}{1 + \gamma k_D \tau [Q]} \tag{9}$$

where τ is the mean lifetime of the excited state in the absence of quenching (i. e. , when [Q] = 0), k_D is the rate constant of complexation of the potential fluorescing species by the quencher Q in the excited state, γ is the probability that the complex will be deactivated rather than dissociate back to the potential fluorescer, and α is the fraction of complex, formed in the ground state, that is excited by direct absorption. If complexation in the ground state is negligible, or if excitation is effected at a wavelength where the complex does not absorb, $\alpha \to 0$ and Equation (9) is reduced to

$$\frac{\phi}{\phi_0} = \frac{1}{1 + k_Q [Q]} \tag{10}$$

where $k_Q = \gamma k_D \tau$. Equation (10) is the well known Stern-Volmer equation [22] which relates the quantum yield of fluorescence to the rate of dynamic quenching and the quencher concentration.

Although quenching of fluorescence is most often regarded as an analytical interference, it also forms the basis of an analytical technique called quenchofluorometry. Quenchofluorometry makes use of the fact that if the intense fluorescence of a reference compound is statically quenched by quantitative reaction with a nonfluorescent analyte of interest, the difference between the fluorescence intensities of the reference compound before and after quenching by the analyte is proportional to the concentration of the analyte. Although this technique has not been employed to anywhere near the extent that direct fluorometry has, it is as sensitive as the direct fluorometry of the reference fluorophore. Moreover, it is as sensitive as most fluorometric methods in which a fluorescing derivative of the analyte must be chemically generated. Dynamic fluorescence quenching is not particularly useful from the quantitative point of view because the occurrence of the quenching during the lifetime of the lowest excited singlet state requires that quencher concentrations be $> 10^{-4}$ M.

III. INSTRUMENTATION AND EXPERIMENTAL
     CONSIDERATIONS [3, 5, 23]

Instrumentation for the measurement of fluorescence consists essentially of (a) a lamp to produce exciting light, (b) a monochromator to disperse the exciting light into its component wavelengths, (c) a sample compartment, (d) a monochromator to disperse the fluorescent light, emitted by the sample, into its component wavelengths, (e) a photodetector to translate the fluorescent light into a measurable electrical signal, and (f) a readout system such as a galvanometer or recorder to determine the intensity of fluorescent light emitted at any given wavelength (Fig. 5). In

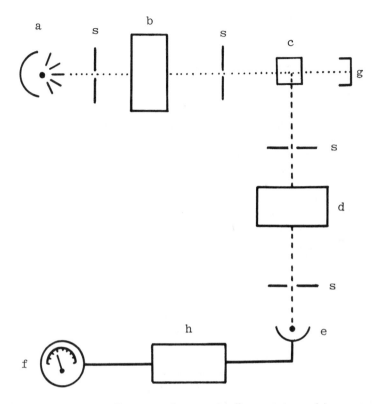

FIG. 5. Schematic diagram of a spectrofluorometer. (a) source of exciting light; (b) excitation monochromator; (c) sample cell; (d) emission monochromator; (e) photodetector; (f) readout system; (g) light-absorbing stop for excitation beam; (h) amplifier for photodetector signal; (s) slits.

addition, slits are usually present on either side of the monochromators to collimate the exciting and fluorescent light and to limit the range of wavelengths (bandpass) of exciting light irradiating the sample and fluorescent light falling on the photodetector. An instrument containing these components is called a spectrofluorometer, a spectrophotofluorometer, or a fluorescence photometer, depending upon the manufacturer's preference. If filters are employed instead of monochromators to restrict the range of wavelengths of light exciting the sample and falling on the detector, the instrument is called a filter fluorometer.

A. Excitation Sources

The excitation sources employed in most commercial spectrofluorometers are either high pressure xenon lamps or low pressure mercury vapor xenon lamps. Xenon lamps provide a continuum of wavelengths throughout the near UV and visible regions of the spectrum and therefore allow a wide range of selectivity in the choice of the proper wavelength of light with which to excite the sample. The choice of excitation wavelength (λ_{exc}) is made by setting the emission monochromator at some wavelength which will allow fluorescence to fall on the detector (λ_f), and scanning the entire spectrum of wavelengths shorter than λ_f with the excitation monochromator. The recording of fluorescence intensity versus excitation wavelength is called an excitation spectrum and displays peaks which roughly correspond to the absorption spectrum of the ground state species absorbing the exciting radiation. The choice of λ_{exc} for analytical purposes is usually made on the basis of maximal fluorescence intensity (for sensitivity) and isolation from the excitation peaks of interfering substances (for selectivity). Below 300 nm the light output of the xenon lamp falls off sharply. This tends to exaggerate the height of the excitation spectrum to appear different from the absorption spectrum. Mercury-xenon lamps produce intense light corresponding to the line emission spectrum of elemental mercury (principal lines are at 254, 313, and 365 nm) but very little light at other wavelengths. Hence, the mercury-xenon lamp does not allow as much freedom in the choice of an excitation wavelength as the xenon lamp. However, many substances have absorption spectra which overlap the mercury emission lines and can therefore be excited. Moreover, the intensity of exciting light produced at the mercury emission lines is generally greater than the intensity of light produced at any given wavelength by a xenon lamp of comparable power rating. Hence, the tradeoff between analytical sensitivity and freedom of choice of exciting wavelength sometimes favors the use of the mercury-xenon lamp.

B. Monochromators

The monochromators employed in commercial spectrofluorometers are either diffraction gratings or quartz prisms. The excitation grating or prism is mounted on a turntable which, when rotated, allows light of different wavelengths (with different angles of dispersion in the monochromator) from the lamp to be focused through a slit and onto the sample. The emission grating or prism is also mounted on a turntable which, when rotated, allows different wavelengths of fluorescent light to be focused through a slit onto the detector. Instruments employing quartz prisms are generally more expensive than those employing diffraction gratings; hence

most commercial instruments employ grating monochromation. The
amount of light passed through the excitation monochromator, onto the
sample, and through the emission monochromator onto the detector depends
upon the angle of dispersion of the light which in turn is governed by the
wavelength of the light and the spacing between lines or grooves on the diffraction grating. As a result, the light passed through the excitation and
emission monochromators does not reflect the true absorption and fluorescence spectra in the wavelength distribution of fluorescence intensities but,
rather, is somewhat distorted by the physical characteristics of the monochromators.

C. Slits

The slits, which focus light onto the monochromators and the detector,
regulate the range of wavelengths which excite the sample and which ultimately pass onto the detector. The smaller the slit widths employed, the
narrower is the range of spectral bandpass and the greater is the analytical
selectivity. For weakly fluorescing samples it is usually necessary to
increase the amount of exciting light falling on the sample and fluorescent
light falling on the detector in order to yield an analytically useful signal.
In this case it may be desirable to increase the slit width, although in
multicomponent samples this generally diminishes selectivity of excitation
and monitoring of fluorescence. In very "dirty" samples of weakly fluorescing analytes such as blood or urine, selectivity is so poor, even with
narrow slits, that physicochemical separation such as solvent extraction
or thin layer chromatography is almost invariably a prerequisite to successful fluorometric analysis. Slits may be either fixed in width, in which
case the changing of slit width entails replacement, or they may be variable,
in which case the spectral bandpass may be varied by turning a micrometer
screw which adjusts the separation of the moveable slit edges. Variable
slits are considerably more expensive than fixed slits but are more convenient for routine work. A major disadvantage of the variable slits is
that with extensive use the knife edges of the slits become worn, resulting
in loss of the slit calibration. This is not a serious drawback in routine
analytical work, but in accurate spectroscopic studies of physicochemical
phenomena the precise knowledge of the excitation and emission slitwidths
may be important.

D. Sample Compartments

Sample compartments contain the cells in which the analytical samples are
excited. They are usually painted with flat black paint to minimize stray

exciting light and are covered, when the instrument is in operation, to exclude external light. In most instruments the sample compartment is arranged so that the fluorescent light emitted by the sample exits from the compartment (to the emission monochromator and detector) at right angles to the line of entry of the exciting light. This arrangement allows for minimal interference by stray exciting light. Since fluorescence is emitted from the sample in all directions, only a fraction of the total fluorescent light is monitored by the detector, the remained being absorbed by the walls of the sample compartment. Sample compartments should be large enough to house accessories such as polarizing prisms or constant temperature accessories which may be employed in specialized fluorescence studies.

Low temperature fluorescence studies may be carried out by inserting into the sample compartment a small Dewar flask with a quartz window or nipple which is aligned with the excitation and emission optics. The Dewar may be filled with liquid nitrogen or another cryogenic fluid. The sample cell is then inserted into the filled Dewar flask so that the sample is exposed to the exciting light through the quartz nipple. Fluorescent light also passes out of the sample to the detector through the quartz nipple. If the sample phosphoresces but does not fluoresce, the latter sample arrangement may also be employed. However, if the sample fluoresces and phosphoresces and it is desired to monitor only the phosphorescence, the fluorescent light may be prevented from reaching the detector by taking advantage of the much greater lifetime of phosphorescence relative to that of fluorescence. A mechanical chopper, consisting of a can with lateral apertures 180° apart, may be inserted into the sample compartment in such a way as to enclose the Dewar flask and its contents. The quartz nipple of the Dewar flask is aligned with the apertures in the side of the can (phosphoroscope). The can may then be rotated at several thousand revolutions per minute with a variable speed motor. Because the aperture in the can are 180° apart and the excitation-emission optics are in a 90° configuration, when one aperture is facing the excitation optics the sample is excited, but emission can only exit at 90° with respect to the emission optics (Fig. 6). Hence, no emitted light falls on the detector. When the can rotates through 90° the exciting light is cut off from the sample. Because of the very short lifetime of fluorescence ($\sim 10^{-8}$ sec) the fluorescent light emitted by the sample has completely vanished during the course of one-quarter turn of the can. However, the phosphorescence, which has a lifetime of from 10^{-4} sec to several seconds, persists as an afterglow and is registered by the detector when the can aperture faces the detector axis. In this way, the phosphorescence spectrum or the phosphorescence excitation spectrum of the sample may be taken exclusive of interfering fluorescence or fluorescence excitation spectra. The rotating can device is the standard phosphoroscope supplied with most commercial instruments. In low temperature fluorescence or phosphorescence work liquid nitrogen is the cryogenic fluid

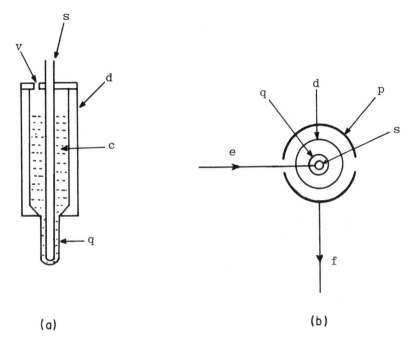

(a)   (b)

FIG. 6. Schematic diagrams of (a) Dewar flask for low temperature fluorescence or phosphorescence studies and (b) top view of sample compartment for phosphorescence studies: c, cryogenic liquid (liquid nitrogen); d, Dewar flask; e, excitation beam; f, emission beam; p, phosphoroscope; q, quartz nipple; s, sample cell; v, vent for vaporized nitrogen.

most often employed. This substance has a tendency to cause spurious luminescence signals as a result of bubbling when the sample is lowered into it. The problem of bubbling can be overcome by adding a small amount of liquid helium to the liquid nitrogen bath.

E. Sample Cells

The sample cells employed in ambient temperature fluorescence spectroscopy are usually 1 cm^2 high quality quartz or fused silica cells. The synthetic fused silica cells are usually superior because they demonstrate less background fluorescence than their counterparts made from naturally occurring quartz. For very small samples, cylindrical quartz microcells are available. However, the curved cell surface is often troublesome, causing a great deal of scattering of the exciting light. Cylindrical micro-cells are also employed in low temperature work because rapid cooling and thawing causes the square cells to crack at the joints. Scattering of excited light is always a problem in low temperature fluorescence spectroscopy, but in phosphorescence spectroscopy the phosphoroscope eliminates most stray exciting light as well as fluorescent light. The emptying and clean-ing of cylindrical microcells often presents a problem; however, this can be circumvented by using a long hypodermic needle attached to a water aspirator.

F. Photodetectors

The detectors employed in fluorescence spectroscopy consist of a multiplier phototube which produces an electrical current upon exposure to light, and an amplifier to increase the small photocurrents produced, to a measur-able level. Phototubes do not respond equally to all wavelengths of light. As a result, the electrical signal put out by a given phototube does not faithfully represent the relative intensity of the wavelength spectrum it receives but rather is biased toward certain wavelength regions of the visible and UV spectrum and therefore causes spectral distortion. Most phototubes in commercially available instruments (e.g., the RCA 1P21, RCA 1P28, and Hitachi R106) have maximum spectral response, from ~300 to 500 nm, and are suitable for the great majority of fluorescence work. However, in the long wavelength region of the spectrum ($\lambda > 550$ nm) the electrical response of these phototubes falls off dramatically, resulting in poor analytical sensitivity. If spectral measurements are to be performed frequently at long wavelengths it is often desirable to employ a special red sensitive phototube such as the Hitachi R136.

G. Signal Readout

Readout systems for fluorescence spectroscopy may be either galvanom-eters, recorders, or oscilloscopes. Galvanometers, the meters supplied with the spectrofluorometers, are convenient for analytical measurements at fixed wavelength but are cumbersome for spectral work, as the spec-trum must be plotted manually from point by point readings on the galvan-ometer. Recorders provide a permanent record of the fluorescence ex-citation or emission spectrum and are two basic types, x-y and x-t. The x-t or strip chart recorder displays fluorescence intensity on the x-axis and wavelength on the t (time)-axis. The t-axis is traversed at a constant rate of speed and may be slaved to the monochromator drive motors which, with the x-t recorders, are also operated at constant scanning rate. Several constant scanning speeds are available on most x-t recorders, allowing spectra to be expanded or compressed to the desired scale. The x-y recorders are usually about twice as expensive as the x-t recorders. As in the x-t recorder the x-axis corresponds to fluorescence intensity which is represented by the deflection of a pen driven by the output from the photodetector. However, the y-axis of the x-y recorder is continuously synchronized with the scanning speed of the monochromators. Thus the slowing down of the monochromator scanning rate in areas of spectroscopic interest or the speeding up of the monochromator scanning rate in spectroscopically uninteresting areas is continuously matched by the scanning rate of the y-axis. This allows an undistorted spectrum to be taken even if different portions of the spectrum were scanned at different rates. Moreover, a spectrum can be made to retrace itself by back-scanning with an x-y recorder. With an x-t recorder the rewinding of the chart is not synchronized with the back-rotation of the monochromators so that the retracing capability is absent. Perhaps the greatest limitation of recorders in general is the rather long response time of the recorder pen (0.1 to 0.5 sec). This limits the rate at which an accurate spectrum can be swept. The oscilloscope circumvents the problem of pen response time by tracing out the spectrum electronically rather than mechanically and in order to obtain a permanent record of the displayed spectrum, some rather elegant photographic apparatus may be required.

H. Filter Instruments

Filter fluorometers are considerably less expensive than spectrofluorometers. However, the spectrofluorometers are considerably more versatile. Because of the use of cutoff or bandpass glass filters which allow passage of broad spectral regions, the selectivity obtainable with the filter instrument is far inferior to that of a monochromated instrument. However, there is, by virtue of the wide bandpass of the filter instrument, much less energy loss in monochromation so that filter instruments often tend to be more sensitive analytically than spectrofluorometers. The filter instruments almost invariably employ the mercury-xenon lamp in preference to the xenon lamp source. Filter fluorometers suffice in many routine laboratory assays such as the determination of pyridoxine metabolites, riboflavin, and quinine. However, it is safe to say that the serious researcher, relying heavily on fluorescence spectroscopy as an analytical technique, would do well to spend the extra money on a spectrofluorometer.

I. Instrumental Distortion of Spectra

Because of the wavelength-variable output of the lamp and responses of the
monochromators and phototube, fluorescence excitation and emission spectra taken on conventional spectrofluorometers are not "true" excitation and
emission spectra (properties of the analyte alone), but rather are apparent
excitation and emission spectra distorted by instrumental response. For
routine quantitative analysis this is usually unimportant. However, the
true fluorescence excitation spectrum is identical to the absorption spectrum of the analyte. The ability to take true excitation spectra is, thus,
analytically very desirable because it facilitates identification of organic
molecules at concentrations far lower than possible by any other means.
The true fluorescence spectrum is necessary for the accurate calculation
of fluorescence quantum yields [from Equation (7)]. Moreover, because
the distortion of the apparent spectrum depends upon the manufacturer of
the spectrofluorometer components as well as upon the age of the lamp and
phototube, true excitation and emission spectra are highly desirable in
order to compare results taken on different instruments. Apparent excitation and emission spectra can be corrected for instrumental response to
yield true excitation and emission spectra by means of commercially available correction accessories which vary from manufacturer to manufacturer
in mode of operation.

J. Measurement of Fluorescence Excitation and
    Emission Spectra

Fluorescence excitation spectra are measured experimentally by manually
adjusting the emission monochromator to the wavelength of maximum fluorescence intensity and recording the output signal (emission signal) as a
function of excitation wavelength λ_{exc}. On an uncorrected spectrofluorometer, the excitation spectrum will depend not only upon the absorption
spectrum of the sample, but also upon the wavelength-variable response
of the instrumental components. This generally means that the uncorrected
excitation spectrum will be similar in appearance to the absorption spectrum but will be skewed to longer wavelength because of the weaker instrumental response at $\lambda_{exc} < 300$ nm. As previously discussed, instrumental
wavelength-variable response can be compensated for, by commercially
available "correction" accessories.

Emission spectra are measured by adjusting the excitation monochromator to the wavelength of maximal excitation (determined from the excitation spectrum) and recording the output signal as a function of emission
wavelength λ_f. On an uncorrected instrument the emission spectrum will

depend not only on the spectroscopic properties of the sample, but also on the wavelength-variable instrumental response. As a result, uncorrected spectra may be used as a qualitative fingerprint of organic materials only for a particular instrument or group of similar instruments. To correct emission spectra, all luminescence signals must compensate for instrumental distortion. Several commercial instruments accomplish this process automatically.

Because fluorescence almost invariably occurs from the lowest excited singlet state, for pure compounds, the shapes of fluorescence spectra are independent of the wavelength of excitation. Conversely, the shape of the excitation spectrum is independent of the wavelength of emission. Corrected excitation spectra are identical to or very similar to the absorption spectra. These facts may be used as criteria of purity for drugs and metabolites.

The effects of the monochromator slit width must be considered when recording spectra. Excitation spectra should be recorded with a sufficiently narrow excitation monochromator slit width to obtain the desired resolution (selectivity), while the emission monochromator slit width may be made considerably wider in order to obtain the intensity required for good sensitivity. Conversely, emission spectra may be recorded with a narrow emission monochromator slit width and a wide excitation monochromator slit width. In either case, the slit widths should not be so wide as to allow the monochromators to pass adjacent interfering bands.

K. Measurement of Fluorescence Quantum Yields

The fluorescence quantum yield ϕ_f of a molecular species may be determined experimentally by comparing the integrated fluorescence intensity I_f (the area under the corrected fluorescence spectrum) and the absorbance at the average wavelength of excitation to the corresponding quantities belonging to a solution of a reference compound of known quantum yield. Quinine bisulfate in $0.1N$ H_2SO_4 has a quantum yield of 0.55 and is the standard most often employed. According to Equation (8), for very dilute solutions of quinine (Q) and of the compound whose quantum yield is to be determined (u), under identical conditions of excitation,

$$\phi_{fu} = \frac{I_{fu}}{I_{fQ}} \frac{A_Q}{A_u} \phi_{fQ} \tag{11}$$

where A_Q and A_u are the absorbances of the test compound and of quinine bisulfate, respectively ($A = \epsilon c \ell$). Reported quantum yield values typically fall between 0.1 and 1.0 for analytically useful determinations.

L. Measurement of Luminescence Lifetime

The decay time of the fluorescence of organic molecules is generally of the order of several nanoseconds, so techniques for its measurement are generally rather elegant and require expensive instrumentation. These include flash tubes, capable of generating subnanosecond light pulses which are used in the stroboscopic method. Commercial flash lamp systems of this type are available (TRW Model 31A Nanosecond Spectral Source, TRW Instruments, El Segundo, Calif. and the Xenon Model 437 Nanopulser and 783A Nanopulse lamp, Xenon Corp., Medford, Mass.).

Phosphorescence lifetimes are much longer than fluorescence lifetimes and are therefore easier to measure. The simplest method is to measure the phosphorescence intensity as a function of time after completer termination of the excitation radiation. For lifetimes longer than about 1.0 sec, a strip chart (x-t) recorder may be used. For faster decay tumes, a wideband oscilloscope is used. Obviously the response time of the readout system must be much smaller than the sample decay time. The mean lifetime is defined as the time required for the measured luminescence signal to decay from any given value to $1/e$ (= 0.368) of that value. The exciting radiation must be cut off quickly; an electrically-operated guillotine shutter is sometimes used. Lifetimes between 10^{-4} and 10^{-1} sec may be measured by using the rotating phosphoroscope can or disc as the shutter and observing the exponential emission light pulses on an oscilloscope. Lifetimes much faster than about 10^{-4} sec may be measured by the stroboscopic technique or by direct observation of the luminescence decay on an oscilloscope following excitation by a short pulse of light.

Most pure organic compounds exhibit first-order (exponential) decays. In such cases a plot of the log luminescence signal vs. time during the decay yields a straight line. Any nonlinearity in this plot is a highly sensitive indication of the presence of impurities and forms the basis of time resolved phosphorimetry.

M. Measurement of Concentration

The measurement of analyte concentration in fluorescence spectroscopy may be accomplished by several distinct experimental methods. The simplest of these, applicable only to intrinsically fluorescent species, is the direct method, which involves the measurement of the fluorescence intensity of the analyte itself, either with or without prior separation from interfering substances. A nonfluorescent or weakly fluorescent substance may be converted into a form more suitable for fluorescence analysis by means of appropriate chemical reactions. Such methods are called chemical methods or indirect methods. If the substance to be determined is non-fluorescent and yet possesses the ability to quench the luminescence of some luminescent compound, the substance may be determined indirectly by the measurement of the reduction in luminescence intensity of the luminescent compound. Such a process would constitute a quenching method. Finally, there are energy transfer methods which involve the absorption of exciting light by a donor species, transfer of the energy from the donor to an acceptor species, and finally, luminescence from the acceptor species.

All of the above methods are relative methods and, as such, require some sort of calibration procedure. The most common calibration method involves the preparation of a series of standard solutions (serial dilutions) of the analyte. These standards are then treated as the unknown samples themselves, according to the particular measurement method used. Thus, in the direct method, the fluorescence intensity of each standard is measured directly. In the chemical method, appropriate reagents are added to each standard, and the mixture is allowed to react before the fluorescence intensity is measured. In the quenching method, suitable reagents are added to each standard before the fluorescence intensity is measured. In the intramolecular energy transfer methods, a suitable acceptor or donor species must be added. The relative fluorescence intensity of each of the standard solutions prepared in the above way is measured, blank-corrected, and plotted vs. the analyte concentration, usually on log-log coordinates. Luminescence analytical curves are typically linear over several decades of concentration, have log-log slopes near unity, and exhibit a plateau region at high analyte concentrations.

Unknown sample solutions are treated and measured in exactly the same way as the standards, and their concentrations are interpolated from the analytical curve. Linear analytical curves are highly desirable because interpolation from a linear plot is relatively easy.

Only in the most ideal analysis will all of the measured light emission from the sample be due to the analyte. The purpose of the blank solution is to correct for absorbing and fluorescing species other than those related to analyte concentration.

All reading of the luminescence signals of samples and standards must be blank-corrected by subtracting the signal reading given by the blank solutions. Several types of blank solutions are used in practice. The ideal or true blank would, in principle, contain everything contained in the unknown samples in the same concentrations as in the unknown samples, except the analyte. A true blank is seldom possible for real analyses in complicated systems. Thus, some approximation to a true blank is usually made. The simplest is a solvent blank, consisting simply of the solvent used to make up the standards and dissolve and dilute the samples. Such a blank would correct only for fluorescent impurities in the solvent and would be suitable only in the direct measurement of a fluorescent compound uncontaminated by fluorescent impurities. More satisfactory is a reagent blank which contains, in addition to the solvent, each of the various reagents in the same concentrations used in the treatment of samples and standards. A reagent blank is useful in the chemical, quenching, and energy-transfer methods since it corrects for absorption by and luminescence of impurities in the added reagents. Neither a solvent blank or a reagent blank, however, corrects for the absorption by and luminescence of contaminants and matrix substances originally in the sample itself. If these interferences cannot be distinguished spectrally, chemical or physicochemical separation may be necessary.

Solvent extraction techniques have been widely used in fluorometric analysis to separate the analyte fluorophore from undesirable interferences. A combination of thin-layer chromatography (TLC) and solvent extraction has also been used to isolate analytes in cases where solvent extraction alone is not sufficient [24]. This involves the following: The analyte is first separated on a TLC plate with an appropriate adsorbent-solvent system, and the spot due to the analyte is detected visually under UV light. Part of the adsorbent on the TLC plate containing the analyte-spot is then scraped off, and the analyte is eluted from it with an appropriate solvent for fluorometric measurement. This method offers a high degree of flexibility and specificity for quantitative analysis. However, the precision of the analysis will depend on the quantitative transfer of adsorbent from the TLC plate in the elution step and the extent of recovery of the analyte from the adsorbent.

Recent developments in the direct quantitation of analytes on TLC plates or on paper chromatograms using scanning chromatogram analyzers has made it possible to eliminate the elution step following the chromatographic separation. This has resulted in greater precision, sensitivity, and time saving [25-27]. The method is usually referred to as "spectrofluorodensitometry" in the case of fluorometric measurement and "spectrophotodensitometry" in the case of UV-visible adsorptiometric measurement. Most of the manufacturers of spectrofluorometers and spectrophotometers supply the scanning chromatogram analyzer accessory. With this accessory a developed chromatoplate containing one or more well separated analyte spots is directly introduced into the scanner. The chromatoplate is then automatically scanned spatially at a desired rate while being excited with light of the appropriate wavelength. The detector detects the fluorescence emission from the chromatoplate at a chosen wavelength and after amplification; this signal is plotted as a function of the chromatoplate scanning rate with the help of a recorder. Some spectrofluorodensitometers and spectrophotodensitometers can be used in reflectance as well as transmission modes. The advantages and disadvantages of quantitative measure-

ments with either of these modes have been extensively discussed [28-34].
These direct scanning techniques have been finding increasing use in the
quantitative analysis of drugs and their metabolites [32-38].

If a separation step is impossible or undesirable, it may be possible to
compensate for the presence of interfering substances by the preparation
of an internal blank which is very nearly a true blank. An internal blank
is produced by adding to the sample, after its fluorescence intensity has
been measured, a nonfluorescent compound which specifically reacts with
the analyte to yield products which are not fluorescent at the excitation and
emission wavelengths used for the analysis. Alternatively, a compound
which specifically quenches the analyte luminescence may be used. If the
instrumental sensitivity should change between the time the analytical
curve is measured and the time that the sample is measured, (e.g., aging
of the excitation lamp, fatigue of the multiplier phototube, etc.), it is possible to correct for this by use of a reference solution. The reference
solution should contain a very stable, easily purified fluorescent species
which absorbs and fluoresces in the approximate wavelength range of interest (e.g., a dilute solution of quinine bisulfate in 0.1 M H_2SO_4). The concentration of the reference species should be on the linear portion of the
curve. After an analytical curve is determined, or during the establishment of the analytical curve, the fluorescence intensity of the reference
solution is also measured. When unknown samples are to be fluorometrically measured at some later time, the instrumental sensitivity is adjusted
to give the same reading originally obtained for the reference solution.
This adjustment is best accomplished by varying the amplifier gain or
phototube voltage rather than the monochromator spectral bandwidth, as
it is the former parameters which alter instrumental sensitivity by their
variance with time.

N. Common Interferences in Luminescence Measurements

1. Raman Bands from Solvents

Solvents containing carbon-hydrogen and oxygen-hydrogen bonds, when
excited with strong radiation, produce Raman bands shifted about 0.3 μm^{-1}
to the lower energy side of the exciting light. These bands can be mistaken
for part of the analyte fluorescence in qualitative fluorometric analysis and
cause serious interference in quantitative fluorometric measurements
when the Raman band of the solvent overlaps the fluorescence band of the
analyte. Unfortunately, most analytically useful solvents contain groups
which give rise to Raman scatter. The analyst must be aware of this
potential interference and should know means of minimizing its effect. It
should be noted that Raman bands are usually weak and do not interfere in
fluorometric measurements at low instrumental sensitivity.

In general, Raman bands can be distinguished from analyte emission by the facts that their wavelengths vary with a change in excitation wavelength and their band width, at constant emission slit, varies with the width of excitation slit. Interference from Raman bands, when present, can be minimized by using a cut-off filter before the emission monochromator to remove all wavelengths below and including the Raman band. Raman bands are not detected in a phosphorescence spectrometer because Raman scatter occurs within the lifetime of a vibration and is blocked by the phosphoroscope.

2. Luminescent Impurities

The fluorescent or phosphorescent impurities present in solvents and those present in reagents used for the preparation of fluorophores and buffers are common sources of interference in fluorometric analysis, especially at low analyte concentration. These interferences can be kept to a minimum by using pure solvents and reagents. Many of these chemicals are now available from commercial suppliers in a degree of purity which is designed for spectral studies. Some solvents can be purified by single or repeated distillation in scrupulously cleaned glassware. For example, ethyl alcohol, hexane, heptane, cyclohexane, isopentane, and ether can be purified by double distillation [3]. Tap water can also be freed from luminescent impurities by double distillation. A higher degree of purification of water can be achieved by first distilling it from alkaline permanganate solution followed by a second distillation. Deionization is also an effective way of purifying water as long as the first portion of the deionized water is rejected. Purified solvents should be stored in scrupulously cleaned glass bottles with aluminum-lined caps.

One of the most serious forms of interference is contamination of glassware and cuvettes, used in fluorometric analysis, with luminescent impurities. This contamination can be minimized by soaking all the glassware in a concentrated nitric acid bath for about 24 h, rinsing with tap water and distilled water, and drying in an oven. For best results nitric acid in the bath should be replaced with fresh nitric acid quite often. Cuvettes should be cleaned in a similar fashion when suspected of contamination. The repeated use of the nitric acid bath for cleaning cuvettes should be avoided, as this may damage the cuvettes. For routine work, the contamination of cuvettes can be minimized by rinsing them at least three times with the sample to be measured. If an ultrasonic cleaner is available, the cuvettes, during rinsing, should be placed in the ultrasonic cleaner for about 30 sec. Prolonged exposure of cuvettes to ultrasonic vibrations should be avoided as this could damage the cuvette joints. Cuvettes should be wiped with lint-free, soft tissue paper each time the cuvette is used. The use of soap or detergents to clean cuvettes should be avoided as these contain highly fluorescent components.

It should be pointed out that most of the plastic and polyethylene lab-ware contains strongly fluorescent impurities which can be leached into the solvents stored in such containers and cause serious interference. It is wise not to use plastic or polyethylene lab-ware for luminescence measurements, especially when high sensitivity is desired.

IV. APPLICATIONS TO DRUG METABOLISM RESEARCH

The quantity of drug present in a dosage form is seldom so small as to require a sensitive analytical method. However, the concentration of drugs and drug metabolites in blood, urine, tissue, and other biological samples are usually extremely low, and fluorometry finds wide application in quantitative studies of rates and mechanisms of drug absorption, metabolism, and excretion. Many compounds of biological origin also fluoresce and therefore are potential interferences in the fluorometric assays of biological samples. Consequently, as a rule, separation of the analytes by extraction or chromatography may be necessary before the fluorescence assay of the desired components can be carried out. In those cases where the drug of interest and its metabolites are separated simultaneously, the drug metabolites will often fluoresce in the same spectral region as the parent drug. This will especially be the case if the metabolic disposition of the drug involves chemical transformation of an alkyl side chain or some other group not intimately coupled with the aromatic portion of the drug (the fluorophore). In this case, physiochemical separation of the drug and its various metabolites becomes necessary if meaningful analytical information is to be obtained. Alternatively, if metabolic transformation of the drug involves chemical transformation of the fluorophore (e.g., aromatic hydroxylation) the spectral properties of the drug and its metabolites will generally be substantially different. For example, phenolic molecules generally absorb and fluoresce at substantially longer wavelength than the nonhydroxylated aromatic molecules. In this case, chemical separation of unmetabolized and metabolized drugs may not be necessary. The differences between excitation and emission spectra of drug and metabolites may allow for sufficient instrumental resolution. Even in those cases where initial fluorometric examination of the solution containing a drug and its metabolites indicates inadequate spectral resolution, it is often possible to vary chemical parameters of the analytical medium, such as pH. If the metabolites contain acidic or basic functional groups not present in the parent drug, selective shifting of the excitation and emission spectra or selective quenching of the fluorescence of certain components of the analytical sample caused by ionization may induce sufficient instrumental resolution to obviate the necessity of physicochemical separation of the drug and its metabolites.

As mentioned earlier, contaminants of biological origin may also complicate fluorometric analysis. However, either on a trial and error basis or if the identity of the fluorescing contaminants is known, chemical modification of the analytical sample may be employed to minimize the interference from the contaminant. For example, tryptophan is often a fluorescing contaminant in biological samples. However, the fluorescence of tryptophan (maximum at 348 nm) is quenched in acid solution at pH below 1 [23] so that cinchonine, which fluoresces in neutral solutions in the same general region as tryptophan but fluoresces intense blue in acid solutions, can be determined unambiguously in the latter media in the presence of tryptophan [39].

From the pharmacological point of view it may be most desirable to employ fluorometry to determine concentrations of unmetabolized drug or any of the various forms of the metabolized drug in biological samples. However, from the analytical point of view there are two circumstances which make it preferable to determine the unmetabolized drug rather than its metabolites. First, the number of drug metabolites whose spectroscopic properties are known is relatively small compared to the number of drugs whose fluorescences have been studied. Second, in most cases the amount of unmetabolized drug recovered from biological samples is generally greater than the amounts of the metabolites present in the sample. In many cases, the quantities of metabolites recoverable from blood or urine samples are so small as to defy estimation even by a method as sensitive as fluorometry.

Fluorometric analytical methods for several common drugs are listed in Tables 1 and 2 (see pp. 236-245). Since there are several books and review published describing the details of fluorometric analysis of these drugs [23, 40-44], the present discussion will be limited to the few examples illustrating the use of different techniques involved in development of a fluorometric method of analysis.

There are two major types of techniques used in fluorometric analysis of drugs: direct and indirect. The direct fluorometric method uses the native fluorescence of the analyte and as such is limited to those drugs and metabolites containing aromatic rings or highly conjugated aliphatic systems. Even in this class of analytes not all members fluoresce. However, compensating for the lack of universality of the directly excited fluorescence is the specificity and great sensitivity of analysis resulting from the fluorescence properties inherent to the analyte of interest. For example, the antidepressant imipramine (Tofranil) and its metabolite desmethylimipramine both have native fluorescence in strongly alkaline solution. In 3 N NaOH both the compounds have excitation maxima at 295 nm and emission maxima at 415 nm. Based on the natural fluorescence of these compounds, Dingell and coworkers [45] have developed a procedure for the fluorometric analysis of imipramine and desmethylimipramine

in biological material. Another example representative of the direct
fluorometric analysis is the assay of lysergic acid diethylamide (LSD) and
its phenolic metabolite. LSD is fluorescent with excitation maxima at 325
nm and emission maxima at 445 nm [46]. Axelrod and coworkers [46]
have devised a method for the analysis of LSD in tissues which can determine as little as 3 ng of the compound per gram of tissue. Aghajanian and
Bing [47] applied the method of Axelrod and coworkers [46] to analyze LSD
in plasma. Szara [48] identified and characterized a phenolic metabolite
of LSD as 13-hydroxy-LSD which showed native fluorescence in 0.2 N acetic
acid. The metabolite can be separated from LSD by prior extraction of
tissue extracts with benzene to remove LSD and analyzed fluorometrically
in 0.2 N acetic acid.

Indirect fluorometric methods are used for analytes which are weakly
fluorescent or nonfluorescent. This method involves either the conversion
of the analyte to a fluorescent derivative, using an appropriate reaction
scheme, or the utilization of the capability of the analyte to influence (enhance or quench) the fluorescence of a fluorescent dye.

Conversion of the analyte to a fluorescent derivative can be achieved
by several techniques. Oxidation, for example, is used to convert pheno-
thiazines into corresponding sulfoxides which are highly fluorescent [49, 50].
Morphine can be analyzed fluorometrically by oxidizing it to fluorescent
pseudomorphine [51]. Several antihistamines yield fluorescent products
on oxidation that can be used for their analysis [52]. Dehydration of car-
diotonic steroids yield fluorescent products, and this reaction is used to
develop several analytical methods for the steroids [53, 54].

Some compounds can be converted to fluorescent derivatives by treating
them with strong mineral acids. For example, morphine gives a highly
fluorescent derivative after being heated in concentrated sulfuric acid.
The reaction product fluoresces when the solution is made alkaline [55].
Codeine and codethyline, when heated in concentrated sulfuric acid and
then making the solution alkaline, show analytically useful fluorescence
[56]. Chlorprothixene, a thioxanthene derivative, gives a fluorescent
product in concentrated phosphoric acid [57]. Reserpine can be converted
to a fluorescent derivative by treating it with nitrous acid [58].

Weakly fluorescent or nonfluorescent primary arylamines and arylhydrazines can be condensed with aldehydes to often yield fluorescent
derivatives. Similarly, aldehydes of analytical interest which generally
do not fluoresce may be condensed with arylhydrazines, such as naphthyl-
hydrazines, or arylamines to yield fluorescent products. A general fluorometric procedure for assaying primary amines using fluorescamine
reagent has been developed by Udenfriend and coworkers [59, 60]. Fluorescamine is a high-sensitivity fluorogenic reagent that reacts directly
with primary amines to form intense fluorophors. Mehta and Schulman

TABLE 1

Fluorometric Methods of Analysis for Some Pharmaceuticals: Direct Methods[a]

Compounds	Solvent	pH	λ_{ex} (nm)	λ_f (nm)	Sensitivity[b]	Ref.
Allylmorphine	Water	1	285	355	Fair	[23]
p-Aminobenzoic acid	Water	8	295	345	Fair	[23]
Aminopterin	Water	7	280, 370	460	Fair	[23]
p-Aminosalicylic acid	Water	11	300	405	Good	[23]
Amobarbital	Water	14	265	410	Fair	[78]
Antimycin A	Water	8	350	420	Fair	[79]
Apomorphin	Ethyl acetate	--	270	370	Fair	[123]
Bromolysergic acid diethylamide	Water	1	315	460	Fair	[23]
Bufotenine	Water	<0	292	520	Fair	[80]
Cinchonidine	Water	1	315	445	Poor	[23]
Cinchonine	Water	1	320	420	Poor	[23]
Codeine	Water	7	285	350	Poor	[81]
Dantrolene	N,N-Dimethyl Formamide-water	--	395	530	Fair	[82]

Desmethylimipramine	Water	14	295	415	Fair	[45, 83, 84]
Diphenylhydramine HCl	Water	2	258	285	Fair	[147]
5,5-Disubstituted oxybarbiturates	0.1 M NaOH	--	267-278	420	Poor	[148]
Eserine	Water	1-7	265, 315	350	Fair	[85]
Estrogens	Water	13	490	546	Fair	[86]
Ethacridine	Water	2	370, 425	515	Good	[87]
5-Fluorocytosine	Water	~13	300	365	Fair	[126]
Gentisic acid	Water	7	315	440	Fair	[23]
Griseofulvin	Water	7	295, 335	450	Good	[23]
Harmine	Water	1	300, 365	400	Good	[23]
Hydroxyamphetamine	Water	1	275	300	Poor	[23]
3-Hydroxy-N-methyl morphinan	Water	1	275	320	Fair	[88]
Imipramine	Water	14	295	415	Fair	[45]
Lysergic acid diethylamide	Water	7	325	365		[88]
	Acid	--	325	445	Good	[46, 47, 89, 90]
Menadione	Ethanol	--	335	480	Fair	[23]
Mephenesin	Water	1	280	315	Fair	[23]

TABLE 1 (Continued)

Compounds	Solvent	pH	λ_{ex} (nm)	λ_f (nm)	Sensitivity[b]	Ref.
Morphine	Water	7	285	350	Fair	[81]
	Water	1	285	350	Fair	[91]
Mycophenolic acid	Water	10	350	438	Fair	[143]
Neocinchophen	Water	7	275, 345	455	Good	[88]
Neosynephrine	Water	1	270	305	Good	[88]
Oxychloroquin	Water	11	335	380	Fair	[88]
Pamaquin	Water	13	300, 370	530	Fair	[88]
Pentobarbital	Water	13	265	440	Fair	[23]
Piperoxan	Water	7	290	325	Fair	[23]
Podophyllotoxin	Water	11	280	325	Good	[23]
Procaine	Water	11	275	345	Good	[23]
Quinacrine	Water	11	285, 420	500	Fair	[23]
Quinidine	Water	1	350	450	Fair	[23, 92]
	Acid	--	360	460		
Quinine	Water	1	250, 350	450	Good	[23]
Rescinnamine	Water	1	310	400	Good	[23]

Salicylic acid	Water	10	310	400	Good	[23, 93]
Sarcolysine	Water	7	260	365	n.i.	[94]
Sotalol–HCl	Alkaline solution	--	250	350	Fair	[120]
	Acidic solution	--	235	309		
Spironolactone	62% v/v H_2SO_4	--	483	525	Good	[124]
Streptomycin	Water	13	366	445	Fair	[95]
Sulfanilamide	Water	3–10	275	350	Fair	[96]
Thiamylal	Water	13	310	530	Fair	[23]
Thiopental	Water	13	315	530	Fair	[23]
Thymoxamine	Water	7–8	295	335	Fair	[142]
		1			
Tribromsalan	Ethyl acetate	--	362	422	Fair	[140]
Warfarin	Methanol	--	290, 342	385	Fair	[23, 97]
Yohimbine	Water	1	270	360	Fair	[23]
Zoxazolamine	Water	11	280	320	Fair	[23]

[a] This table is not meant to be exhaustive, but to show representative methods of analysis in drug research. Readers are urged to consult the original references for procedural details of the analytical methods listed.

[b] Sensitivity: good, < 0.01 ppm; fair, 0.01 to 0.1 ppm; poor, > 0.1 ppm.

n.i., not indicated.

TABLE 2

Fluorometric Methods of Analysis for Some Pharmaceuticals: Indirect Methods[a]

Compounds	Reagent and reaction	λ_{ex} (nm)	λ_f (nm)	Sensitivity[b]	Ref.
Acetylsalicylic acid	Hydrolysis to salicylic acid 1% acetic acid-chloroform	313 280	442 335	Good Good	[93, 98] [99, 100]
Actinomycin D	Oxidation with H_2O_2	370	420	Fair	[101]
Aliphatic amines (primary and secondary)	Reaction with 9-isothiocyanato-acridine	See ref.	See ref.	See ref.	[129]
	Condensation with fluorescamine	See ref.	See ref.	See ref.	[146]
5-Alkyl-2-thiohydantoine	2,6-Dichloroquinone chlorimide	365	520	Poor	[102]
Alloxan	Condensation with o-phenylene-diamine	405	520	Good	[23]
n-Allylnormorphine	Heating with conc. H_2SO_4	365	420	Fair	[55]
p-Aminobenzoic acid	Condensation with fluorescamine	405	500	Good	[146]
7-Aminoclonazepam	Condensation with fluorescamine	412	505	Fair	[146]
7-Amino-3-hydroxy-clonazepam	Condensation with fluorescamine	412	505	Fair	[146]
p-Aminosalicylic acid	Condensation with fluorescamine	405	495	Fair	[146]
Amphetamine	Reaction with 9-isothiocyanato-acridine	300	520	Fair	[129]

Compound	Method				Ref.
Amphetamine sulfate	Condensation with fluorescamine	395	490	Fair	[146]
Ampicillin	Acidic hydrolysis in presence of formaldehyde	346	422	Good	[119]
Aristolochic acid	Reduction with sodium hydrosulfite	340	n.i.	Fair	[141]
Atabrine	Caffeine-0.05 M H_2SO_4	365	540	Good	[103]
Atropine	Coupling with eosine γ	365	556	Poor	[71]
Bethanidine	Coupling with eosine γ	535	560	Good	[135]
Bromridazine	Oxidation with H_2O_2	340	380	Poor	[104]
Carbidopa	Condensation with p-dimethyl-aminobenzaldehyde in $CHCl_3$	466	546	Fair	[130]
Carphenazine	Oxidation with H_2O_2	370	475	Poor	[104]
Chloridazine	Oxidation with H_2O_2	340	380	Poor	[104]
Chlorothen	Coupling with cyanogen bromide	345	414	Fair	[52]
Chlorpromazine	Oxidation with H_2O_2 reaction with 9-bromomethyl acridine followed by UV irradiation	340 350	385 474	Fair Fair	[105, 106] [136]
Chlorpromazine metabolites	Coupling with dimethylamino-naphthyl sulfonyl chloride	320-358	460-535	Good	[118]
Chlorphenothiazine	Oxidation with $KMnO_4$ in O_2N H_2SO_4	360	440	Fair	[49, 50]

TABLE 2 (Continued)

Compounds	Reagent and reaction	λ_{ex} (nm)	λ_f (nm)	Sensitivity[b]	Ref.
Chlorprothixene	Oxidation with H_2O_2	345	410	Poor	[104]
Digitalis alkaloids	HCl–glycerol heating with strong acid acetic anhydride and CF_3 COOH	UV UV 470	Green Green 500	Fair	[107] [54] [108]
Dihydroisoquinolines	Chemical or photo–oxidation	335	380	Fair	[128]
Diphenylhydramine	Coupling with tinopal GS	365	450	Poor	[68]
Diphenylhydantoin	Oxidation with alkaline $KMnO_4$	360	490	Poor	[144]
Emetine	Iodine in alkali	436	570, 620	Fair	[109]
Epinephrine	Conversion to trihydroxyindole	455	540	Good	[23]
Flurazepam and metabolites	Acid hydrolysis followed by conversion to 9–acridone with K_2CO_3 – DMF	See ref.	See ref.	See ref.	[122]
Heroine	Heating with conc. H_2SO_4	365	420	Good	[55]
Hydrazine	Condensation with p–dimethyl–aminobenzaldehyde	466	546	Good	[149]
5–Hydroxytryptophan	Condensation with o–phthaldi–aldehyde	360	480	Good	[150]

Isoniazide	Condensation with salicyl-aldehyde	392	478	Good	[110] [111] [133]
Isosulfisoxazole	Condensation with fluorescamine	400	495	Good	[146]
Mescaline	Condensation with formaldehyde and NH_3	375	515	Good	[112]
Metaraminol	Condensation with o-phthaldehyde	370	500	Good	[62]
Methapyrilene	Coupling with cyanogen bromide	350	412	Good	[52]
Methotrexate	Oxidation with $KMnO_4$	280, 370	450	Fair	[23]
3-Methoxy-4-hydroxy-phenylalanine	Condensation with fluorescamine	390	480	Fair	[138]
Methyltestosterone	Reaction with ascorbic acid – HCl	470	530	Good	[125]
Morphine	Heating with conc. H_2SO_4	365	420	Good	[51, 55]
Oxytetracycline	Complexation with Mg^{2+} alkaline degradation	390	520	Fair	[65]
		337	410	Fair	[127]
Pancuronium bromide	Coupling with rose bengal	340	490, 550	Fair	[145]
Penicillin	Coupling with 2-methoxy-6-chloro-9β-aminoethylacridine	420	500	Fair	[23]
Pheniramine	Coupling with cyanogen bromide	275	434	Poor	[52]
Phenothiazines	Oxidation with H_2O_2	See ref.	See ref.	Poor	[106]
Phenylpropanolamine	Condensation with fluorescamine	395	490	Fair	[146]

TABLE 2 (Continued)

Compounds	Reagent and reaction	λ_{ex} (nm)	λ_f (nm)	Sensitivity[b]	Ref.
Procainamide	Condensation with fluorescamine	400	498	Fair	[134]
		400	485	Fair	[139]
Procaine HCl	Condensation with fluorescamine	400	485	Good	[146]
Pyribenzamine	Coupling with cyanogen bromide	370	460	Poor	[23, 113]
Quinapyramine	Coupling with eosin	365	550	Good	[114]
Reserpine	Oxidation	350	440	Good	[23, 115]
Rifampicin	Oxidation with H_2O_2	370	480	Fair	[137]
Salicylamide metabolites	Acid hydrolysis	310	435	--	[121]
Streptomycin	Coupling with β-naphthoquin-one-4-sulfonate	365	445	Fair	[87]
Sulfadiazine Sulfadoxidine					
Sulfamethoxazole Sulfanilamide Sulfisoxazole	Condensation with fluorescamine	400	495	Good	[146]
Sulfonamides	Coupling with 4,5-methylene-dioxyphthaldehyde	320, 327	375, 425	Good	[116]

Tetracycline	Complexation with calcium and barbituric acid	405	530	Good	[67]
Tetrahydroisoquinolines	Chemical- or photo-oxidation	370	458	Fair	[128]
Thioridazine	Oxidation with H_2O_2	365	440	Good	[105, 106, 132]
Trimethoprim	Oxidation with $KMnO_4$	275	350	Fair	[117]
		275	345	Fair	[131]
d-Tubocurarine	Coupling with Rose Bengal	570	590	Good	[69]

[a]This table is not meant to be exhaustive, but to show representative methods of analysis in drug research. Readers are urged to consult the original references for procedural details of the analytical methods listed.

[b]Sensitivity: good, < 0.01 ppm; fair, 0.01 to 0.1 ppm; poor, > 0.1 ppm.

n.i., not indicated

[61] applied the procedure of Udenfriend to the determination of amphetamine. Metaraminol, a potent sympathomimetic agent related m-hydroxy-
phenylethylamine analogs, can be analyzed fluorometrically based on condensation with aldehydes [62, 63]. α-Methyldopamine and α-methylnor-
epinephrine can be determined fluorometrically by a condensation method
developed by Schümann and coworkers [64].

Chelation of the analyte with certain metal ions yields analytically useful fluorescent chelates. For example, the magnesium chelates of tetracyclines are highly fluorescent, and some tetracycline-metal complexes
have been used for the fluorometric analysis of tetracyclines [65, 66]. Kohn
[67] has developed a highly sensitive and specific methof for the tetracycline
antibiotics (with the exception of oxytetracycline) based on the ability of the
tetracycline to form extractable mixed complexes with calcium and barbiturates.

Drugs that have basic groups can interact with water soluble acidic fluorescent dyes, such as Eosin, to form neutral complexes which will be extractable into organic solvents. Since the polar dye will not be extracted
into the organic solvent, the fluorescence of the extract will be a measure
of the concentration of the basic drug. Glazko and coworkers [68] have
investigated a variety of acid dyes and conditions for their application to
the assay of basic drugs. For example, the nonfluorescent antihistamine,
diphenylhydramine (Benadryl) can be assayed by using the dye Tinopal GS
[68]. d-Tubocurarine can be analyzed fluorometrically by using the dye
Rose Bengal [69]. Generally, when an organic base-dye complex is formed,
the spectral characteristics of the dye are changed. This change can be
utilized for the fluorometric assay of the complex. Laugel [70] has developed such a procedure for the assay of basic drugs. Ogawa and coworkers
[71] have used Eosin Y to measure atropine by complex formation in chloroform according to the procedure of Laugel [70].

Some drugs may interact with intensely fluorescent dyes and quench the
fluorescence of the latter. The extent of quenching can be quantitatively
related to the concentration of the quencher. For example, Sturgeon and
Schulman [72] have developed a quenchofluorometric method of analysis of
arylamine type drugs using the intensely fluorescent Bratton-Marshall
reagent, N-(1-naphthyl)ethylenediamine. When a weakly or nonfluorescent
arylamine is first diazotized and then condensed with Bratton-Marshall
reagent, a nonfluorescent diazo derivative results, thereby quenching the
fluorescence of the reagent. Thus, by quantitating the disappearance of
the fluorescence of Bratton-Marshall reagent, the concentration of arylamine can be determined [72].

The indirect method has the general advantage over the direct method in that, provided that a suitable reactant can be found to produce a fluorescent derivative, virtually any drug or metabolite having functional groups can be made amenable to fluorometric analysis. However, it should be borne in mind that derivatization methods are most often applicable to classes of analytes rather than specific analytes and that the fluorescence of the derivative usually arises from an electronic transition localized on the derivatizing reagent. As a result, the gain in generality of this method is partially offset by the sacrifice of the analytical selectivity. Moreover, because the derivatization reaction is at least bimolecular in the great majority of cases, the maximum obtainable fluorescence intensity from the derivative will be limited by the concentration of the analyte, not only in the same sense as is directly excited fluorescence, but also by the completeness of the derivatization reaction. The latter will generally decrease as the analyte concentration decreases. Consequently, indirect fluorometry will in many cases be less sensitive than direct fluorometry.

Up to the present, the discussion of the application of fluorometry to drug metabolism research has been confined to the determination of absolute amount of drug or metabolite recovered from a biological sample. However, the most elegant metabolic studies may entail the need for information about the relative fraction of drugs in true solution in the interstitial and the intracellular fluids and bound to cellular and extracellular structures, such as proteins, nucleic acids, and membranes. Some drugs containing aromatic rings demonstrate changes in their fluorescent properties upon passing from aqueous solution to a bound condition on cellular structures. Some molecules which do not fluoresce in aqueous solution become fluorescent upon binding. Others which fluoresce in fluid solution may have their fluorescences quenched upon binding. Still others may have their fluorescences shifted in energy, enhanced in intensity, or only partially quenched upon binding. The reason for the alterations of the fluorescence properties of these compounds upon binding has been a subject of much research interest. Although it is generally conceded that changes in the intensity and energy characterisitcs of the fluorescences of these molecules upon binding are due to environmental effects, the specific nature of these effects is the subject of much controversy. Arguments involving viscosity [73], hydrogen bonding [73], environmental dielectric strength [74], and excited state proton transfer [75] have been invoked, but no one of these adequately explains all of the observed effects. For the present discussion it will suffice to say that changes in the fluorescence spectrum occurring as a result of drug binding can be quantitatively related to the relative fractions of bound and unbound drugs. The exact form of the quantitative relation will depend upon whether the fluorescence intensity at the analytical wavelength is measurable for both bound and unbound forms of the molecule [76] or only for one of these categories [77].

V. A LOOK TOWARD THE FUTURE

Although analytical fluorescence spectroscopy has been employed in the study of drugs and drug metabolites for several decades, the field is not stagnant. Current research in the areas of molecular interactions, new reagents for preparing fluorescent derivatives of weakly fluorescent or nonfluorescent analytes, and new instrumental techniques promise to yield unprecedented selectivity and sensitivity in fluorometric analysis.

Among the most exciting instrumental developments which may soon find their way into investigative applications are laser excited fluorescence, time-resolved fluorometry, selective-modulation fluorometry, and micro-spectrofluorometry.

A. Laser-excited Fluorometry [151]

The laser is an excitation source which produces an extremely intense burst of highly monochromatic light. Because of the great intensity of the laser-produced light it is possible to excite virtually all the molecules in the optical path of the exciting light. With a convenient light source such as a xenon arc lamp, only a small fraction of the potentially fluorescent molecules in the optical path are excited at any instant of time. As a result, the laser enables the generation of measurable fluorescence from analytes having moderate to high quantum yields of fluorescence which are present in concentrations too low to be observed by conventional means. Although laser-excitation cannot alter the fraction of excited molecules which fluoresce, it can greatly increase the absolute number of molecules which are deactivated by fluorescence. Hence, the laser may substantially increase the number of molecular species which are amenable to analysis by fluorometry.

The highly monochromatic nature of laser radiation also means that the excitation spectra of several molecular species which are substantially overlapping can be resolved. Thus, selectivity of an order which is not obtainable with conventional broad-banded excitation sources and mono-chromators is also a desirable feature of laser-excited fluorescence. The principal difficulties with the present state of the art of laser-excited fluorescence spectroscopy are its high cost ($15,000 just for the excitation source) and the limited number of substances which demonstrate the lasing phenomenon (population inversion followed by light stimulated emission). The paucity of substances which emit UV radiation is especially acute, visible lasers being far more common. This is an especially serious limitation in drug analysis because most drugs which fluoresce are ex-cited by UV frequencies. However, in the future it is to be expected that the range of application of laser-excited fluorescence will be substantially expanded.

B. Time-resolved Fluorometry [152]

In the current practice of analytical fluorometry, selectivity, the resolution of the fluorescence of a substance of analytical interest from the emission of interfering substances, is achieved either by manipulation of the chemistry of the sample or by resolution of the excitation or emission spectra of the analyte and interferences by means of monochromators. In many cases such resolution is inadequate for analytical purposes, and time-consuming chemical separations are then required prior to the measurement of fluorescences. However, in many cases it is possible, in the event of several overlapping fluorescences, to achieve spectral resolution by means of the measurement of the differing decay-time characteristics of the overlapping fluorescences. This is accomplished by exciting the sample with a pulsed excitation source whose rise and decay time is shorter than the lifetime of the lowest excited singlet state of the analyte of interest. The fluorescence observed from the sample will then show the composite decay characteristics of all fluorescing species whose decay times are longer than that of the pulsed source. If the decay characteristics of the pulsed source and those of the sample are respectively fed into the two channels of a dual beam oscilloscope, the decay curve from the source can be used to calibrate the time-axis of the oscilloscope screen while the decay curve from the sample can be taken as representative of the decay characterisitcs of the sample. If the decay-times of the fluorescing components of the sample are different (even though their fluorescence spectra may overlap), a plot of the logarithm of the intensity of fluorescence of the sample (calibrated against suitable standards) against the decay time, will yield several straight line segments. This plot is similar to that employed in radiochemical analysis for the resolution of nuclides of differing lifetimes. Each straight-line segment corresponds to the decay of a different fluorescing component of the sample, those demonstrating the steepest slopes having the shortest decay times. The extrapolation of each line segment to the intensity (concentration) axis will yield the concentration of the corresponding fluorescing species. The identity of each species can be established by comparing the time-axis intercept of each line segment with the decay-time characteristics of the fluorescence of a pure sample of each analyte. In this way the concentrations of several species, whose fluorescences overlap, can be determined without chemical separation. The principal difficulties of this method lie with the currently primitive instrumentation available for lifetime measurement and the need for computerization in cases where several fluorescing materials of only slightly differing lifetime of fluorescence are present.

C. Selective-modulation Fluorometry

A recently established method alternative to time-resolution for the determination of fluorescing analytes whose excitation or emission spectra
overlap is selective-modulation fluorometry [153]. In this method either
the excitation wavelength is modulated (scanned rapidly back and forth over
a small wavelength interval) and the fluorescence spectrum scanned in toto,
or the fluorescence wavelength is modulated and the excitation monochromator scanned. This technique produces essentially a difference fluorescence
or excitation spectrum which by means of frequency-selective electronics
(a lock-in amplifier) and judicious choice of the modulation interval enables
the emissions of the fluorescing components to be measured independently.
Presumably, future demand for this instrumentation will bring the cost of
the sophisticated electronics down to the point where it can enjoy wide
application in analytical laboratories.

D. Microspectrofluorometry

Fluorescence microscopy has been employed for some time in clinical
chemistry for qualitative immunofluorescent identification of pathogens
and in the identification of cellular structures by fluorescent staining techniques. However, recently the development and commercial availability
of monochromated microspectrofluorometers capable of quantitative measurement by means of phototubes has become a reality [152].

The microspectrofluorometer is, in essence, a fluorescence spectrometer coupled to a dark-field microscope. The microscope stage serves as
the sample compartment and is flooded by exciting light coming through the
excitation monochromator of the spectrometer. The fluorescence from a
specimen on the microscope stage is focused through the optics of the
microscope and may be observed visually through the ocular or passed
through an emission monochromator to a photodetector and onto a suitable
readout device. The dark-field optical arrangement of the microscope
prevents the exciting light which floods the microscope stage from being
transmitted through the barrel of the microscope and thereby eliminates
this intense light as a source of interference. Modern microspectrofluorometers can be employed to take excitation and emission spectra of cross-
sections as small as 1 μm in diameter. Consequently, this device is useful not only for the fluorometric analysis of small tissue samples, but also
for the quantification of drugs in specific parts of single cells. Moreover,
the ability to record excitation and emission spectra with the microspectrofluorometer is potentially of great use in studying the nature of the interactions of drugs and metabolites with specific cellular structures. Although

the technology of microspectrofluorometry is at a relatively advanced state, it has yet to be applied to pharmaceutical problems. Presumably, this situation will change in the next few years.

ACKNOWLEDGMENT

This work was supported in part by the College of Pharmacy, University of Kentucky, Lexington, Kentucky, where SGS was employed as a visiting professor during the spring of 1976.

The authors are grateful to Ms. Lauren Brewster, Ms. Mickey Mills, and Miss Vicki Cooper for typing the manuscript.

REFERENCES

1.   J. D. Winefordner, W. J. McCarthy, and P. A. St. John, in Methods of Biochemical Analysis, Vol. 15 (D. Glick, ed.), Wiley (interscience), New York, 1967.

2.   J. D. Winefordner, P. A. St. John, and W. J. McCarthy, in Fluorescence Assay in Biology and Medicine, Vol. 2 (S. Udenfriend, ed.), Academic Press, New York, 1969, Chap. 2.

3.   J. D. Winefordner, S. G. Schulman, and T. C. O'Haver, Luminescence Spectrometry in Analytical Chemistry, Wiley (Interscience), New York, 1972.

4.   D. M. Hercules, in Fluorescence and Phosphorescence Analysis (D. M. Hercules, ed.), Wiley (Interscience), New York, 1966, Chap. 1.

5.   C. A. Parker, Photoluminescence of Solutions, American Elsevier, New York, 1968.

6.   A. J. Pesce, C. G. Rosen, and T. L. Pasby, Fluorescence Spectroscopy, Dekker, New York, 1971, Chaps. 1, 2.

7.   G. H. Schenk, Absorption of Light and Ultraviolet Radiation: Fluorescence and Phosphorescence Emission, Allyn and Bacon, Boston, 1973.

8.   S. G. Schulman and J. D. Winefordner, Talanta, 17, 607 (1970).

9.   E. L. Wehry and L. B. Rogers, in Fluorescence and Phosphorescence Analysis (D. M. Hercules, ed.), Wiley (Interscience), New York, 1966, Chap. 3.

10. N. Mataga and T. Kubota, Molecular Interactions and Electronic Spectra, Dekker, New York, 1970.

11. S. G. Schulman and W. L. Paul, Fluorescence News, 7, (4), 25, (1973).

12. S. G. Schulman, Fluorescence News, 7, (5), 33 (1973).
13. S. G. Schulman, in Physical Methods in Heterocyclic Chemistry, Vol. 7 (A. R. Katritzky, ed.), Academic Press, New York, 1974.
14. E. L. Wehry, Fluorescence News, 6, (3), 1 (1972).
15. S. G. Schulman, Fluorescence News, 6, (4), 1 (1972).
16. A. Weller, Progr. React. Kin., 1, 187 (1961).
17. E. Vander Donckt, Progr. React. Kin., 5, 274 (1970).
18. S. G. Schulman, Rev. Anal. Chem., 1, 85 (1971).
19. S. G. Schulman, in Modern Fluorescence Spectroscopy, Vol. 2 (E. L. Wehry, ed.), Plenum, New York, 1976.
20. N. J. Turro, Molecular Photochemistry, W. A. Benjamin, New York, 1967, Chap. 5.
21. I. B. Berlman, Energy Transfer Parameters of Aromatic Compounds, Academic Press, New York, 1973.
22. O. Stern and M. Volmer, Z. Physik, 20, 183 (1919).
23. S. Udenfriend, Fluorescence Assay in Biology and Medicine, Academic Press, New York, 1962.
24. H. Gänshirt, in Thin Layer Chromatography, 2nd ed. (E. Stahl, ed.), Springer-Verlag, New York, 1969.
25. G. Pataki, Chromatographia, 1, 492 (1968).
26. V. Novacek, Amer. Lab., 1, 27 (1969).
27. M. S. Lefar and A. D. Lewis, Anal. Chem., 42, 79A (1970).
28. J. C. Touchstone, S. S. Levin, and T. Matawec, Anal. Chem., 43, 858 (1971).
29. H. Zücher, G. Pataki, J. Borko, and R. W. Frei, J. Chromatogr., 43, 457 (1969).
30. V. Pollack and A. A. Boulton, J. Chromatogr., 45, 200 (1969); 50, 30 (1970).
31. H. Jork, J. Chromatogr., 48, 372 (1970).
32. J. Petryka, J. Chromatogr., 50, 447 (1970).
33. J. C. Touchstone, T. Murawec, M. Kasparow, and A. K. Balin, J. Chromatogr. Sci., 8, 81 (1970).
34. V. M. Novacek, Amer. Lab., 5, 85 (1973).
35. R. W. Frei and J. F. Lawrence, J. Chromatogr., 61, 174 (1971).
36. R. W. Frei, J. F. Lawrence, and D. S. Le Gay, Analyst (London), 98, 9 (1973).
37. C. W. Sigel and M. E. Grace, J. Chromatogr., 80, 111 (1973).
38. J. A. F. de Silva, I. Bekersky, and C. V. Puglisi, J. Pharm. Sci., 63, 1837 (1974).
39. B. B. Brodie, S. Udenfriend, W. Dill, and G. Downing, J. Biol. Chem., 168, 311 (1947).
40. S. Udenfriend, Fluorescence Assay in Biology and Medicine, Vol. II, Academic Press, New York, 1969.
41. J. A. F. de Silva, J. Forensic Sci., 14, 184 (1969).
42. D. W. Cornish, D. M. Grossman, A. L. Jacobs, A. F. Michaelis, and B. Salsitz, Anal. Chem., 45, 22IR (1973).

43. A. Weissler, Anal. Chem., 46, 500R (1974).
44. G. G. Guilbault, Practical Fluorescence: Theory, Methods and Techniques, Dekker, New York, 1973.
45. J. V. Dingell, F. Salser, and J. R. Gilette, J. Pharmacol. Exp. Ther., 143, 14 (1964).
46. J. Axelrod, R. O. Brady, B. Witkop, and E. V. Evarts, Ann. N. Y. Acad. Sci., 66, 435 (1957).
47. G. K. Aghajanian and H. L. Bing, Clin. Pharmacol. Ther., 5, 611 (1964).
48. S. Szara, Life Sci. (Oxford), 9, 662 (1963).
49. T. J. Mellinger and C. E. Keeler, Anal. Chem., 35, 554 (1963).
50. T. J. Mellinger and C. F. Keeler, Anal. Chem., 36, 1840 (1964).
51. H. Kupferberg, A. Burkhalter, and E. L. Way, J. Pharmacol. Exp. Ther., 145, 247 (1964).
52. R. E. Jensen and R. T. Pflaum, J. Pharm. Sci., 53, 835 (1964).
53. M. Frèrejacque and P. De Graeve, Ann. Pharm. Fr., 21, 509 (1963).
54. D. Wells, B. Katzung, and F. H. Meyers, J. Pharm. Pharmacol., 13, 389 (1961).
55. G. Nadeau and G. Sobolewski, Can. J. Biochem. Physiol., 36, 625 (1958).
56. P. H. Balatre, M. Traisnel, and J. R. Delcambre, Ann. Pharm. Fr., 19, 171 (1961).
57. T. J. Mellinger, E. M. Mellinger, and W. T. Smith, Amer. J. Psychiat., 120, 1111 (1964).
58. R. P. Haycock, P. B. Sheth, and W. J. Mader, J. Pharm. Sci., 48, 479 (1959).
59. S. Udenfriend, S. Stein, P. Bohlen, W. Dairman, W. Leimgruber, and M. Wiegele, Science, 178, 871 (1973).
60. S. Stein, P. Bohlen, K. Imaj, J. Stone, and S. Udenfriend, Fluorescence News, 7, 9 (1973).
61. A. C. Mehta and S. G. Schulman, J. Pharm. Sci., 63, 1150 (1974).
62. P. A. Shore and H. S. Alpers, Life Sci. (Oxford), 3, 551 (1964).
63. W. F. Coulson, A. D. Smith, and J. B. Jepson, Anal. Biochem., 10, 101 (1965).
64. H. J. Schümann, H. Grobecker, and K. Schmidt, Arch. Exp. Pathol. Pharmakol., 251, 48 (1965).
65. K. H. Ibsen, R. L. Saunders, and M. R. Urist, Anal. Biochem., 5, 505 (1963).
66. R. G. Kelly, H. A. Floyd, and K. D. Hoyt, Antimicrobial Agents and Chemotherapy, American Society of Microbiologists, Ann Arbor, Michigan, 1966, p. 666.
67. K. W. Kohn, Anal. Chem., 33, 862 (1961).
68. A. J. Glazko, W. A. Dill, and R. L. Fransway, Fed. Proc., 21, 269 (1962).

69. E. N. Cohen, J. Lab. Clin. Med., 61, 338 (1963).

70. M. P. Laugel, Compt. Rend. Acad. Sci., 255, 692 (1962).

71. S. Ogawa, M. Morita, K. Nishiura, and K. Fujisawa, J. Pharm. Soc. (Japan) (Yakugaku Zasshi), 85, 650 (1965).

72. R. J. Sturgeon and S. G. Schulman, Anal. Chim. Acta, 75, 225 (1975).

73. W. O. McClure and G. M. Edelman, Biochem., 5, 1908 (1966).

74. D. C. Turner and L. Brand, Biochem., 7, 3381 (1968).

75. L. Styrer, J. Amer. Chem. Soc., 88, 5708 (1966).

76. D. V. Naik, W. L. Paul, and S. G. Schulman, J. Pharm. Sci., 64, 1677 (1975).

77. D. V. Naik, W. L. Paul, R. M. Threatte, and S. G. Schulman, Anal. Chem., 47, 267 (1975).

78. J. E. Swagzdis and T. L. Flanagan, Anal. Biochem., 7, 147 (1964).

79. S. N. Sehgal and C. Vezina, Anal. Biochem., 21, 266 (1967).

80. J. W. Bridges and R. T. Williams, Biochem. J., 107, 225 (1968).

81. R. Brandt, S. Ehrlich-Rogozinsky, and N. D. Cheronis, Microchem. J., 5, 215 (1961).

82. R. D. Hollifield and John D. Conklin, J. Pharm. Sci., 62, 271 (1973).

83. J. Gilette, J. Dingell, F. Sulser, R. Kuntzman, and B. Brodie, Experientia, 17, 377 (1961).

84. N. A. Small, Clin. Chim. Acta, 8, 803 (1963).

85. R. Williams, in Spectrofluorimetric Techniques in Biology, NATO Advanced Study Institute, Milan, 1964, p. 233.

86. H. Strickler and P. Stanchak, Clin. Chem., 15, 137 (1969).

87. B. Issekutz and P. Hajdu, Arzneim.-Forsch., 16, 645 (1966).

88. S. Udenfriend, D. Duggan, B. Vasta, and B. Brodie, J. Pharmacol. Exp. Ther., 120, 26 (1957).

89. K. Genest and C. G. Farmilo, J. Pharm. Pharmacol., 16, 250 (1964).

90. L. A. Dal Cortivo, J. R. Broich, A. Dihrberg, and B. Newman, Anal. Chem., 38, 1959 (1966).

91. R. Bowman, P. Caulfield, and S. Udenfriend, Science, 122, 32 (1955).

92. A. Edgar and M. Sokolov, J. Lab. Clin. Med., 36, 478 (1950).

93. W. E. Lange and S. A. Bell, J. Pharm. Sci., 55, 386 (1966).

94. M. Chirigos and J. A. R. Mead, Anal. Biochem., 7, 259 (1964).

95. F. Faure and P. Blanquet, Clin. Chim. Acta, 9, 292 (1964).

96. R. Williams, in Spectrofluorimetric Techniques in Biology, NATO Advanced Study Institute, Milan, 1964, p. 247.

97. M. Corn and R. Berberich, Clin. Chem., 13, 126 (1967).

98. V. F. Cotty and H. M. Ederma, J. Pharm. Sci., 55, 837 (1966).

99. P. A. Harris and S. Riegelman, J. Pharm. Sci., 56, 713 (1967).

100. C. Miles and G. Schenk, Anal. Chem., 42, 656 (1970).

101.   J. Finkel and K. Knapp, Anal. Biochem., 25, 465 (1968).

102.   M. E. Auerbach and E. Angell, J. Pharm. Pharmacol., 10, 776 (1958).

103.   W. Jusko, J. Pharm. Sci., 60, 728 (1971).

104.   J. B. Ragland and V. J. Kinross-Wright, Anal. Chem., 36, 1356 (1964).

105.   J. B. Ragland and V. J. Kinross-Wright, Anal. Biochem., 12, 60 (1965).

106.   S. L. Tomsett, Acta Pharmacol. Toxicol., 26, 298 (1967).

107.   K. B. Jensen, Acta Pharmacol. Toxicol., 8, 101 (1952).

108.   I. M. Jakovljevic, Anal. Chem., 35, 1513 (1963).

109.   T. Ichimura, Bunseki Kagaku, 10, 623 (1961); Chem. Abstr. 56, 1530e (1962).

110.   J. H. Peters, Amer. Rev. Resp. Dis., 81, 485 (1960).

111.   E. M. Scott and R. C. Wright, J. Lab. Clin. Med., 70, 335 (1967).

112.   N. Seiler and M. Wiechmann, Z. Phys. Chem. (Leipzig), 337, 229 (1964).

113.   E. Pearlman, J. Pharmacol. Exp. Ther., 95, 465 (1949).

114.   A. Spinks, Biochem. J., 47, 299 (1950).

115.   F. Tishler, P. B. Sheth, and M. B. Giamimo, J. Ass. Offic. Agric. Chem., 46, 448 (1963).

116.   T. Amano, Yakugaku Zasshi, 85, 1049 (1965).

117.   D. Schwartz, B. Koechlin, and R. Weinfeld, Chemotherapia, 14, 22 (1969).

118.   P. N. Kaul, M. W. Conway, M. L. Clark, and J. Huffine, J. Pharm. Sci., 59, 1745 (1970).

119.   W. J. Jusko, J. Pharm. Sci., 60, 728 (1971).

120.   E. R. Garrett and K. Schnelle, J. Pharm. Sci., 60, 833 (1971).

121.   S. A. Varesh, F. S. Hom, and J. J. Miskel, J. Pharm. Sci., 60, 1092 (1971).

122.   J. A. F. de Silva and N. Strojny, J. Pharm. Sci., 60, 1303 (1971).

123.   W. Kent Van Tyle and A. M. Burkman, J. Pharm. Sci., 60, 1736 (1971).

124.   W. Sadee, M. Dagcioglu, and S. Riegelman, J. Pharm. Sci., 61, 1126 (1972).

125.   D. Alkalay, L. Khemani, and M. F. Bartlett, J. Pharm. Sci., 61, 1746 (1972).

126.   D. Wade and G. Sudlow, J. Pharm. Sci., 62, 828 (1973).

127.   B. Scales and D. A. Assinder, J. Pharm. Sci., 62, 913 (1973).

128.   J. A. F. de Silva, N. Strojny, and N. Munno, J. Pharm. Sci., 62, 1066 (1973).

129.   A. de Leenheer, J. E. Sinsheimer, and J. H. Burekhatter, J. Pharm. Sci., 62, 1370 (1973).

130. S. Vickers and E. K. Stuart, J. Pharm. Sci., 62, 1550 (1973).
131. S. A. Kaplan, R. E. Weinfield, and T. L. Lee, J. Pharm. Sci., 62, 1865 (1973).
132. N. R. West, M. P. Rosenblum, H. Sprince, S. Gold, D. H. Boehme, and W. H. Vogel, J. Pharm. Sci., 63, 417 (1974).
133. H. G. Boxenbaum and S. Riegelman, J. Pharm. Sci., 63, 1191 (1974).
134. J. Sterling, S. Cox, and W. G. Haney, J. Pharm. Sci., 63, 1744 (1974).
135. C. N. Corder, T. S. Klaniecki, R. H. McDonald, and C. Berlin, J. Pharm. Sci., 64, 785 (1975).
136. R. E. Lehr and P. N. Raul, J. Pharm. Sci., 64, 950 (1975).
137. J. M. Finkel, R. F. Pittillo, L. B. Mellett, Chemotherapia, 16, 380 (1971).
138. L. K. Cheng, M. Levitt, and H. L. Fung, J. Pharm. Sci., 64, 839 (1975).
139. H. S. I. Tan and C. Beiser, J. Pharm. Sci., 64, 1207 (1975).
140. H. S. C. Hong, R. T. Steltenkaup, and N. L. Smith, J. Pharm. Sci., 64, 2007 (1975).
141. R. V. Rao, Y. Tanrikut, and K. Rillion, J. Pharm. Sci., 64, 345 (1975).
142. A. G. Arbab and P. Turner, J. Pharm. Pharmacol., 23, 719 (1971).
143. R. J. Bopp, R. E. Schirmer, and D. B. Meyers, J. Pharm. Sci., 61, 1750 (1972).
144. W. A. Dill and A. J. Glazko, Clin. Chem., 18, 675 (1972).
145. V. W. Kersten, D. K. F. Meijer, and S. Agoston, Clin. Chim. Acta, 49, 61 (1973).
146. J. A. F. de Silva and N. Strojny, Anal. Chem., 47, 714 (1975).
147. D. R. Wirz, D. L. Wilson, and G. H. Schenk, Anal. Chem., 46, 896 (1974).
148. L. A. Gifford, W. P. Hayes, L. A. King, J. N. Miller, D. T. Burns, and J. W. Bridges, Anal. Chem., 46, 94 (1974).
149. S. Vickers and E. K. Stuart, Anal. Chem., 46, 138 (1974).
150. K. H. Tachiki and M. H. Aprison, Anal. Chem., 47, 7 (1975).
151. B. W. Smith, F. W. Plankey, N. Omnetto, L. P. Hart, and J. D. Winefordner, Spectrochim. Acta, 30A, 1459 (1974).
152. A. A. Thaer and M. Sernetz (eds.), Fluorescence Techniques in Cell Biology, Springer-Verlag, New York, 1973.
153. T. C. O'Haver and W. M. Parks, Anal. Chem., 46, 1886 (1974).

Chapter 5

NONRADIOACTIVE IMMUNOASSAYS

Joseph Haimovich and Michael Sela*

Department of Chemical Immunology
The Weizmann Institute of Science
Rehovot, Israel

I. INTRODUCTION

Highly specific, sensitive, and simple immunoassays for the quantitative determination of drugs and other antigens are now widely used in clinical and research laboratories. Radioimmunoassay (RIA) is undoubtedly used most frequently. It is discussed in several other chapters with consideration to the general problems in the development of any immunoassay such as the search for high affinity antibodies and the development of highly

---

*Established Investigator of The Chief Scientist's Bureau, Ministry of Health.

specific antisera. This chapter will therefore concern itself solely with the particular characteristics and usefulness of nonradioactive immunoassays, and will exclude the spin-label immunoassay which is detailed in Chapter 7 of Volume 1 of this series.

In principle, every antibody-antigen reaction can be developed into a quantitative assay for the determination of antigens, but the need for sensitivity may limit the choice, although a nonsensitive assay may still be useful if a particular antigen is in adequate body fluid concentration. However, in general, an assay must quantify antigens at the concentrations of ng/ml and lower where particular antigens of clinical importance are found in body fluids. The enzymoimmunoassays and viroimmunoassays are nonradioactive immunoassays that are most adequate for this purpose.

II. VIROIMMUNOASSAY

A. General Considerations

The inactivation of bacteriophages is an extremely sensitive assay for the determination of anti-bacteriophage antibodies due to the ability of bacteriophages to reproduce. One single phage particle with a mass as small as 10^{-14} mg (6×10^6 daltons is the mass of ϕX174 bacteriophage) can show up and be recorded as a macroscopically visible plaque on a layer of bacteria. This process is prevented when antibodies attach to bacteriophages [1].

In order to use this assay for the detection of antibodies of any desired specificity, bacteriophages are chemically modified by the attachment of a particular antigen to their protein coat. The requirement of a viable phage restricts the chemical reactions that can be used for the coupling process. Nevertheless, even if only a small fraction of the phage population remains alive after the coupling process, the conjugate preparation is still suitable for the assay since inactivation of bacteriophages as well as inactivation of modified bacteriophages proceeds with pseudo first-order kinetics. This is due to the fact that the antibody greatly exceeds the number of phages, even at extremely low concentrations of antibody and in the presence of excess dead phage.

The use of inhibition of inactivation of chemically modified bacteriophages for analytical purposes is termed viroimmunoassay (VIA).

The first successful attachments to bacteriophages were those of the nitroiodophenylacetyl group [2] and of poly(amino acids) [3]. Since the first introduction of the assay in 1966, a great number of additional chemical substances were coupled chemically to bacteriophages and the conjugates were successfully used in assays for the detection of antibodies [4].

As in other immunological assays, the specificity of the reaction is proved by blocking the activity of the antibodies upon the addition of the particular antigen for which specificity is sought. Thus, the specificity of inactivation of 2,4-dinitrophenyl-bacteriophage was proven when 2,4-dinitrophenyl lysine prevented inactivation. The extent of inhibition of inactivation of modified bacteriophages depends on the concentration of inhibitor. Therefore, a calibration curve of the extent of inhibition as a function of the inhibitor concentration provides a means for quantitative determination of antigens. A schematic presentation of the principles of inactivation and inhibition of inactivation is given in Figure 1. The inactivation of penicilloyl-T4 and inhibition of the inactivation with penicillin and penicilloyl-caproic acid are given as examples in Figures 2 and 3.

Haimovich et al. [5] developed conditions to successfully couple proteins to bacteriophages with bifunctional reagents which made possible the assay of proteins and peptides by the inhibition of inactivation of protein-bacteriophage conjugates as an alternative to RIA in quantifying substances of clinical importance. RIA was compared with VIA for the quantitative determination of proteins, specifically insulin. The results are given in Table 1 (page 263) [6]. The methods were compared for steroids [7] and prostaglandins [8,9] (Fig. 4, page 264), and the sensitivity of VIA equaled or bettered RIA, especially when performed at 0°C.

In contrast to RIA, VIA has the advantages that it does not demand hazardous radioactive materials and there is no need to separate "bound" and "unbound" reactants. The "labeled" reagents, the chemically modified bacteriophages, are stable for years and thus avoid the repeated preparation and calibration of reactants. The equipment needed for VIA is minimal: a controlled temperature bath and a 37°C incubator. Of course VIA can be automated with the automatic plaque counters and dilutors presently commercially available.

The main drawback of the VIA is the necessity to find the optimal conditions for the preparation of the antigen-bacteriophage conjugates. As already pointed out, the coupling process must maintain the viability of 0.1 to 1% of the conjugated phage and render it susceptible to inactivation by antibodies. The determination of the optimal concentrations of reactants (phage, bifunctional reagent, and antigen) and the optimal time of reaction and pH is a time- and antigen-consuming task. Thus, expensive and rare antigens are not proper choices for VIA.

The conditions for the preparation of protein-bacteriophage conjugates reported in the literature and the concentration of antigen required for 20, 50, and 80% inhibition of inactivation of the conjugates are summarized in Table 2 (pages 265-266). Experience has shown that antigens of relatively high molecular weights, e.g., IgG and albumins, are difficult to prepare, and the procedures are not precisely reproducible. Consider them as

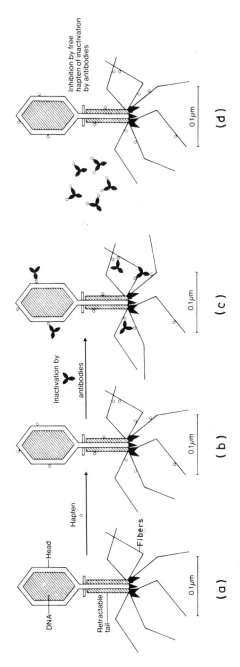

FIG. 1. Schematic presentation of (a) bacteriophage T4, (b) the attachment of a hapten to bacteriophage T4, (c) the inactivation of the resulting hapten–bacteriophage conjugate with anti-hapten antibody, and (d) the inhibition of such inactivation by means of the free hapten. The phage is modeled after Kourilsky [69] and Kellenberger [70]. (Reprinted from Ref. 34 p. 64 by courtesy of Sandoz Ltd., Basle.)

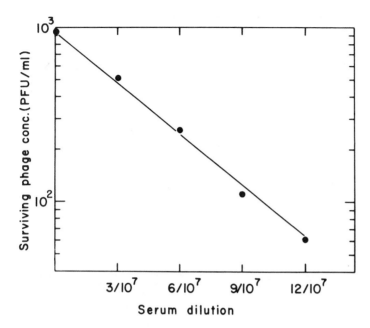

FIG. 2. Inactivation of penicilloyl bacteriophage T4 by anti-penicilloyl serum. The reaction mixtures were incubated for 3 h at 37°C. (Reprinted from Ref. 4 by courtesy of Academic Press Inc., New York).

guidelines and vary the conditions for proper optimization. Preparations of conjugates of low molecular weight proteins and polypeptidic hormones, e.g., lysozyme, however, are reproducible. In fact, a positive control experiment with lysozyme is used to check for the quality of reagents when coupling conditions for a new protein are sought. Coupling with glutaraldehyde is more reproducible than coupling with toluene-2,4-diisocyanate.

An interesting approach to overcome the difficulty of binding high molecular weight proteins to bacteriophages was undertaken in a study on carcinoembrionic antigen, CEA [10]. Rather than coupling the whole molecule of CEA, a small molecular weight peptide with the N-terminal 11 amino acids of the CEA molecule was covalently bound to bacteriophage T4. This was in turn successfully inactivated by antibodies specific for the particular peptide. The peptide, crude preparations of CEA, and the sera of patients with colonic cancer inhibited the inactivation. This synthetic approach where a peptide with a particular antigenic determinant of a large protein molecule is bound to a bacteriophage is very promising.

There are too few reports on the practical application of the VIA for the quantitative determination of antigens. In addition to insulin [6], human

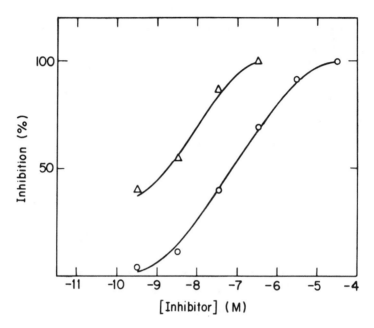

FIG. 3. Inhibition of the inactivation of penicilloyl bacteriophage T4 by anti-penicilloyl serum with penicillin G (○) and penicilloyl-ε-aminocaproic acid (△). (Reprinted from Ref. 4 by courtesy of Academic Press Inc., New York.)

lysozyme was determined in tears, saliva, serum, and urine and compared well with results obtained by enzymatic assays [11]. Tyrosinase was determined in culture of Neurospora and compared well with enzymatic activity [12]. Nerve growth factor was determined in mouse fibroblast cultures [13].

Other substances of diagnostic importance were successfully coupled to bacteriophages. These included drugs and hormones such as penicillin [14], oxazolone [15], steroids [7,16], prostaglandin [8,9], and plant hormones [17,18], and the coupling of low molecular weight drugs to bacteriophages was easier than the coupling of proteins. In all cases studied, the coupling was performed via amino groups on the bacteriophage protein coat. This occurs spontaneously with oxazolone and penicillin at moderately alkaline pH. Other drugs studied were first converted into a mixed anhydride derivative by carbodiimide and then added to bacteriophages at moderately alkaline pH. These procedures were reproducible. Unfortunately, there are no reports on these VIA assays in biological fluids in the presence of potentially interfering other substances.

TABLE 1

Determination of Insulin Concentration in Human Sera
by Inhibition of Inactivation of Insulin-bacteriophage
Conjugate and by Radioimmunoassay[a]

| Serum no. | Insulin concentration (μ units/ml) | |
	Phage	RIA
7295	34	40
7296	150	187
7297	250	>200
7433	13	24
7435	126	138
7504	15	5
7505	170	66
7571	350	>200
7830	42	35
8115	33	26
8119	310	>200

[a]Reprinted from Ref. 6 p. 128 by courtesy of Elsevier
Publishing Co., Amsterdam.

Fuchs et al. [18] determined abscisic acid in plant extracts using
abscisic acid-bacteriophage conjugates and compared the results with a
bioassay. They concluded that the VIA was not affected by the presence
of other hormones and had better reproducibility.

In the previously discussed studies, the VIA was based on covalently
linked antigen-bacteriophage conjugates. A modification was introduced
by Taussig [19] who reacted a native bacteriophage with an Fab fragment
preparation of anti-phage antibody at concentrations that bound to the phage
but did not substantially inactivate. Inactivation was effected subsequently
by antibodies against determinants present on the Fab fragment. Maron
and Dray used this "immunologically modified bacteriophage" technique,
detected anti-allotype antibodies and assayed immunoglobulin of a particular
allotype in cell cultures by inhibition of the inactivation [20]. They found
good correlation with RIA.

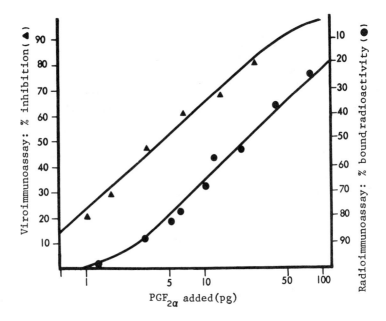

FIG. 4.   Comparison of immunoassays of Prostaglandin $F_{2\alpha}$ ($PGF_{2\alpha}$):
●, RIA; ▲, VIA.   (Reprinted from Ref. 9, p. 19 by courtesy of Geron-X
Inc., Los Altos, California.)

The assay was generalized for antigens by coupling them to antiphage
Fab and inactivating the immunologically modified bacteriophage with antibodies against the antigen coupled to the Fab. Amos et al. [21] and Gurari
et al. [22], detected anti-aspirin and anti-nucleic acid antibodies, respectively, by this procedure but did not report on their quantification. In
principle this could be done readily by adding the "free" antigens to the
assay reaction mixture.

Both chemically and immunologically modified bacteriophage assays are
based on assaying the viability of the modified phages in the presence of
antibodies and antigens as a probe for the free and bound antigen. The
sensitivity of the reaction stems from the fact that very little antibody is
necessary for the process of inactivation, and therefore very little antigen
is necessary for blocking the antibody. However, since the assay is based
on the viability of the phage it also suffers from the disadvantage of being
affected by factors that may nonspecifically influence this viability. Thus,
the assays are very difficult to perform with undiluted sera since the phages
can be spontaneously inactivated by the sera used as inhibitors. This inactivation may be due to the presence of "natural" anti-phage antibodies in
serum samples. As the sensitivity of the assay is very high, this phenom-

TABLE 2

Coupling of Proteins to Bacteriophage and Inhibition of Inactivation by "Free" Protein

Protein coupled to bacteriophage	Protein (mg/ml)[a]	Bifunctional reagent (% v/v)[a]	Concentration of protein for the following % inhibition (ng/ml)			Reference
			20	50	80	
TDIC[b]						
RNase	7	0.008	0.4	3	100	[5, 6]
BSA	11	0.2		ND[d]		[5, 6]
RSA	17	0.6	2	8	60	[5, 6]
Rabbit IgG	9	0.016	0.03	0.2	2	[5, 6]
Lysozyme	21	0.0025	0.2	1	8	[5, 6]
Insulin	17	0.2	0.03	0.1	0.3	[5, 6]
Papain	7	0.01		ND		[24]
Chymopapain	8.6	0.6		ND		[24]
Glutaraldehyde						
RNase	4.5	0.01	0.2	2	50	[5, 6]
Lysozyme	10	0.01	0.1	1	5	[5, 6]

TABLE 2 (Continued)

Protein coupled to bacteriophage	Protein (mg/ml)[a]	Bifunctional reagent (% v/v)[a]	Concentration of protein for the following % inhibition (ng/ml)			Reference
			20	50	80	
Naja naja siamensis toxin	4	0.01	0.1	1	100	[29]
Nerve growth factor	4	0.01		10		[13]
Tyrosinase	15	0.02	40	80	200	[12]
Human calcitonin	13	0.06	2	ND		[30]
Staph. nuclease	4	0.01	2	20	150	[31]
Angiotensin	11	0.036		2		[32]
F_2DNB[c]						
Poly-L-proline	25	0.45		ND		[33]

[a]Final concentration in the reaction mixture. F_2DNB concentration in w/v.

[b]2,4-Tolylene diisocyanate.

[c]1,3-Difluoro-4,6-dinitrobenzene.

[d]ND, not determined.

enon can usually be overcome by diluting the sera at least ten-fold and assaying at a minimal background inactivation.

A recently published VIA of high sensitivity for dinitrophenyl (DNP) derivatives of lysine and BSA [23] resembled RIA. The bacteriophages were used to tag the antigen in a manner similar to the radioactive tag on antigens in RIA. The bound tagged antigen or the modified phage-antibody complex was recorded upon plating after separation from the unbound tagged antigen by an immunoadsorbent. Antigen resembling that coupled to the bacteriophage will inhibit the binding of the phage to the immunoadsorbent and its subsequent development into a plaque. The assay had previously been used for the detection of anti-phage antibodies [24]. Its principle is presented in Figure 5. The assay has a great potential in determining antigens as it is based on detecting antibody modified bacteriophage com-

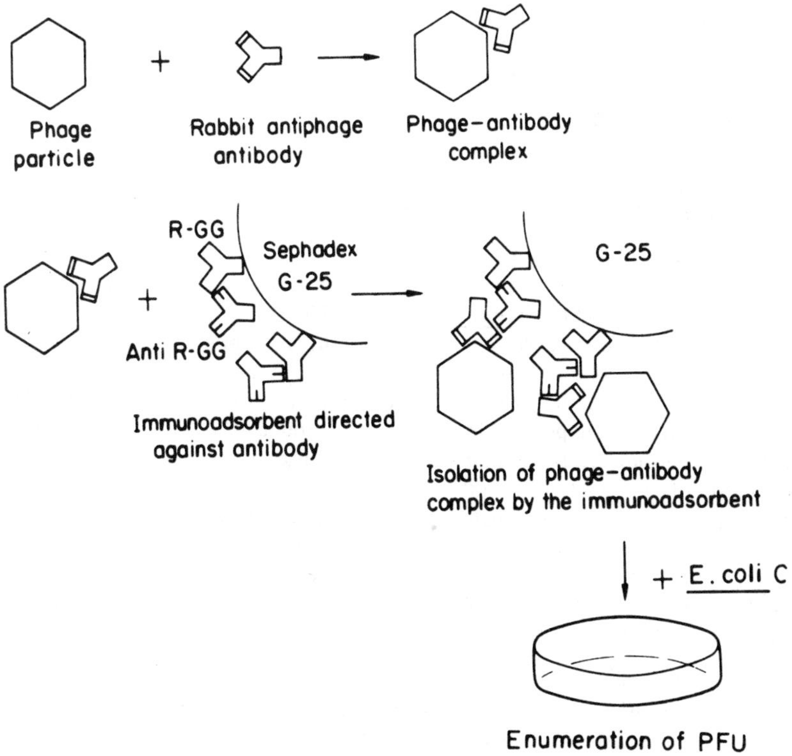

FIG. 5. Schematic representation of anti-phage antibody assay using the immunoadsorbent technique. (Reprinted from Ref. 24 p. 367 by courtesy of Pergamon Press Ltd., England.)

plexes that are not necessarily inactivated. It is reasonable to assume that coupling of antigens to bacteriophages occurs all over the phage's protein coat, whereas only those at or near the site on the phage responsible for adsorption to the bacterium are involved in inactivation of the phage upon the binding of antibodies. Thus, suitable conditions for coupling antigens to any part of the bacteriophage may be easier to find than reaction conditions that must leave the phage viable but nevertheless susceptible to inactivation by antibodies that must bind to the region on the phage crucial for its adsorption to the bacterium. However, calibration curves for antigen determination were not presented and results [23] were inconsistent. It should be remembered that in many systems the sensitivity borderline is dictated by the affinity of the antibody preparation used for the assay and not by the sensitivity of the label. This is also true in RIA. Certainly, very sensitive assays are also vulnerable to errors and nonspecific deviations that affect reliability and reproducibility. Further experiments are needed to evaluate the usefulness of the above immunoadsorbent VIA for diagnostic purposes.

B. Detailed Procedures for the Performance of Viroimmunoassay

1. Preparation of Bacteriophages

Bacteriophage T4 is grown in liquid medium by the procedure described by Adams [1] and purified according to Putnam et al. [25]. In brief, this consists of growing <u>Escherichia coli</u> B at 37°C in tryptone broth (10 g Bacto-Tryptone and 5 g NaCl per liter broth) to a density of $A_{650} = 0.7$; infecting with T4 at low multiplicity (1-2 $\times$ 10^{10} plaque forming units (PFU)/ liter bacterial culture). The bacteria are grown for an additional 2 h, then centrifuged and resuspended in a minimal amount of tryptone broth. Chloroform is added (about 10-20% of the suspension volume) and the bacterial suspension is stirred vigorously for about 10 min on a magnetic stirrer. This liberates the bacteriophage. The yield obtained is usually 10^{14} PFU per liter bacterial culture. Purification is obtained by several sequential differential centrifugations at 20,000 g, discarding the supernatant and 5,000 g, and discarding the pellet. The purity is checked by the ratio of A_{260}/A_{280} which should reach 1.3 to 1.4 and by the concentration in PFU/ ml for a solution of a particular A_{260}. A solution of $A_{260}^{1\ cm} = 1.0$ should contain about 10^{11} PFU/ml. Stock solutions of bacteriophage T4 are kept in 0.05 M phosphate pH 6.8 (PB) at 4°C. They are stable for years.

Bacteriophage ϕX174 is prepared according to Sinsheimer [26]. In brief, a culture of <u>E. coli</u> C at a density of 4 to 5 $\times$ 10^8/ml that has been grown at 37°C in TPG3A medium [26] with aeration is infected with ϕX174 at a multiplicity of 3 phages/bacterium. Half an hour later, 10 ml of 0.1

M disodium versenate is added and the pH is adjusted to pH 7.0. The culture is grown for 5 to 7 h reaching a concentration of about 10^{12} PFU/ml. Purification of ϕX174 is achieved by adding 126 ml of 20% sodium dextran sulfate 500 and 400 ml of 40% polyethylene glycol to a 2-liter phage culture. The culture is shaken well and left for 48 h at 4°C. Most of the phage will concentrate in an interface layer which is collected, centrifuged for 10 to 15 min at 10,000 g, and the supernatant discarded. The pellet is resuspended in 10 ml 0.01 M Tris-acetate, pH 8.0 and sedimented again, then resuspended in 15 ml saturated (4°C) sodium borate and stirred for 15 to 18 h at 4°C. After centrifugation, the supernatant is collected and the pellet re-extracted with 5 ml saturated sodium borate. To the ϕX174 solution in borate is added 1/10 volume of 50 g/liter Tryptone and CsCl (0.625 g CsCl per 1 g of solution) to raise the density to 1.41. The phage is banded by centrifuging in a Spinco Model L centrifuge in the 40 rotor at 37,000 rpm for 24 h at 6°C and removed by pipetting it out. Pure ϕX174 solution of an $A_{260} = 1.3$ contains 10^{13} phage particles. Using the above procedures, 50 to 60% of the phage is viable. Purified phage is dialyzed against sodium borate and stored at 4°C.

2. Preparation of Chemically Modified Bacteriophages

The following are examples for the preparation of several antigen-bacteriophage conjugates. Preparation of other conjugates is described in detail in the literature [2-23, 28-33].

a. Penicilloyl-T4 [14]

A solution of bacteriophage T4 in 0.3 M carbonate buffer pH 9.5 containing 10^{11} PFU/ml is prepared by diluting a concentrated stock solution of T4 ($1-2 \times 10^{13}$ PFU/ml) into the above buffer. Penicillin is added to a final concentration of 100 mg/ml, the solution is allowed to stand at 37°C for 10 to 24 h, is then dialyzed against PB, and stored at 4°C.

b. 17β-Estradiol-T4 [16] and prostaglandin-T4 [8]

Ten mg of 17β-estradiol-6-carboxymethoxime or prostaglandin $F_{2\alpha}$ are activated with 10 mg N, N'-dicyclohexylcarbodiimide by stirring in 0.3 ml dioxane for 30 min at room temperature. After centrifugation, 0.1 ml of the supernatant is added slowly with continuous stirring to 0.6 ml of T4 solution (10^{12} PFU/ml PB). The reaction is stopped after 10 min at room temperature by the addition of 50 ml 0.05 M phosphate pH 6.8 containing 20 μg/ml of gelatin (PBG) and dialysis against PB.

c. Protein-T4 [5]

Bacteriophage T4 and protein solutions are mixed to a final concentration of 10^{13} PFU/ml. The optimal concentration of the particular proteins given in Table 2. Several of these concentrations should be used in the attempt to couple new proteins with bacteriophage T4. Volumes as low as

5 μl of each bacteriophage and protein solution can be used for proteins that are precious; otherwise, volumes of 0.1 to 0.3 ml are convenient. Glutaraldehyde or toluene-2, 4-diisocyanate are added in turn. The optimal concentrations of the bifunctional reagents for the coupling of several proteins and polypeptidic hormones to bacteriophage T4 are given in Table 2. The mixture is allowed to stand for 1 h at room temperature and is then brought to 10 ml with PBG. The protein-bacteriophage conjugate is separated from the unreacted protein by two successive centrifugations for 1 h at 20, 000 g.

   3.   Inactivation of Penicilloyl Bacteriophage T4
        by Anti-penicilloyl Serum

0.2 ml of penicilloyl-T4 solution (3×10^3 PFU/ml) and 0.2 ml aliquots from serial dilutions of anti-penicilloyl serum are added to a series of test tubes (12 $\times$ 100 mm). (Smaller volumes of phage and antibody solutions may be used if necessary.) The mixtures are kept at 37°C for 1 to 5 h. Soft agar (2.5 ml kept at 46°C) and bacteria (3×10^8 of E. coli B) are added to the reaction mixtures which are poured in turn on top of "bottom agar" containing Petri dishes. The bottom agar contains 10 g Bacto-Tryptone, 12 g Bacto-Agar, 8 g NaCl, 2 g sodium citrate, and 3 g glucose dissolved in 1 liter H_2O. Soft agar contains the same ingredients except for Bacto-Agar which is 7 g/liter. The plates are incubated for 8 to 20 h at 37°C and the number of plaques are counted. Figure 2 (page 261) shows the results of a typical experiment.

   4.   Determination of Penicillin by the Inhibition of
        Inactivation of Penicilloyl Bacteriophage T4 (VIA)

The inhibitor penicillin G or penicilloyl-ϵ-aminocaproic acid (0.2 ml) is added to a series of tubes containing 0.2 ml of antipenicilloyl serum described in Figure 2 (at a dilution of 3.6×10^{-6}) to a final concentration of 10^{-4} to 10^{-9} M. Buffer is added to control tubes instead of inhibitor. The mixtures are kept at 37°C for 30 min. Penicilloyl-T4 is added (0.2 ml containing about 600 PFU) and the mixtures kept at 37°C for an additional 3 h and plated.

   By preincubating the antibodies with the inhibitor, the extent of inactivation of penicilloyl-T4, compared to that obtained in the absence of inhibitor, is reduced and corresponds to an extent characteristic of a lower concentration of free antibody. For example, penicilloyl-T4 at an initial concentration of 10^3 PFU/ml was reduced to a concentration of 60 PFU/ml when reacted for 3 h at 37°C with anti-penicilloyl serum at a final dilution of 12:10^7 (Fig. 2). By preincubating the antiserum at the same final dilution with penicillin G at a final concentration of 3×10^{-7} M, the extent of inactivation was reduced so that the concentration of viable phage dropped to only 200 PFU/ml. This extent of inactivation corresponds to that obtained

by only 60% of the initial concentration of antibody (see Fig. 2) and is
therefore considered to be due to 40% inhibition of the antibodies by the
inhibitor. Obviously, 100% inhibition results in no inactivation of the
penicilloyl-T4 by the antiserum added.

The results of an inhibition experiment performed as described above
are summarized in Figure 3 (page 262).

For the detection and quantitation of penicillin G, the same procedure
is employed with 0.2 ml of the sample to be tested. The amount of penicillin G in the sample tested is determined by the extent of inhibition
achieved and with the aid of the results summarized in Figure 3.

5. Determination of Protein Concentration by the
    Inhibition of Inactivation of Protein-bacteriophage
    Conjugates

Inhibition of inactivation of protein-T4 is performed in a similar way as
for penicilloyl-T4 except that protein and antibodies are reacted for longer
times prior to the addition of phage (20 h at 4°C and an additional 2 h at
37°C). Also, the complex inactivation method [27] is used for the assay.
In this method 0.1 ml of anti-Ig of the species from which the anti-protein
is obtained is added at a dilution of 1:100 to 1:1,000, and incubation is
continued for 8 to 10 min prior to plating.

III. ENZYMOIMMUNOASSAY

A. General Considerations

The enzymoimmunoassay (EIA) technique is very similar in principle to
that of the RIA except that the antigen or the antibody in question is labeled
with an enzyme rather than an isotope. The labeled reagent is detected
in turn by an enzymatic reaction, usually with a substrate that changes
into a product with an increase in light absorbance or fluorescence. The
use of immunoadsorbent-coupled antigens or antibodies and the use of
different enzymes make for a versatile assay.

Avrameas and Guilbert [35,36] coupled the enzyme peroxidase to human
and rat IgG. Anti-IgG, rendered insoluble with ethyl chloroformate, bound
the enzyme-labeled IgG unless nonlabeled IgG was added first to a calibrated
amount of insoluble anti-IgG. The amount of enzyme-labeled IgG remaining in the supernatant increased, therefore, with the increase of nonlabeled
IgG added. The assay was accurate in the range of 20 to 200 ng of IgG in
samples of 0.1 ml. A modification of the above procedure was performed
by the same authors: Labeled and unlabeled IgG were allowed to react

with antibodies in solution, and the complexes were precipitated with insoluble antibodies against the anti-IgG. The amount of enzyme-labeled IgG remaining in the supernatant in this indirect method was directly related to the amount of nonlabeled IgG added, and the assay proved to be more accurate than the direct procedure.

Van Weemen and Schuurs [37] developed an identical assay (both direct and indirect) with peroxidase coupled to human chorionic gonadotropin (HCG). The hormone was accurately determined at concentrations of 0.1 to 1.0 IU/ml, and there was good correlation between the EIA and a hemagglutination inhibition assay for HCG. (See Section IV.) The assay proved useful in the diagnosis of pregnancy.

Engvall and Perlmann [38] developed a similar EIA. Alkaline phosphatase was linked to IgG, and nonlabeled IgG competed with the labeled antigen for binding to anti-IgG bound to an immunoadsorbent. The assay was denoted ELISA (enzyme-linked immunoadsorbent assay). Determination of antigen was accurate in the range of 10 to 100 ng in 0.1 ml of antigen solution added.

The three EIA's described had in common the principle of labeling an antigen with an enzyme, and thereby detecting the ability of an unlabeled antigen to compete with the enzyme-labeled one for binding to an antibody (either in solution or solid phase linked). The principle is very similar to a RIA in which antigens are labeled with a radioisotope.

Rubenstein et al. [39] and Rowley et al. [40] developed EIA's that were entirely different in principle. The enzyme served not just as a tag for quantitation of antigen, but as an active molecule to which other determinants are coupled. Antibodies that bound to the determinants on the enzyme inactivated the catalytic activity of the enzyme. Antigen in solution, identical or similar to the one coupled to the enzyme, will block the antibodies and prevent them from inactivating the enzyme. As the authors pointed out, their assay is similar in its principle to the inhibition of inactivation of antigen-phage conjugates. Also, similar to the VIA, their EIA does not require the separation between bound- and free-labeled antigen. The assay was successfully used for the quantitative determination of morphine and related substances at threshold concentrations of about 10^{-9} M. The enzymes used for the assay were lysozyme [39] and malate dehydrogenase [40].

In some EIAs, antibodies rather than antigens are labeled with enzymes. Maiolini et al. [41] labeled anti-α-fetoprotein (AFP) with glucose oxidase and measured its activity after binding to insolubilized AFP. Addition of soluble AFP decreased the amount of enzyme-labeled antibody bound to the insoluble AFP. Antigen at 1 to 10 ng/ml was determined.

Other enzymoimmunoassays are based on a "sandwich" procedure in which antibodies are insolubilized (either by adsorption to polystyrene tubes or coupled to immunoadsorbents). Antigen is added to the insoluble antibody and enzyme-labeled antibody (or antibody and enzyme-labeled anti-antibody) is added to the complex. The more antigen coupled in the first step, the more labeled antibody is bound to the complex. However, only polyvalent antigens can be detected by the sandwich technique. This kind of EIA was employed for the determination of α-fetoprotein [42, 43] a pregnancy-associated α-macroglobulin [44] and IgG [45]. Of particular interest is the assay for IgG in which the enzyme β-galactosidase was coupled to anti-IgG. The enzymatic activity was measured using a substrate which gave a fluorescent product which permitted the quantitative determination of 0.2 ng IgG.

Insulin was also determined with an insulin-β-galactosidase complex in the regular competitive assay and by determination of product fluorescence [46]. The same RIA commercial kit (Pharmacia) was used to bind enzyme-labeled insulin. Both methods had equivalent sensitivity.

In summary, EIA is a promising alternative assay to RIA. It has advantages of utilizing reagents that are stable for long periods of time and less expensive equipment. The sensitivity and accuracy are similar to RIA, especially when fluorescence, rather than light absorbance, is measured.

B. Detailed Procedures for the Performance
   of Enzymoimmunoassay

   1. Enzyme-linked Immunosorbent Assay (ELISA) [38]

The globulin fraction of sheep anti-rabbit IgG is coupled to CNBr activated [47] microcrystalline cellulose. The immunoadsorbent containing 0.5% protein is stored at 4°C in 0.9% NaCl containing 0.5% Tween 20 and NaN$_3$ as preservative. Alkaline phosphatase (ALP) is conjugated to rabbit IgG by the use of glutaraldehyde [48]. Samples of 0.1 ml IgG of known concentrations and samples of tested solutions are added to 0.1 ml of a proper dilution of ALP-IgG conjugate and mixed with 1 ml of immunoadsorbent suspension capable of binding 50% of the conugate. Dilutions are made in 0.15 M NaCl-0.01 M phosphate pH 7.2 (PBS) containing 1% human serum albumin. The samples are incubated for 16 h at 8°C in a roller drum, spun down, and washed twice with 5 ml PBS containing 0.05% Tween 20. The enzymatic activity of adsorbed conjugates is determined by adding 2.5 ml of 2.5 mM p-nitrophenylphosphate in 0.05 M sodium carbonate pH 9.8 containing 1 mM MgCl$_2$ and incubating for 4 h at 23°C with rotation. The reaction is stopped with 0.1 ml 3 M NaOH and the absorbance of the centrifuged samples is measured at 400 nm. A dose-response curve is obtained with decreasing amounts of bound conjugate as a function of the increase in concentration of inhibitory IgG.

2. "Homogeneous" EIA [39]

Carboxymethyl morphine (CMM) is coupled to lysozyme by reacting CMM-
isobutyl chloroformate mixed anhydride [49] with lysozyme in aqueous solution at pH 9.5 to 10.0 and dialysis against water. The IgG fraction of rabbit anti-morphine is added to the conjugate, and this results in inhibition
of the enzymic activity of the conjugate. After calibration of the amount
of antibody necessary to inhibit about 95% of the enzyme activity, free
morphine is added at increasing concentrations, thus increasing the enzyme
activity by blocking the available antibodies. Enzyme activity is measured
by the ratio of lysis of Micrococcus luteus tested by the change in light
transmission [50].

IV. OTHER IMMUNOASSAYS

Any antibody-antigen reaction can be developed into a quantitative assay
for antigens. These assays are of two types: (1) direct detection of antigens by antibodies and (2) inhibition of an antibody-antigen reaction with
either polyvalent or monovalent antigens.

   The direct reaction between antibodies and multideterminant antigens
in solution causes the precipitation of both reactants when mixed at the
proper ratio. This characteristic was the basis of the quantitative precipitin analysis for the determination of antibodies [51]. Determination
of both antibodies and antigens as well as evaluation of the specificity of
the reactants can be done by precipitin reactions in gels [52]. When precipitin reactions in gels are performed such that antigen diffuses into an
antibody-containing gel, the distance at which the precipitation occurs depends on the amount of antigen added to the well [53]. This "radial immunodiffusion" assay can serve for the detection and quantitation of antigens
with the aid of calibrated antigen solutions of known concentrations. The
sensitivity of the assay is poor (approximately 1 μg), can be easily visual-
ized, but can be increased when the antigen is an enzyme so that visualiza-
tion of the precipitate is effected by an enzymatic assay [54]. Higher sensitivity was also obtained when antigen was radioactively labeled [55].

   An assay similar to radial immunodiffusion was developed by Laurell
[56], the "rocket" technique. As in the radial immunodiffusion, the antigen is placed in a well cut in an antibody-containing agarose gel. However,
the antigen is electrophoresed at pH 8.6 where the antibodies do not move
in the gel, but the antigens form a rocket-shaped precipitin line. The
sensitivity is equivalent to radial immunodiffusion. Obviously, the above
quantitative immune precipitin assays in gels are suitable only for polyvalent antigens that form precipitates when reacting with antibodies. Most
of the important drugs for which immunoassays are developed belong to

the group of antigens that do not form precipitates. Due to this fact and
to their low sensitivity, the above assays have not been commonly used for
determination of drugs.

However, low molecular weight substances resembling the antigenic
determinants on polyvalent hapten-protein conjugates can inhibit precipitin
reactions. This fact is the basis of a nephelometric inhibition immunoassay (NINIA) [57] in which precipitates of antibody and antigens are determined by the turbidity of the solutions where the turbidity is inhibited
by the addition of small molecular weight inhibitors that bind to the antibody. The reactions were performed by adding small volumes of inhibitor
solutions such as dinitrophenol (15 μg/ml) and 11-hydroxyprogesterone
(4 μg/ml); tubes were dried and diluted sera were added and checked for
turbidity. The amounts of progesterone significantly detected were in the
range of 10 to 100 ng.

Complement fixation is an old sensitive assay for the determination of
antibody-antigen reactions [58]. The assay has been used for the determination of chloramphenicol [59]. Anti-chloramphenicol was reacted with
chloramphenicol conjugated to rabbit serum albumin, and the consumption
of the complement added was measured by the usual hemolysis assay.
Addition of chloramphenicol to the reaction mixture blocked the antibody
and prevented the fixation of the complement. One ng of the drug sufficed
for significant inhibition. With improvement of the assay (not described
in the article) the author estimated that the assay could detect amounts as
small as 10^{-5} μg. In a similar fashion, Van Vunakis et al. [60] developed
an assay for the drugs: 3,4,5-trimethoxyphenylethylamine, 3,4-dimeth-
oxyphenylethylamine, and 2,5-dimethoxy-4-methylamphetamine. Antibodies against each of these drugs were inhibited by the drugs. Amounts
required for 50% inhibition of complement fixation were about 2 to 5 μg
for the homologous system (inhibition by the drug used for immunization)
and much higher when the inhibitors were the structurally similar compounds. Although the sensitivity of the reaction was relatively low, its
specificity was very high, enabling the distinction between the similar substances.

The passive hemagglutination assay [61] was also successfully used for
quantitative determination of antigenic drugs. Adler and Liu [62] developed an assay for the determination of morphine. Anti-morphine raised
by injection of carboxymethyl morphine (CMM) conjugated to BSA, was
reacted with CMM-coated tanned sheep red blood cells (SRBC). Addition
of the free drug inhibited the reaction. Concentration of 1 ng/ml was inhibitory. Methadone, the chemically nonrelated substance used in clinical
treatment of addicts, was inhibitory only at concentrations 10^3- to 10^4-fold
higher. The same assay was developed for the reverse system with anti-
methadone antibodies [63], in which morphine was far less inhibitory.
The authors pointed out that inhibition of passive hemagglutination was a

better assay for methadone than the nonimmunological thin-layer chromatography (TLC) technique.

The assay for the detection of heroin was checked in a clinical survey of drug addicts. It was concluded that the assay was more suitable than the less sensitive and more confusing TLC assay [64].

Hemagglutination inhibition was also used for the determination of glutethimide (Doriden). The threshold concentration detected was 50 ng per 0.1 ml test sample. Phenobarbital and the structurally related diphenylhydantoin were far less inhibitory [65].

Passive immune hemolysis is similar in principle to passive hemagglutination except that antigen-treated erythrocytes are lysed rather than agglutinated by antibodies. This assay can also be inhibited by the free antigen. The assay has been used for the detection of penicillin in protein-free serum ultrafiltrates [66]. Concentrations in the range of 3 to 3,000 μg/ml sodium penicillin G were significantly determined.

An interesting assay for the direct determination of antigens was recently developed by Molinaro and Dray [67]. In this assay antibodies rather than antigens are coupled to erythrocytes, and agglutination or hemolysis is brought about by the direct reaction with the specific antigen. When reacted with cells, the coated erythrocytes are able to form rosettes around antigen bearing cells. The assay was used for the determination of allotypes of immunoglobulins. A concentration of 0.2 ng/ml was inhibitory. The assay is applicable to any polyvalent antigen. Small molecular weight monovalent ligands, on the other hand (such as most of the drugs), cannot be detected in this way.

A recently published unusual assay [68] consists of a quartz cell that is illuminated by a beam of light from a helium–cadmium laser at an angle that causes total internal reflection so that the light penetrates only slightly into the solution. The quartz cell is coated with antigen, and the solution contains fluoresceinated antibody that binds to the antigen and fluoresces unless free antigen is added to the solution and inhibits the antibodies from binding to the antigen on the quartz surface. Morphine at relatively high concentrations (2×10^{-7} M) was detected in this way.

REFERENCES

1. M. H. Adams, Bacteriophages, Wiley (Interscience), New York, 1969.
2. O. Mäkelä, Immunology, 10, 81 (1966).
3. J. Haimovich and M. Sela, J. Immunol., 97, 338 (1966).

4. J. Haimovich and M. Sela, in Methods in Immunology and Immuno-chemistry, Vol. IV (C. A. Williams and M. W. Chase, eds.), Academic Press, New York, in press.
5. J. Haimovich, E. Hurwitz, N. Novik, and M. Sela, Biochim. Biophys. Acta, 207, 115 (1970).
6. J. Haimovich, E. Hurwitz, N. Novik, and M. Sela, Biochim. Biophys. Acta, 207, 125 (1970).
7. J. M. Andrieu, S. Mamas, and F. Dray, in Radioimmunoassay and Related Procedures in Medicine, IAEA, Vienna, 1974, pp. 47-55.
8. F. Dray, E. Maron, S. A. Tillson, and M. Sela, Anal. Biochem., 50, 399 (1972).
9. J. M. Andrieu, S. Mamas, and F. Dray, Prostaglandins, 6, 15 (1974).
10. R. Arnon, M. Bustin, E. Calef, S. Chaitchik, J. Haimovich, N. Novik, and M. Sela, Proc. Nat. Acad. Sci. U.S., 73, 2123 (1976).
11. E. Maron and B. Bonavida, Biochim. Biophys. Acta, 229, 273 (1971).
12. T. Katan, R. Arnon, and E. Galun, Eur. J. Biochem., 59, 387 (1975).
13. J. Oger, B. G. W. Arnason, N. Pantazis, J. Lehrich, and M. Young, Proc. Nat. Acad. Sci. U.S., 71, 1554 (1974).
14. J. Haimovich, M. Sela, J. M. Dewdney, and F. R. Batchelor, Nature, 214, 1369 (1967).
15. S. Jormalainen, J. Aird, and O. Mäkelä, Immunochemistry, 8, 450 (1971).
16. J. M. Andrieu, S. Mamas, and F. Dray, Eur. J. Immunol., 4, 417 (1974).
17. S. Fuchs, J. Haimovich, and Y. Fuchs, Eur. J. Biochem., 18, 384 (1971).
18. Y. Fuchs, S. Mayak, and S. Fuchs, Planta, 103, 117 (1972).
19. M. J. Taussig, Immunology, 18, 323 (1970).
20. E. Maron and S. Dray, J. Immunol. Meth., 3, 347 (1973).
21. H. E. Amos, D. W. Wilson, M. J. Taussig, and S. J. Carlton, Clin. Exp. Immunol., 8, 563 (1971).
22. D. Gurari, B. Bonavida, M. J. Taussig, S. Fuchs, and M. Sela, Eur. J. Biochem., 26, 247 (1972).
23. S. Pestka, A. Rosenfeld, and R. Harris, Immunochemistry, 11, 213 (1974).
24. V. T. Skvortsov, Immunochemistry, 9, 366 (1972).
25. F. W. Putnam, L. M. Kozloff, and J. C. Neil, J. Biol. Chem., 179, 303 (1949).
26. R. L. Sinsheimer in Procedures in Nucleic Acid Research (G. L. Cantoni and D. R. Davies, eds.), Harper and Row, New York, 1966, pp. 569-576.
27. W. M. Krummel and J. W. Uhr, J. Immunol., 102, 772 (1969).
28. J. Eder and R. Arnon, Immunochemistry, 10, 535 (1973).

29. A. Aharonov, D. Gurari, and S. Fuchs, Eur. J. Biochem., 45, 297 (1974).

30. A. W. Steiner and F. M. Dietrich, Z. Immun.-Forsch., 145, 275 (1973).

31. S. Fuchs, M. Sela, and C. B. Anfinsen, Arch. Biochem. Biophys., 154, 601 (1973).

32. E. Hurwitz, F. M. Dietrich, and M. Sela, Eur. J. Biochem., 17, 273 (1970).

33. D. Gurari, H. Ungar-Waron, and M. Sela, Eur. J. Immunol., 3, 196 (1973).

34. M. Sela, Triangle, 11, 61 (1972).

35. S. Avrameas and B. Guilbert, C. R. Acad. Sci., 275, 2705 (1971).

36. S. Avrameas and B. Guilbert, Biochemie, 54, 837 (1972).

37. B. K. Van Weeman and A. H. W. M. Schuurs, FEBS Lett., 15, 232 (1971).

38. E. Engvall and P. Perlman, Immunochemistry, 8, 871 (1971).

39. K. E. Rubenstein, R. S. Schneider, and E. F. Ullman, Biochem. Biophys. Res. Commun., 47, 846 (1972).

40. G. L. Rowley, K. E. Rubenstein, J. Hisjen, and E. F. Ullman, J. Biol. Chem., 250, 2759 (1975).

41. R. Maiolini, B. Ferrua, and R. Masseyeff, J. Immunol. Meth., 6, 355 (1975).

42. L. Belanger, C. Sylvestro, and D. Dufour, Clin. Chim. Acta, 48, 15 (1973).

43. R. Maiolini and R. Masseyeff, J. Immunol. Meth., 8, 223 (1975).

44. W. H. Stimson and J. M. Sinclair, FEBS Lett., 47, 190 (1974).

45. K. Kato, Y. Hamaguchi, H. Fukui, and E. Ishikawa, J. Biochem., 78, 423 (1975).

46. K. Kato, Y. Hamaguchi, H. Fukui, and E. Ishikawa, J. Biochem., 78, 235 (1975).

47. R. Axen, J. Porath, and S. Ernbach, Nature, 214, 1302 (1967).

48. S. Avrameas, Immunochemistry, 6, 43 (1969).

49. R. K. Leute, H. F. Ullman, A. Goldstein, and L. A. Herzenberg, Nature, 236, 93 (1972).

50. D. Shugar, Biochim. Biophys. Acta, 92, 412 (1964).

51. M. Heidelberger and F. E. Kendall, J. Exp. Med., 55, 555 (1932).

52. O. Oucterloni, Acta Pathol. Microbiol. Scand., 32, 231 (1953).

53. G. Mancini, A. O. Carbonara, and J. F. Heremans, Immunochemistry, 2, 235 (1965).

54. B. Geiger, R. Navon, Y. Ben-Yoseph, and R. Arnon, Eur. J. Biochem., 56, 311 (1975).

55. R. Jalanti and C. S. Henney, J. Immunol. Meth., 1, 123 (1972).

56. C. B. Laurell, Anal. Biochem., 15, 45 (1966).

57. C. L. Cambiaso, H. A. Ricconi, P. L. Masson, and J. F. Heremans, J. Immunol. Meth., 5, 293 (1974).

58. L. Levine in Handbook of Experimental Immunology (D. M. Wier, ed.), Blackwell, Oxford, 1967, pp. 707-719.
59. R. N. Hamburger, Science, 152, 203 (1966).
60. H. Van Vunakis, H. Brandvica, P. Benda, and L. Levine, Biochem. Pharmacol., 18, 393 (1969).
61. W. H. Herbert in Handbook of Experimental Immunology (D. M. Weit, ed.), Blackwell, Oxford, 1967, pp. 720-744.
62. F. L. Adler and C.-T. Liu, J. Immunol., 106, 1684 (1971).
63. C.-T. Liu and F. L. Adler, J. Immunol., 111, 472 (1973).
64. D. H. Catlin, F. L. Adler, and C.-T. Liu, Clin. Immunol. Immunopath., 1, 446 (1973).
65. J. C. Valentour, W. W. Harold, A. B. Stavistsky, G. Kananen, and I. Sunshine, Clin. Chim. Acta, 43, 65 (1973).
66. G. H. Wiedermann, H. Stemberger, H.-P. Werner, and D. Kraft, Z. Immun. Forsch., 143, 491 (1972).
67. G. A. Molinaro and S. Dray, Nature, 248, 515 (1974).
68. M. N. Kronick and W. A. Little, J. Immunol. Meth., 8, 235 (1975).
69. P. Kourilsky, Triangle, 10, 11 (1971).
70. E. Kellenberger, Advan. Virus. Res., 8, 7 (1961).

Chapter 6

ANALYSIS OF GLUCURONIC ACID CONJUGATES

Jelka Tomašić*

Section on Carbohydrates
Laboratory of Chemistry, NIAMDD
National Institutes of Health
Bethesda, Maryland

*Present address: Tracer Laboratory, Rudjer Bošković Institute,
Zagreb, Yugoslavia.

I. INTRODUCTION

Conjugation with D-glucuronic acid is one of the principal mechanisms of drug metabolism taking place in humans and animals, and is the final step in metabolic transformations [1-4]. Functional groups such as hydroxyl, carboxyl, amino, and sulfhydryl in the molecules of drugs or endogenous compounds undergo conjugation with D-glucuronic acid. For relatively nonpolar compounds, conversion into more polar metabolites is often a prerequisite for conjugation with glucuronic acid. Polar groups are introduced by oxidation, reduction, dealkylation, and hydrolysis by appropriate enzymes of the body.

The presence of activated D-glucuronic acid in the form of uridine 5'-(D-glucopyranosyluronic acid pyrophosphate) (uridine diphosphoglucuronic acid; UDPGA) is necessary for glucuronidation [5]. The UDPGA is easily generated from glucose via UDP-glucose by the action of the specific enzyme UDPG-dehydrogenase. Transfer of glucuronic acid from the glucuronyl donor UDPGA to the aglycone is catalyzed by a microsomal enzyme, glucuronyl transferase, in the following reaction:

$$\text{UDP-}\alpha\text{-D-glucuronic acid} + \text{R-H} \rightarrow \text{R-}\beta\text{-D-glucuronic acid} + \text{UDP}$$

The reaction is stereospecific and the conjugates of glucuronic acid always have the β-D configuration. The pyranoside structure has been assigned to, and proved for, naturally occurring glucuronic acid conjugates [3, 6-8]. The conjugates formed are usually referred to as glucuronides, glucosiduronic acids, glucopyranosyluronic acids, and glucosiduronates. In this chapter, the term glucuronide will be employed to conform with customary biochemical usage as a convenient trivial name for glycosides of D-glucuronic acid that are systematically named as D-glucosiduronic acids. The 1-acyl esters of D-glucuronic acids are not included in the term glucuronide. The term glucuronate should be used only for derivatives in which the C-6 carboxyl group is esterified or for salts of glucuronic acid, and glucosiduronate for salts and esters of glycosidic conjugates.

The endogenous conjugating agent glucuronic acid has an active hydroxyl group at C-1. The conjugation with various drugs and endogenous compounds results in the formation of several classes of conjugates: D-glucosiduronic acids (trivial name, glucuronides), 1-O-acylglucuronic acids (incorrect trivial name, ester "glucuronides"), glucopyranosylamineuronic acids (trivial name, N-glucuronides), and 1-thioglucopyranosiduronic acids (trivial name, S-glucuronides).

In the case of the glucuronides, three groups are distinguished: the ether glucuronides, the enol type of conjugates, and the conjugates of N-hydroxy compounds. Ether glucuronides are formed from primary, secondary, and tertiary alcohols and phenols, the most significant group being the steroid glucosiduronic acids. In general, glucuronides of the ether type are stable in alkaline solutions, but they differ in stability in acid. Due to their stability, conjugates of this type have proved to be suitable compounds for the study of configuration and molecular structure. Numerous ether glucuronides have been isolated from biological material, and many have been synthesized [3, 9].

Conjugates of the enol type are represented by derivatives of some steroids and pseudoacids, where the aglycone is conjugated with glucuronic acid through an enolized ketone group [10]. A common characteristic of enolglucosiduronic acids is instability in alkaline solutions. N-Hydroxy compounds with glucuronic acid form alkali-sensitive N-substituted glucuronides. A few compounds belonging to this group have recently been synthesized or isolated from biological material [11]. They became the compounds of interest after the discovery that metabolism of such carcinogenic substances as N-2-fluorenylacetamide results in the formation of O-glucuronides of N-hydroxy compounds [12].

Compounds containing a carboxyl group undergo conjugation with glucuronic acid to form 1-O-acylglucuronic acids. This group includes the conjugates of various anti-inflammatory drugs and indolic acids. The usual procedures for the isolation and synthesis of these conjugates are hampered by their marked instability in alkaline solution. Although a few isolates from biological material had been reported previously [13, 14], a successful synthesis has been reported recently [15-17].

N-Glucuronides result from the reaction of glucuronic acid with foreign compounds containing an aromatic or aliphatic amino group, a sulfonamide or carbamoyl group, or a heterocyclic nitrogen atom [3, 18]. The resulting conjugates differ significantly in their stability in acid solution, the stability depending upon the nature of the aglycone and the mode and site of linkage of the glucuronic acid moiety to the aglycone. Conjugates of aromatic amines are acid labile, whereas conjugates formed from drugs containing the carbamoyl group and from sulfonamides exhibit considerable stability in acid [19].

S-Glucuronides originate from reactions of glucuronic acid with compounds containing the sulfhydryl group. They are stable both to alkali and acid, and successful syntheses, biosyntheses, and isolations have been reported [3, 20]. However, in comparison to ether glucuronides, only a very limited number of S-glucuronides have been found in biological material.

A group-specific enzyme, β-D-glucuronidase, has been isolated from various mammalian and bacterial sources, as well as from invertebrates, plants, and fungi [21, 22]. All glucuronic acid conjugates except N-glucuronides of aromatic and aliphatic amines are enzymatically hydrolyzed by β-D-glucuronidase, yielding the free aglycone and glucuronic acid. Only the β-D-glycosidic linkage is cleaved by β-D-glucuronidase, and α-D-anomers are not affected. The reaction is strongly inhibited by D-glucaro-1, 4-lactone.

Conjugation with glucuronic acid results in the formation of strongly acidic compounds, entirely ionized at physiological pH values, thus enabling the excretion of a compound in the urine and bile. Ionized conjugates are prevented from permeating through cell membranes, and they are mainly confined to the extracellular fluids, urine, bile, and blood [4]. The route of excretion is determined by various chemical factors such as the molecular weight, the molecular structure, and the polarity of the glucuronide [23]. It has generally been assumed that glucuronides of low molecular weight are excreted mainly in the urine. High molecular weight (over 300) and relatively lipophilic behavior of conjugates are prerequisites for extensive biliary excretion. Glucuronides of intermediate molecular weight are usually excreted by both routes.

Conjugates excreted in urine are eliminated from the body, whereas the metabolites excreted in bile can be eliminated in feces, but can also undergo enterohepatic circulation prior to final excretion in the urine [24].

Since conjugation with glucuronic acid is usually the final step in the metabolism, conjugates are excreted either in the bile or in the urine and feces. In addition, due to enterohepatic circulation, minor quantities of glucuronides exist in blood. In vitro studies are frequently performed on homogenates of liver, kidneys, intestine, etc. Consequently, analysis of glucuronides consists of various isolation and separation procedures, chemical reactions, and enzymic hydrolysis which are applied to bile, urine, feces, blood, and tissue homogenates. Regardless of the nature of the conjugate and the biological material examined, the major difficulty is the possible interference of the other natural constituents present. Only a very limited number of glucuronide determinations can be directly conducted on physiological fluids. For more accurate results, the isolation and separation of glucuronides from other metabolites prior to their identification and characterization is required. The choice of methods depends on the specificity and accuracy requirements. The highest accuracy is achieved in experiments with labeled drugs. Studies with labeled compounds have to be performed in order to obtain quantitative data on metabolic patterns and routes of excretion.

Hydrolysis with β-glucuronidase is an essential step in the analysis of glucuronides, and is performed either directly on the biological material or on a purified product. Combined experiments with the inhibitor D-glucaro-1,4-lactone are highly recommended, since some enzyme preparations contain impurities such as sulfatases, and may lead to false results.

The fate of administered drugs is often unpredictable due to possible metabolic changes prior to conjugation and excretion. Since a relatively simple parent drug can give rise to various derivatives, it is of the utmost importance to identify and prove the structure of the aglycone liberated by enzymic, acidic, or alkaline hydrolysis. Such studies are also greatly facilitated by the use of labeled parent drugs.

The first glucuronic acid conjugates isolated from biological material were identified by derivatization and comparison with synthetic samples. Methyl esterification of the carboxyl group in the glucuronic acid moiety, followed by acetylation of the free hydroxyl groups, often yielded crystalline derivatives, suitable for analysis and comparison with authentic specimens. The structures of numerous glucuronic acid conjugates were proved in this way. Derivatization of the glucuronic acid moiety in the conjugate molecule facilitated and enabled the application of the various instrumental techniques used today for the identification or characterization of glucuronides.

Conclusive evidence for the structure of a particular glucuronic acid conjugate should be deduced from physicochemical data concerning the structure of the aglycone, the presence of glucuronic acid moiety, and the mode and position of linkage of the aglycone to the glucuronic acid. When possible, the structural assignment should be confirmed by direct comparison with a synthetic sample.

Possibilities for the direct estimation of glucuronic acid conjugates are discussed in Section II. Section III deals with the isolation procedures most frequently used, and Section IV with methods for the separation and characterization of glucuronic acid conjugates. Hydrolysis with β-D-glucuronidase will be covered in the Section V.

II. DIRECT ASSAY OF GLUCURONIC ACID CONJUGATES
IN BIOLOGICAL MATERIAL

Direct estimation of glucuronic acid conjugates in urine, blood, bile, or the supernatant liquors of tissue homogenates is usually hampered by the presence of (1) large proportions of normal excretion products, which interfere with determination procedures for glucuronides, and (2) low concentrations of drug metabolites in unconcentrated physiological fluids.

Existing methods that are suitable for direct assays fall into several groups. The first is based on differential analysis of glucuronides and free glucuronic acid, employing naphthoresorcinol or carbazole for colorimetric determination of the glucuronic acid equivalent in the glucuronide moiety. Interfering free glucuronic acid is either selectively oxidized or degraded in alkali. This limits the application of such methods to alkali-stable ether glucuronides. The estimation of 1-O-acylglucuronic acids can be accomplished by specific reaction of these esters with hydroxamic acids.

The method most frequently used is chromatography on an analytical or preparative scale. Prerequisites for successful application and accuracy are suitable standards for comparison purposes and, preferably, the use of radiolabeled parent drugs.

Instrumental techniques, gas chromatography, and high-pressure liquid chromatography offer new possibilities for fast and very accurate isolation and characterization of glucuronic acid conjugates from biological material in one step.

A. Methods Based on Reaction of Naphthoresorcinol
and Carbazole with Glucuronic Acid

The modified naphthoresorcinol reaction, introduced in 1908 by Tollens [25], has been used for qualitative and quantitative assays of glucuronic acid. The blue pigment formed in the reaction between naphthoresorcinol and glucuronic acid is extracted into an organic solvent, and the amount of complex formed is estimated colorimetrically. As the reaction is performed in the presence of a strong acid, it can be applied to glucuronic acid conjugates since the glycosidic linkage is cleaved by acid. If the reagent is added to the mixture of free and conjugated glucuronic acid, the value for total glucuronic acid is obtained. There is a great probability that free glucuronic acid will be present in physiological fluids. In order to obtain the value for conjugated glucuronic acid, the free acid should be eliminated prior to the addition of naphthoresorcinol. In 1955, Fishman and Green [26] proposed a method based on the selective oxidation of free glucuronic acid (and other oxidizable, interfering substances) by alkaline iodine solution. The glucuronides present were resistant to oxidation. In subsequent reaction with naphthoresorcinol, the amount of conjugated glucuronic acid was obtained, since the D-glucaric acid formed from the free glucuronic acid did not react. The amount of free glucuronic acid was calculated from the difference between the total and the conjugated glucuronic acid. The carbazole reaction of Dische [27] can be successfully used in the differential analysis of free glucuronic acid and glucosiduronic acids [28] instead of naphthoresorcinol.

Oxidation with iodine is conducted under alkaline conditions (pH 10.1), and its use is limited to alkali-stable glucosiduronic acids.

The accuracy of the method is affected by large proportions of glucose that may also be present in physiological fluids. The problem of D-glucose interference in the naphthoresorcinol reaction was solved by pretreating the deproteinized human blood sample with D-glucose oxidase [29].

A slightly modified Fishman method [30] used iodine for oxidation and naphthoresorcinol for glucuronic acid estimation, but no comment was made on the possible interference by D-glucose.

Recently, Mazzuchin et al. [31] reported modification with alkaline degradation of the free glucuronic acid instead of oxidation by iodine. Glucose was selectively oxidized by glucose oxidase prior to assay of the glucuronic acid. The authors elaborated the procedure in detail, and studied the accuracy and reproducibility of the naphthoresorcinol method. The use of NaOH for the degradation of glucuronic acid limited the applicability of the procedure to ether glucuronides.

The use of existing methods based on naphthoresorcinol and carbazole reaction enables the quantitative assay of glucuronic acid conjugates in physiological fluids with reasonable accuracy. However, these methods have the common disadvantage that they do not distinguish between the individual metabolites and do not provide data on the nature of the aglycone.

B. Chemical Estimation of 1-O-Acylglucuronic Acids

Alkali-labile ester "glucuronides" react with hydroxylamine to form characteristic hydroxamic acids. Free glucuronic acid and conjugates with nonacyl groups do not give hydroxamic acids. This provides the possibility to selectively determine ester glucuronides directly in biological material.

Schachter [32] elaborated the method for estimation of various 1-O-acyl-glucuronic acids in urine. Stable hydroxamates of aglycones were formed upon the addition of hydroxylamine at neutral pH and room temperature, followed by the addition of acidic ferric chloride solution. The separation of colored derivatives from reaction mixtures by extraction with ether offered the possibility for further characterization and subsequent identification of metabolites, if suitable reference compounds were available. Schachter examined ether extracts by paper chromatography, comparing hydroxamates from urine with synthetic samples. Data on urinary excretion patterns in man for benzoyl, salicyl, and probenecid acyl conjugates were reported. In a subsequent paper, the estimation of the acyl conjugate of salicylic acid in plasma and urine was described [33]. A modification was applied to estimate a probenecid acyl conjugate [34].

C. Chromatographic Methods

Paper and thin-layer chromatography have found extensive application in the analysis of glucuronic acid conjugates due to their simplicity, inexpensiveness, and speed. Chromatographic assays of biological material without prior purification are affected by the presence of endogenous constituents in physiological fluids and extracts.

For accurate results in chromatographic assays the radioactive parent drug and corresponding standards for comparison purposes should be available. The use of labeled parent drug permits distinction between a metabolite and naturally occurring constituents in the material examined. At the same time, location of labeled metabolites by radioactive scanning eliminates the possible errors in the estimation of R_f values. Severe changes in R_f frequently occur due to the interference of pigments, salts, and other constituents of biological materials.

Presumptive evidence of identity for various glucuronic acid conjugates have been reported based on direct comparison of several chromatographic parameters with those of standards. Usually, several cochromatographies of physiological fluids in various solvent systems are needed for satisfactory results. The use of labeled drugs has the additional advantage that scanning of chromatograms permits the quantitation of metabolites according to the radioactivity detected.

Qualitative detection of glucuronic acid conjugates on paper or thin-layer chromatograms is in most cases performed by spraying with the naphthoresorcinol reagent. Acid present in the reagent mixture, combined with heating of the chromatogram, hydrolyzes the conjugate, and liberated glucuronic acid is revealed as a blue spot. Trichloroacetic acid [3, 35], or phosphoric acid [19, 36] are most frequently used with naphthoresorcinol. A periodate - benzidine spray was used for the detection of glucuronic acid conjugates of salicylic acid [14].

Paper chromatography has been used to determine species differences in the metabolic patterns of labeled parent drugs [37]. Examples are the urinary excretion of benzoic acid in man and 20 other animal species [37] and the fate of phenol [38], naphthol, morphine, and phenacetin [35].

Paper chromatography was also used for the estimation of metabolites of the insecticide 2, 2-dichlorovinyl-dimethyl phosphate, including 2, 2-dichloro-ethyl glucuronide [39], urinary metabolites of prontosil {4-[(2, 4-diaminophenyl)-azo] benzenesulfonamide}, including a labile N-glucuronide [40], urinary metabolites of phenacetin [41], and biliary thyroxine glucuronide [42].

Recently, Atef and Nilsen [43] estimated and quantified sulfadiazine-N^4 glucuronide in goat urine, plasma, and milk by paper chromatography. Paper and thin-layer chromatography can be extended for preparative purposes. Glucuronic acid conjugates separated on paper or TLC can be eluted from paper strips and characterized. Direct isolation from biological material has been reported for thyroxine glucuronide from bile [44, 45], for various S-glucuronides from supernatant liquors of incubation mixtures [20] and for lorazepam glucuronide extracted from urine and plasma [46].

Preparative chromatography was employed for the final purification of glucuronic acid conjugates. Yoshimura et al. [47] reported the preparation of morphine-6 glucuronide. Wood et al. [48] discussed the final separation of tolamolol {1-[2-(4-carbamoylphenoxy)ethylamino]-3-(2-methylphenoxy)propan-2-ol} metabolites after concentration on XAD-2 resin and partial separation on silica gel columns.

III. ISOLATION OF GLUCURONIC ACID CONJUGATES
   FROM BIOLOGICAL MATERIAL

Methods for the isolation of polar metabolites from biological fluids should be considered as the initial steps in glucuronide analysis, not as self-sufficient and complete procedures. The isolated product is frequently a mixture of conjugated and nonconjugated polar metabolites that include both glucuronides and sulfates and contain salts, pigments, and other endogenous constituents present in the biological material examined. Although the proportion of impurities can be lessened to some extent by the proper combination of isolation techniques, the final products are usually complex mixtures which require further purification, separation, and characterization. The choice of a suitable method for isolation will depend upon the type and stability of the particular glucuronide and on the instruments and chemicals available. Regardless of the technique chosen, it is worthwhile to start with the extraction of nonpolar metabolites and unchanged parent compounds. Extraction with organic solvents at neutral pH would remove nonpolar compounds and facilitate the handling of other compounds.

Instrumental isolation procedures, such as high-pressure liquid chromatography and gas chromatography, which also provide separation and characterization, will be described in Section IV.

A. Extraction with Organic Solvents

Concentration of glucuronic acid conjugates from biological material by extraction with organic solvents is a normal first step in isolation and separation procedures. Unconjugated compounds and relatively nonpolar metabolites can be extracted at neutral values and low ionic strength. Acidic polar metabolites require lower pH values and the addition of inorganic salts for satisfactory results. It is possible to extract polar metabolite such as glucuronides with the proper adjustment of pH and ionic strength of physiological fluids.

Organic solvents such as 1-butanol, ethyl acetate, and ethanol-ether are frequently employed for glucuronide extraction. n-Butanol isolated a mixture containing N-dedimethylchlorpromazine glucuronide by continuous extraction from urine [49], and extracted retinyl glucuronide and 1-O-retinoylglucuronic acid from bile and incubation mixtures [50]. Ether-ethanol was used for extraction of the O-glucuronide of N-hydroxy-2-acetamidofluorene from bile [12].

The best results are obtained with step-wise extraction procedures. Unchanged drugs and unconjugated metabolites are removed first, followed by the acidification of the remaining aqueous layer and the addition of inorganic salts such as ammonium sulfate. Examples are the isolation of indomethacin glucuronide from human urine [51], probenecid glucuronides from bile, urine, and plasma [52, 53], and metabolites of the anti-inflammatory drug 4-[3-(dimethylamino)propyl]-3,4-dihydro-2-(1-hydroxyethyl)-3-phenyl-2H-1,4-benzothiazine from urine and incubation mixtures [54]. Tetrahydrocortisone glucuronide and estrone and 17β-estradiol glucuronides [55, 56] were extracted from incubation mixtures with 1-butanol. The fate of pentaerythritol nitrates in rats was extensively studied [57, 59] by isolation of the corresponding glucuronides from bile, plasma, urine, and supernatant liquors of tissue homogenates after extraction with ethyl acetate subsequent to the removal of unconjugated drug and metabolites.

Extraction with organic solvents has several limitations. It is not convenient for large volumes of physiological fluids, and it does not always provide good recoveries. The choice of solvent is important. A solvent most commonly used is 1-butanol; it has a high boiling point and a tendency to form emulsions. Ether-ethanol mixtures are highly inflammable.

B. Precipitation of Glucuronides as Their Lead Salts

The lead salt technique was first reported by Kamil et al. [60] as a successful method for the isolation of glucuronic acid conjugates from urine. Saturated normal lead acetate was added to urine at pH 4. The first precipitate was discarded, the supernatant liquor brought to pH 8, and saturated aqueous basic lead acetate added in excess. Lead was removed by treatment of the resulting precipitate in methanol or water suspension with H_2S, yielding the free glucuronide in the supernatant liquor.

It is possible that some glucuronides will be precipitated with normal lead acetate. Thus both normal and basic lead precipitates should be checked for glucuronic acid content by the naphthoresorcinol or carbazole method. The lead salt technique was very frequently employed prior to the elaboration of column chromatography. Since 1951, Williams and his collaborators have reported a series of studies in detoxication [13, 61-65, 209]. Numerous ether glucuronides and "ester glucuronides" were isolated, characterized, and identified by such relatively simple procedures as solvent extraction, the lead salt technique, and conversion into crystalline salts and derivatives. Alternative applications of solvent extraction and lead salt techniques were necessary when glucuronides were not completely precipitated as lead salts, even under alkaline conditions. Ester glucuronides of salicylic acid [63] and p-aminosalicylic acid [14] were isolated as lead salts from urine. A meprobamate metabolite, an N-glucuronide, was obtained as a gum [66] after treatment with basic lead acetate, and as the crystalline Na salt [67].

The lead salt technique has been applied to the isolation of conjugates of N-hydroxy compounds, N-2-fluorenylacethydroxamic acid [68] and N-acetyl-N-phenylhydroxylamine [69]. This method has been applied to the isolation of a new apigenin glucuronide from pyrethrum flowers [70], the purification of thiamphenicol glucuronide isolated by preparative, thin-layer chromatography from urine and bile [71], and the isolation of biosynthetically prepared N-acetyl-p-aminophenyl glucuronide [41]. The method's obvious advantage is that it employs mild conditions that permit the isolation of alkali- and acid-labile glucuronic acid conjugates. In the isolated product, interfering compounds are minimized and crystalline conjugates or derivatives can be readily prepared. Unfortunately, the overall recovery of the glucuronide component is usually poor.

C. Adsorption on Activated Charcoal

Concentration of glucuronic acid conjugates from urine by use of activated charcoal is a method of choice for large quantities of urine. It is applicable to glucuronic acid conjugates with aglycones such as steroids, aromatic compounds, and alkaloids that meet the requirements for adsorption on charcoal. Acetic acid and ammonia, with or without polar organic solvents, are usual eluants for glucuronic acid conjugates.

Arcos and Lieberman [72] studied the adsorption process for steroid glucuronides and evaluated the quantitative ratios of charcoal and urine, the effect of temperature on binding, and the efficiency of various solvents as eluting agents. They claimed that the structure of the conjugate was not altered by the processes of adsorption and desorption.

Applications have been the isolation of sulfathiazole-N glucuronide from human urine by charcoal extraction of metabolite prior to chromatography on ion-exchange resins [73], and charcoal adsorption as the first isolation step for morphine and metabolites from bile and urine of rabbits [47] and urine from cats [74]. Chloramphenicol glucuronide [75] and lorazepam and oxazepam glucuronides [76] have been isolated from urine by charcoal adsorption.

Adsorption on charcoal, like most of the procedures described in this section, is a nonspecific process yielding complex mixtures that require further separation.

D. Adsorption on XAD Resins

Amberlite XAD resin is a nonionic, three-dimensional styrene - divinyl-benzene copolymer having a high surface area. Its most significant property is the adsorption of water soluble, organic species from aqueous solutions. Gustafson et al. [77] extensively studied XAD resin adsorption of various molecular structures. Hydrophobic methylene groups or aromatic rings enhanced adsorption, and a distinct separation of organic components from inorganic salts was achieved. Bradlow [78] reported a successful and simple isolation procedure using neutral XAD-2 resin for the extraction of steroid glucuronides from urine. Two liters of urine were processed on 1 kg of resin. Extensive washing with water removed inorganic material and urea and amino acids. Subsequent elution with methanol yielded glucuronides, pigments, unconjugated metabolites, and other endogenous constituents of biological material. The advantages were quantitative recoveries of glucuronic acid conjugates.

XAD-2 was used subsequently for the isolation of steroid metabolites such as estrone-3 glucosiduronic acid and 17β-estradiol-3 glucosiduronic acid [79], 17-estradiol glucosiduronic acid [80], corticosteroid metabolites [81], estrogen conjugates [82], glucuronosulfates of cortisol [83], aldosterone-18 and tetrahydroaldosterone glucuronide [84], norgestrel glucuronide [85], testosterone-17 glucosiduronic acid [86], and the 3-glucuronide 17-acetylglucosaminide of 17α-estradiol [87].

Amberlite XAD-2 effectively separated narcotic drugs and their metabolites from urinary constituents [88]. Weissman et al. [89] demonstrated that adsorption on XAD-2 can isolate metabolites of narcotics, analgesics, symphatomimetics, hypnotics, and sedatives. Morphine-3 glucuronide [90] and hydromorphone and dihydromorphine glucuronides [91] were isolated in this way. Isolation of conjugated compounds from cow's milk was accomplished with XAD-4 resin [92]. Metabolites of lorazepam and oxazepam [93], of the larvicide 4-nitro-3-(trifluoromethyl)phenol [94], of analgesic H-88 [1-(3-fluoromethyl)phenyl-3-(2-hydroxyethyl)quinazoline-2,4(1H,3H)-dione] [95], of tolamolol {1-[2-(4-carbamoylphenoxy)ethyl-amino]-3-(2-methylphenoxy)propan-2-ol} [48] and of viloxazine [2-(2-ethoxyphenoxymethyl)-2,3,5,6-tetrahydro-1,4-oxazine] [96] were also processed on Amberlite XAD-2.

The use of nonionic resins permits simple, rapid, inexpensive, and essentially quantitative isolation of organic material, including glucuronic acid conjugates from large volumes of biological fluids. Performed at neutral pH values, it is applicable to all groups of glucuronides, and is unlikely to cause undesirable alterations in the structure of glucuronic acid conjugates.

E. Isolation by Gel Filtration on Sephadex

Sephadexes G-10 and G-25 are molecular sieves in the isolation of glucuronic acid conjugates. In the process of gel filtration, constituents of urine of low molecular weight are retained on Sephadex. Continuous elution with water yields glucuronic acid conjugates, separated from material of high molecular weight and from salts.

Estrogen conjugates were preliminarily purified [97] and processed from Sephadex filtration of urine [98]. The isolation of steroids from large volumes of urine was described by Cohen and Oran [99]. Estrogen conjugates precipitated with ammonium sulfate were processed on Sephadex G-25 columns. Pyridinethione glucuronide (S-type conjugate) was isolated from rabbit urine by filtration of Sephadex G-10, followed by ion-exchange chromatography [100]. The conjugate of N-hydroxy-4-aminobiphenyl was isolated from urine by using Sephadex G-10 for initial fractionation prior to chromatography on Sephadex LH-20 [101].

This procedure with mild conditions yields urinary glucuronic acid conjugates free from salts and does not demand inherent stability. In spite of its simplicity and generally good performance, the method is still not frequently used for the isolation of glucuronides.

F. Ion-exchange Chromatography

The glucuronide carboxyl group suggests the use of ion-exchange resins. Conjugates of relatively simple aglycones would undergo anionic exchange due to the dissociable carboxyl group in the glucuronic acid moiety. In the more complex conjugates, both the aglycone and glucuronic acid residue would contribute to separation on ion-exchange resins. Conjugates with dissociable nitrogen or other functional groups in the aglycone will undergo anionic and cationic exchange processes. The proper combination of acidic and basic resins should provide the partial elimination of various ionizable and nonionizable impurities.

1. Ion-exchange Resins

Isolation procedures employing ion-exchange resins are usually performed in two steps. Most of the conjugates will be retained on basic resins in the formate, carbonate, or acetate form, and will subsequently be eluted with buffers containing corresponding anions. The conjugate 2,2,2-trifluoroethyl glucuronide was eluted with water from Dowex-50 (H^+) and subsequently submitted to an anion-exchange process on Dowex-1 (OH^-) [102]. For more complex glucuronides, such as sulfadimethoxine glucuronide [19], apomorphine glucuronide [103], and dopamine glucuronide [104], more elaborate systems were used. Due to the properties of nitrogen in aglycones, conjugates were retained on basic as well as on acidic resins. Washing with water eliminated impurities in each step, and elution with appropriate buffers yielded conjugates. Morphine and its conjugates were recovered [105] after processing the supernatant liquors of brain homogenates on a cation-exchange resin (Dowex-50, H^+) prior to separation on thin-layer chromatograms. Complete purification was achieved, with difficulty, due to the presence of such ionizable substances as amino acids. The isolate of crude sulfamethoxine glucuronide [19] still contained 60% impurities, mostly amino acids.

The ion-exchange resins usually employed in the isolation of glucuronides act as strong acids and bases, and should, therefore, be applied only to stable glucuronic acid conjugates.

2. DEAE-Cellulose and DEAE-Sephadex

The use of DEAE-cellulose and DEAE-Sephadex has also been reported. The 2-diethylaminoethyl group is a weakly basic ion-exchanger that separates labile glucuronic acid conjugates without affecting the glycosidic linkage.

Various aryl glucosiduronic acids were recovered from incubation mixtures by using chromatography on DEAE-cellulose [106]. A bile sample was chromatographed directly on DEAE-cellulose in the acetate form, and the mixture containing the O-glucuronide of N-hydroxy-2-acetamidofluorene was eluted with acetic acid [12]. Preliminary purification of 5,6-dihydro-5,6-dihydroxycarbaryl glucuronide from urine [107] and quantitative separation of radioactive diphenylhydantoin and its p-hydroxylated metabolites from plasma [108] was effected on DEAE-cellulose.

DEAE-Sephadex was used for the isolation of ethyl glucuronide from urine [109] for the separation of urinary constituents after administration of safrol (4-allyl-1,2-methylenedioxybenzene) [110], and the metabolites of estrogen from supernatant liquors of liver and kidney homogenates [111, 112]. The supernatant liquor from incubation mixtures, containing acyl conjugate of 3-hydroxyanthranilic acid, was processed [113], and the same procedure was applied to isolate the acyl conjugate from urine [114]. The glucuronide of N-hydroxy-4-acetamidobiphenyl was isolated and purified from rat bile by chromatography on DEAE-Sephadex (acetate form) and subsequent, repeated chromatography on Sephadex G-10 [101].

3. Liquid Ion-exchangers

The use of liquid ion-exchangers for the isolation of polar metabolites was recently introduced by Hofman [115], who suggested the same technique for the extraction of steroid glucosiduronic acid. Liquid ion-exchangers are long-chain aliphatic amines such as methyltricaprylylammonium chloride, trioctylamine, tetraheptylammonium chloride (THAC), and a few branched-chain, aliphatic primary and secondary amines (Amberlite LA-2 and XLA-3). The use of liquid ion-exchangers offers the possibility for the extraction of polar organic compounds from water into organic solvent. The extraction is enhanced by the addition of ammonium sulfate or inorganic salts to the aqueous phase. Mattox et al. [116, 117] extensively studied the applicability of various liquid ion-exchangers to the extraction of glucosiduronic acids of various steroids differing in polarity. Methods for paper chromatography of steroid conjugates using tetraheptylammonium chloride in the mobile phase in combination with chloroform - formamide, toluene, or ethyl acetate were also reported [118]. The addition of THAC to the mobile phase increased the mobility of polar glucosiduronic acids, and permitted their separation.

IV. SEPARATION AND CHARACTERIZATION OF
     GLUCURONIC ACID CONJUGATES

This discussion will be confined mainly to chromatographic and instrumental
procedures for the separation and characterization of glucuronic acid conjugates.

Chromatography on DEAE- and LH-Sephadex separated partially purified
sulfuric acid and glucuronic acid conjugates. Glucuronic acid conjugates
can be further separated by counter-current distribution, partition chromatography, or paper and thin-layer chromatography, and are of particular
value in the analysis of steroid conjugates. Simple and inexpensive separations by paper or thin-layer chromatography are frequently final steps
in the purification of glucuronic acid conjugates.

High-resolution liquid chromatography can separate glucuronides with
UV-absorbing aglycones. Glucuronic acid conjugates converted to sufficiently volatile derivatives can be separated by gas chromatography, provided that the derivatives employed are stable on high-temperature columns.

Physicochemical methods for the characterization of glucuronides include
gas chromatography, mass spectrometry, and NMR, UV, and IR spectroscopy. Conversion into a suitable stable crystalline derivative, preferably
the methyl ester or triacetate, is helpful. Evidence for the structure of a
particular conjugate is usually based on a spectral data and chromatographic behavior.

The methods to determine the position of attachment of the glucosyluronic group to the steroid residue are also discussed.

A. Group Separation of Sulfuric Acid and Glucuronic
    Acid Conjugates

Conjugation with sulfuric acid is a widely encountered metabolic pathway
that frequently parallels glucuronic acid conjugation. The occurrence of
double conjugates has been demonstrated in the steroid series: estrogen
sulfoglucosiduronic acid [119, 120] and 5α-androstane-3α, 17β-diol dicon-
jugate [86]. Most of the methods elaborated for the group separation of
sulfuric acid and glucuronic acid conjugates are related to steroids.

In a separation based on differential hydrolysis of biological fluids or
isolated conjugates [86], hydrolysis with β-D-glucuronidase is followed
by extraction of steroid aglycones and subsequent characterization. The
sulfate conjugates in the remaining aqueous phase are submitted to acid
or sulfatase hydrolysis. The liberated aglycones are further extracted
and characterized.

More accurate methods separate intact conjugates. Goertz et al. [121] described a method utilizing the specific reaction of sulfuric esters with Methylene Blue. After extraction of unconjugated steroids, Methylene Blue (Vlitos reagent) was added to the mixture. The complex with sulfate conjugates was extracted with chloroform and the glucuronic acid conjugates which did not react with Methylene Blue remained in the aqueous phase. It was claimed that excess reagent did not affect the enzymic hydrolysis of the remaining glucosiduronic acids.

Chromatographic separation can be based on differences in the polarities of the nonsteroidal part of the molecule. Jirku and Levitz [122] separated the biliary and urinary conjugates of estrone 3-sulfate by chromatography on alumina; sulfates were separated from glucosiduronic acid and sulfoglucosiduronic acids. The latter were further separated by partition chromatography on Celite.

Hobkirk et al. [119] reported the successful chromatographic separation of various estrone and 17β-estradiol conjugates on DEAE-Sephadex A-25 by using gradient elution with NaCl. The elution patterns exhibited several distinct zones; free steroids were followed by glucosiduronic acids, sulfates, and sulfoglucosiduronic acids. This procedure, in combination with pre-purification of biological fluids on XAD resins, separated numerous steroid conjugates, including those of estrogen [79, 80, 120], aldosterone [84], estrone [82], and urinary metabolites of the totally synthetic steroid DL-norgestrel [85]. Further separation of the components in glucosiduronic acids group was effected by partition on Celite, repeated fractionation on DEAE-Sephadex, or paper chromatography [123, 124].

The lipophilic properties of Sephadex LH-20 were convenient for the separation of various steroid conjugates. Elution with chloroform - methanol containing sodium chloride resulted in distinct resolution. Glucuronides were eluted first, followed by sulfates and sulfoglucosiduronic acids. The elution volume of a particular conjugate varied with the concentration of chloroform and sodium chloride. Proper adjustment of the solvent-to-salt ratio in the eluant enabled good separation of structurally similar conjugates. The extraction of free steroids prior to chromatography has been reported in many cases, such as in the use of Sephadex LH-20 for the separation of glucosiduronic acids and sulfates of various C_{19} and C_{21} steroids [125, 126] and the separation of endogenous steroid conjugates from the bile of human fetuses [127]. The separation of steroid metabolites in urine was improved by processing urine on Sephadex G-25 prior to group separation [128]. The same procedure was used for the separation of estriol conjugates [129]. Estriol-16α-glucuronide was purified on XAD-2 resin and Sephadex G-25, followed by chromatography on Sephadex LH-20 [130]. The resolution of biliary testosterone metabolites was effected on XAD-2 resin, followed by chromatography on Sephadex LH-20 [86].

In 1964, Kornel [131] suggested the use of high-voltage paper electrophoresis for group separation of corticosteroid conjugates, since glucuronic
acid conjugates differ in mobility from steroid sulfates, monosulfates from
disulfates, and monoglucuronides from diglucuronides. The effectiveness
of separation is dependent upon the pH, the choice of buffer, and the cur-
rent-potential gradient. This method separated corticosteroid metabolites
in human urine [81] and corticosteroid conjugates in human plasma [83].
A complete separation and purification of metabolites present in the sample could be achieved by several successive electrophoretic runs.

Thin-layer and paper chromatography are applicable to group separation,
such as in the TLC separation of indoxyl glucuronide and sulfate after the
administration of labeled indole [132]. Steroid conjugates are not suitable
for standard chromatography on paper or in TLC. Only partial separation
of sulfates from glucosiduronic acids and sulfoglucosiduronic acids could
be achieved, since only the sulfate conjugates exhibited sufficient mobility
[133]. The mobility of steroidal glucosiduronic acids can be enhanced by
the addition of a liquid ion-exchanger (such as THAC) to the mobile phase
and KCl to the stationary phase of conventional chromatographic systems
[116]. Mattox et al. [134] considered the effects of various chromatographic parameters upon the separation of steroid conjugates. The conjugates exhibiting the same chromatographic mobility in a particular system containing a liquid ion-exchanger could be separated if the concentration of the counter-ion in the stationary phase were adjusted properly. The
R_f values for the various conjugates in several chromatographic systems
are presented in the Appendix.

B. Separation by Counter-current Distribution (CCD)

Separation by CCD is based on the difference in distribution coefficients
exhibited by components of a mixture after successive transfers between
two immiscible solvents. Applications and limitations in the separation
of steroid conjugates are discussed in the literature [120, 135, 136].

Notwithstanding the laborious and time-consuming aspects of this method,
it frequently is the only way for the successful separation of conjugates of
structurally similar aglycones and purification of the crude glucosiduronic
acid preparations to remove polar contaminants. Processing the conjugates in liquid phases avoids eventual irreversible adsorption on stationary
phases. The use of labeled compound facilitates the detection and tracing
of metabolites and enhances the accuracy.

Systematic resolutions of metabolites or conjugates originating from a
single administered steroid were described with several solvent systems
for the labeled estriol 3-sulfate 16-glucosiduronic acid [137], 16-epiestriol
[138], and testosterone [139].

Mattox et al. [140] presented partition coefficients of six conjugates of synthetic corticosteroid glucosiduronic acids in eleven solvent systems. These data should help to choose the proper solvent system for the separation of corticosteroid conjugates.

Glucosiduronic acids of the mono-, di-, and trinitrates of pentaerythritol [58] were separated from bile and urine extracts by distribution between an aqueous phase (saturated ammonium sulfate) and an organic phase (ethyl acetate - ethanol). CCD between the two phases of the 1-butanol - acetic acid - water system isolated hydromorphone and dihydromorphine glucuronides [91]. The processing lowered the amounts of polar organic contaminants in the mixture, but failed to resolve the two conjugates. Final separation was achieved by subsequent chromatography on aluminum oxide.

Successful separation of 1-O-acylglucuronic acids under these mild conditions of distribution were effected [51]. Conjugates of indomethacin [1-(p-chlorobenzoyl)-5-methoxy-2-methylindole-3-acetic acid], dechlorobenzoylindomethacin, and O-demethylindomethacin were separated in the two phases of a system containing phosphate buffer, ethyl acetate, and sec-butyl alcohol. CCD usually provides only partial resolution into components differing in purity, but permits more effective further purification. Radioactive homogeneity for the glucuronides of pentaerythritol nitrates was estimated to be in the range of ~95 to 99%, whereas the purity of preparations of indomethacin and related glucosiduronic acids varied from 55 to 85%.

C. High-resolution Liquid Chromatography

UV absorbing constituents from urine can be separated with high-resolution liquid chromtaographic systems. A high-pressure anion-exchange chromatograph developed at the Oak Ridge National Laboratory separated numerous components from urine which are described in the succession of reports mentioned below. The resolutions were conducted by utilizing an anion-exchange resin (Dowex-1 X-8, Bio-Rad A-15, or Bio-Rad A-27) and ammonium acetate - acetic acid buffer as the eluant. The separate components were monitored by their UV absorption.

Several glucuronic acid conjugates bearing an UV-absorbing aglycone have been detected in biological fluids such as the two metabolites of phenacetin, conjugates of 4-hydroxyacetanilide, and 4-hydroxy-3-methoxy acetanilide [141]. Glucosiduronic acids were verified by hydrolysis with β-D-glucuronidase. Further identification of these conjugates was attempted [142], but the TMS derivatives decomposed on gas chromatography (GC), and the underivatized samples were not sufficiently volatile for both

GC and MS analysis. 1-O-(4-acetylaminobenzoyl)glucuronic acid, the metabolite of administered 4-aminobenzoic acid, was detected [143] by this technique [142]. The most extensive and detailed study of UV-absorbing urinary glucuronic acid conjugates was reported by Mrochek and Rainey [144]. The isolation and separation of nine ether types and three ester types of conjugates from the urine of normal and pathological subjects were performed on Bio-Rad A-27 on a preparative scale. Isolated samples were converted into the TMS derivatives, and these were submitted to GC-MS analysis.

The mild conditions employed for processing the urine in a high-pressure liquid chromatography system permits separation of labile glucuronic acid conjugates. However, UV monitoring limits the application to conjugates having a UV-absorbing aglycone or 1-O-acyl group.

D. Gas Chromatography (GC)

Glucuronic acid conjugates are polar polyfunctional molecules that usually undergo thermal degradation in GC systems prior to volatilization. It is therefore necessary to prepare volatile, thermally stable derivatives. Frequent procedures are to replace an active hydrogen atom in the carboxyl and hydroxyl groups in the sugar moiety by methyl, acetyl, or trimethylsilyl (TMS) groups. Acetylation and trimethylsilylation are two-step procedures that follow the preparation of the methyl ester of a glucuronide (usually with diazomethane). Acetylation of the hydroxyl groups is performed either with acetic acid anhydride and methanesulfonic acid [106, 145] or with acetic acid and pyridine [146]. Methyl esters of glucuronides can be trimethylsilylated in pyridine with chlorotrimethylsilane (CTMS) and hexamethyldisilazane [76, 109, 146]. Per(trimethylsilyl)ated glucuronic acid conjugates were prepared with CTMS and trifluoro-bis(trimethylsilyl)-acetamide [144].

In a series of papers, Thompson et al. [147-151] described a one-step procedure for the methylation of glucuronides. Permethylation with dimethylsulfinylsodium (Me_2SO^-) and methyl iodide was applicable to purified conjugates, but was equally successful with whole bile. GC analysis of permethylated bile distinctly revealed the presence of conjugates absent from control bile, and allowed for the separation and characterization of glucuronides. All the conjugates examined and estimated were glucuronides of the ether type; no comment was made on the possibility of applying the method to the other types of glucuronic acid conjugates.

The stability of volatile derivatives and the accuracy of GC analysis is often affected by the type of linkage and by the type of aglycone. Imanari and Tamura [146] studied the stability of methyl triacetates and TMS derivatives of ether, N-, and S-glucuronides and 1-O-acylglucuronic acids and the applicability of GC to the analysis of various derivatives. Glucuronides with simple aglycones of low molecular weight gave fairly stable derivatives, whereas higher molecular weight glucuronides showed a tendency to decompose as methyl triacetates, but were quite stable as TMS derivatives. N-Glucuronides were not suitable for GC analysis, and did not give stable derivatives, except for uracil and thymine derivatives.

Derivatives of 1-O-acylglucuronic acids were generally unsuitable for gas chromatography. Only the TMS derivative of isoketopinic acid was stable and exhibited a single peak in a gas chromatogram [146]. Mrochek and Rainey [144] studied three 1-O-acylglucuronic acids and observed partial cleavage of the ester bond, even during the trimethylsilylation procedure. Complete deconjugation occurred on GC for 1-O-(4-acetamido-benzoyl)glucuronic acid and 1-O-(indol-3-ylacetyl)glucuronic acid and partial deconjugation for 1-O-(indol-3-ylcarboxyl)glucuronic acid.

Knaak et al. [106] discussed the applicability of acetylation and trimethylsilylation for the preparation of derivatives for GC analysis. Ether glucuronides were synthesized in vitro, isolated, and partially purified. The acetylation procedure proved to be more suitable and quantitative for such conjugates which contain contaminants than trimethylsilylation. Direct trimethylsilylation after methylation was not quantitative, due to the interfering contaminants. The authors recommended trimethylsilylation as the method of choice for highly purified conjugates only.

The proper adjustment of GC column parameters and temperature and a suitable choice of the stationary phase can achieve distinct separations of high molecular compounds (such as glucuronides) without interference from compounds of low molecular weight. Examples of GC variables, suitable for glucuronide separation, are listed in Table 1 (choice of inert support, liquid phase, and column temperature). Compounds separated and detected on GC columns are characterized and identified on the basis of the retention data: retention time and relative retention time.

The retention data of glucuronide derivatives are usually compared with the parameters obtained from known reference compounds analyzed under identical conditions. The reference compounds most often employed are saturated hydrocarbons of high molecular weight. Retention data may be expressed in terms of methylene units (MU), based on comparison of retention times for sample and long-chain alkanes [152]. MU values for some glucuronides are also listed in Table 1.

If two samples exhibit the same MU value or retention time, a variation of liquid phase or temperature may reveal the difference between them, or confirm the assumption that the two compounds are identical.

TABLE 1

Data for Gas-Liquid Chromatography of Glucuronic Acid Conjugates

Glucosiduronic acid	Derivative		Inert support	Liquid phase	Temperature (°C)	MU values	Ref.
	Ester	Ether					
Ethyl β-	Me	TMS	Gas Chrom P	10% F-60	90-250 2/min	19.86	[109]
Ethyl α-	Me	TMS	Gas Chrom P	10% F-60	2/min	19.70	[109]
Methyl β-	Me	TMS	Gas Chrom P	10% F-60	2/min	19.53	[109]
Safrol-1'-yl[a]	Me	TMS	Gas Chrom P	1% SE-30	180 2/min	27.0	[110]
Monohydroxyetho-suximide[b]	Me	TMS	Gas Chrom P	1% SE-30	From 160 2/min	26.3	[153]
Naphthalene-1-yl	Me	TMS	Gas Chrom Q	5% SE-30	300		[106]
Oxazepam[c]-3-yl	Me	TMS	Gas Chrom Q	3% OV-17	320		[76]
Lorazepam[d]-3-yl	Me	TMS	Gas Chrom Q	3% OV-17	320		
Morphine-3-yl	TMS	TMS	Chromosorb	3% OV-1	100-325 10/min	36.38	[144]
Morphine-3-yl	TMS	TMS	Chromosorb	3% OV-17	10/min	38.81	[144]
p-Tolyl	TMS	TMS	Chromosorb	3% OV-1	10/min	24.65	[144]
p-Tolyl	TMS	TMS	Chromosorb	3% OV-17	10/min	25.55	[144]

5-Hydroxyindole-6-yl	TMS	TMS	Chromosorb	3% OV-1	10/min	32.36	[144]
5-Hydroxyindole-6-yl	TMS	TMS	Chromosorb	3% OV-17	10/min	34.10	[144]
p-Cresyl	Me	Ac	Gas Chrom P	1% SE-30	220		[146]
Phenyl 1-thio-	Me	Ac	Gas Chrom P	1% SE-30	200		[146]
5-HPPH[e]-4'-yl	Me	Me	Chromosorb W	3% OV-1	From 100 5/min		[151]
2-Methyl-1,4-naphtho-hydroquinone[f]	Me	Me	Gas Chrom P	1% OV-1	105-230 10/min		[148]
1-O-Acylglucuronic acid							
Indole-3-ylacetyl	TMS	TMS	Chromosorb	3% OV-1	100-325 10/min	31.32	[144]
"Isoketopinoyl"	Me	TMS	Anakrom	1% NGS	220		[146]

[a] 4-(1-Hydroxyallyl)-1,2-methylenedioxybenzene.
[b] Monohydroxy derivative of 2-ethyl-2-methylsuccinimide; position of hydroxyl group not determined.
[c] 7-Chloro-1,3-dihydro-3-hydroxy-5-phenyl-2H-1,4-benzodiazepin-2-one.
[d] 7-Chloro-1,3-dihydro-3-hydroxy-5-(o-chlorophenyl)-2H-1,4-benzodiazepin-2-one.
[e] 5-(4-Hydroxyphenyl)-5-phenylhydantoin.
[f] Attached position of glucosyluronic group not determined (1 or 4).

E. Mass Spectral Analysis (MS)

MS analysis is a technique used for the characterization and identification
of various natural products and metabolites. The molecule is fragmented
by various ionization techniques such as electron impact, chemical ionization, charge exchange, and field desorption. The resulting fragmentation
patterns provide evidence for the structure of a conjugate and its molecular
weight, and information concerning the nature of the aglycone and the type
of linkage. Structural features characteristic of glucuronides can be deduced from mass spectra even without comparison with standards.

   The fragmentation of glucuronic acid conjugates is influenced by various
functional groups and the type of aglycone, but the final shape of the fragmentation pattern depends on the ionization technique used. The widely
used ionization and fragmentation by electron impact gives spectra relatively rich in small fragments, but with small amounts of molecular ion or
no molecular ion at all. Such spectra reveal characteristic masses associated with fragmentation of the derivatized glucuronic acid moiety to fingerprint the conjugates as glucuronides, but do not give direct information
as to molecular weight.

   Gentler ionization techniques are chemical ionization and charge exchange. Chemical ionization is achieved by adding a proton-transfer reagent (such as methane or isobutane) to the carrier gas and sample mixture. The yield of molecular ion in the spectra generated in this way was
enhanced [93]. Charge-exchange mass spectra [154] obtained with a mixture of NO/N_2 also exhibited enhancement in molecular ion and less extensive fragmentation of the molecule.

   A new possibility for glucuronide analysis is field-desorption mass
spectrometry (FDMS). This technique was used to analyze an underivatized steroid glucuronide (estriol-16α-glucuronide), which was unstable
under electron-impact conditions, but revealed intensive molecular ion
when submitted to FDMS [130]. Schulten and Games [213] applied FDMS
to structural studies of various glycosides, including the highly polar sodium
salt of testosterone glucuronide. The technique was applicable only to purified conjugates because a direct introduction system was used. The possible advantage of FDMS is in the analysis of underivatized glucuronic acid
conjugates. Fragmentation techniques need derivatized conjugates of adequate volatility such as TMS ethers, triacetate methyl esters, or permethylated conjugates. They are prepared as described in Section IV. D.
The combined GC-MS system is especially convenient for mixtures containing glucuronides when the derivatized conjugates are stable and do not
decompose on high-temperature chromatographic columns. Even with stable derivatives, mass spectra recorded after GC separation are not always
satisfactory. Direct insertion of the sample into the source of the mass

spectrometer has permitted the detection of molecular ions generated by the electron-impact technique [155]. The use of the combined GC-MS system did not always provide molecular ions, probably owing to the enhanced thermal excitation.

Characteristic masses in the spectra of derivatized glucuronides provide evidence for the structure of glucuronic acid conjugates. Paulson et al. [145] reported a comparative study on the mass spectra of aryl glucuronides, glucosides, galactosides, and galacturonides in the form of methyl ester triacetates. Aryl glucosiduronic acids were distinctly differentiated from any other type of conjugate examined, and from derivatized glucuronic acid. Characteristic ions at m/e 317, 257, 215, 197, 173, 155, and 127 due to the derivatized glucuronic acid moiety were common to aryl glucuronides, regardless of the aglycone. These peaks are absent from or less intense in the spectra of glucosides and galactosides. Galacturonides do not exhibit a peak at m/e 257, and the relative intensities of the other characteristic peaks were markedly different. The structures of the metabolites of an anti-inflammatory drug (H-88) were confirmed, and one metabolite was identified as a glucuronide by use of mass spectrometry [95]. The MS of the methyl ester triacetate exhibited the molecular ion and characteristic peaks generated from the glucuronic acid moiety (m/e 333 and 317). The structures of biliary metabolites of estrone in the rat were deduced from various physicochemical data, including MS [156]. Methyl esters of tri-O-acetyl derivatives of 2-methoxyestrone-3 glucuronide, estrone-3 glucuronide, and four other steroid conjugates exhibited molecular-ion peaks and peaks at m/e 317 in their mass spectra. Billets et al. [155] examined the mass spectra of a series of TMS derivatives of aromatic and aliphatic ether glucuronides and derived the general principles for the identification of glucuronic acid conjugates using ions not commonly found in the fragmentation of silylated carbohydrates. Cleavage of the aglycone led to the formation of ions at m/e 407 (Me esters) and 465 (TMS esters). Further elimination of Me_3SiOH resulted in ions at 317 (Me esters) and 375 (TMS esters). Ions at m/e 204 and 217 were common to all silylated carbohydrates. Frequently an intense peak at M - 15 (loss of methyl group) occurred in the spectra. Fragmentation in the trimethylsilyl groups resulted in peaks M - 73 ($-Me_3Si$), M - 90 ($-Me_3SiOH$), and M - 105 (M - 15, M - 90).

The TMS derivatives of some glucuronides and characteristic ions detected in their mass spectra are listed in Table 2. The applicability of mass spectral analysis to permethylated ether glucuronides was studied by Thompson and Desiderio [147] with steroid glucuronides and phenyramidol {α-[(2-pyridylamino)methyl]benzyl} glucuronide. Intact glucuronides were permethylated with Me_2SO^- and MeI, and the products used for MS analysis through the direct introduction system. Satisfactory spectra with meaningful fragmentation patterns were obtained with nanomolar quantities.

TABLE 2

Characteristic Masses Detected in the Mass Spectra of TMS Derivatives of Some Glucosiduronic Acids

Glucosiduronic acid	Derivative		m/e												Ref.
	Ester	Ether	M^+	M-15	M-73	M-90	M-105	465	407	375	333	317	217	204	
6-Bromonaphthalene- 2-yl	Me	TMS	+	+	+		+		+			+	+	+	[155]
Chloramphenicol	Me	TMS		+		+	+		+			+	+	+	[155]
Safrole-1-yl[a]	Me	TMS	+										+	+	[110]
Ethyl	Me	TMS		+								+	+	+	[109]
Monohydroxyetho- succimide[b]	Me	TMS	+	+	+		+		+			+	+	+	[153]
Oxazepam[c]-3-yl	Me	TMS	+	+		+	+		+			+	+	+	[76]
Lorazepam[d]-3-yl	Me	TMS	+	+		+	+		+			+	+	+	[76]
Quinolin-8-yl	TMS	TMS	+		+	+	+	+		+	+		+	+	[155]
5-Hydroxyindol- 6-yl	Me	TMS	+	+				+			+	+	+	+	[144]

For an explanation of footnotes a, b, c, and d, see Table 1.

The authors indicated a few characteristic ions arising from the glucuronic acid moiety that are common to all spectra of permethylated glucuronides: m/e 101, 141, 169, 201, and 233 (in spectra of permethylated aliphatic ether glucuronides) or 232 (in spectra of permethylated phenolic ether glucuronides). The peak at m/e 201 was for the most important ion in the identification of permethylated glucuronic acid conjugates. This provided the possibility of differentiating between glucuronides and glucosides, since permethylated glucosides do not exhibit this ion in their mass spectra. Extensive fragmentation of the examined steroid glucuronides was observed, and molecular ions were not always detected in their spectra. Phenyramidol glucuronide exhibited M^+ and other ions attributed to the cleavages of the glucuronic acid moiety.

Thompson et al. [149] elaborated a convenient method for the direct detection and identification of glucuronides in bile. Permethylation of bile was followed by GLC separation and subsequent analysis by mass spectrometry. The differences between the sample and control bile were estimated first by GC and then by MS analysis. In some cases, permethylated glucuronides underwent thermal decomposition on high-temperature GC columns and, therefore, the direct-introduction system should be applied. The presence of endogenous compounds in permethylated bile did not affect the interpretation of the mass spectra of glucuronides.

The method has been successfully applied for the identification of numerous glucuronides formed in bile in in vivo and in vitro experiments [148, 150, 151]. Some of the characteristic ions detected in the spectra of permethylated glucuronides are listed in Table 3.

F. Nuclear Magnetic Resonance Spectroscopy (NMR)

NMR spectroscopy has been of limited value in the elucidation of the structure of glucuronic acid conjugates. It provides fingerprint patterns that can be used comparatively and information concerning protons, but the spectra of glucosiduronic acids usually exhibit a multitude of proton signals, and thus result in unrecognizable patterns.

Case [157] pointed out that NMR spectroscopic analysis of glucuronides is hampered by the need for large sample quantities and by the low solubility of the conjugates in suitable solvents.

Derivatized glucuronic acid conjugates are more convenient for NMR analysis. The NMR spectra of acetylated apigenin glucosiduronic acid [70] revealed the presence of three acetyl groups on the glucuronic acid moiety. The 3-glucuronide 17-(2-acetamido-2-deoxy glucoside) of 17α-estradiol [87] was characterized through the physicochemical data for the acetylated

TABLE 3

Characteristic Masses Detected in the Mass Spectra of Permethylated Glucosiduronic Acids

Permethylated glucosiduronic acids	M+	M − CH$_3$OH	m/e 232 (233)	201	169	141	101	Ref.
Phenyramidol[a]-1-yl	+	+		+	+	+	+	[147]
Testosterone-17β-yl				+	+	+	+	[147]
4-Hydroxybiphenyl	+	+	+	+	+	+	+	[149]
5-HPPH[b]-4'-yl		+	+	+	+	+	+	[149]
Chloramphenicol-3-yl			+	+	+	+	+	[149]
2-Methyl-1,4-naphthoquinone[c]	+	+		+	+	+	+	[148]
3-(2-Hydroxyphenoxy)-1-propanol-2-yl	+	+	+	+	+	+	+	[150]

[a] α-[(2-Pyridylamino)methyl]benzyl alcohol.

[b] 5-(4-Hydroxyphenyl)-5-phenylhydantoin.

[c] Position of attachment of glucosiduronic group (1 or 4) not determined.

methyl ester. The NMR spectra supported the structure assigned. A codeine conjugate isolated from dog urine [90] was characterized as codeine-6 glucosiduronic acid. The NMR spectra indicated the presence of aromatic vinylene protons and of O- and N-methyl groups in the conjugate. Biliary metabolites of estrone in rat were characterized [156] by direct comparison with synthetic methyl glucosiduronates triacetates. Physicochemical data used for characterization and comparison purposes included NMR spectral data.

G. IR Spectroscopy

IR spectroscopy is a widely used, inexpensive technique for characterization and comparison if authentic specimens are available. The compound must be purified, but lability is not a significant problem. The presence of functionalities such as carbonyl, hydroxyl, and groups characteristic for aglycones can be confirmed.

H. Determination of the Position of Attachment of the Glucosyluronic Group to the Aglycone

Biotransformation of various drugs often results in conjugation of free hydroxyl groups with glucuronic acid. Compounds with two or more free hydroxyl groups may give rise to various conjugates in which the glucuronic acid moiety may be attached at different positions on the aglycone molecule.

In the steroid series, the problem of conjugates of closely related structures is frequently encountered, and proper identification of each particular metabolite is necessary. The methods usually employed are: comparison with a synthetic sample; or conversion into a derivative, followed by hydrolysis, and identification of the aglycone. Since synthetic samples of steroid glucosiduronic acids are not always available, the alternative is to characterize the aglycone through a derivatized conjugate. Methyl ether groups are most convenient for derivatization since the glycosidic linkage can be selectively hydrolyzed in their presence.

All hydroxyl groups, however, are not equally susceptible to methylation. The phenolic group in steroid molecules and the carboxyl group in the glucuronic acid moiety are readily converted into the methyl ether or ester, respectively, with diazomethane [7]. Selective methylation of the phenolic group occurred in steroid molecules with dimethyl sulfate in borate buffer [158]. Exhaustive methylation with diazomethane (boron trifluoride as the catalyst) yielded a completely methylated conjugate [7]. Methyl iodide in

N, N-dimethylformamide plus barium oxide and hydroxide gave complete methylation in one step [159].

Hydrolysis with dilute HCl yields an aglycone with one free hydroxyl group, arising from the cleavage of the glycosidic bond. The derivatized aglycone is characterized from its physicochemical properties and spectral data. The most accurate methods for aglycone identification are with labeled compounds. The aglycone from the labeled parent drug should be mixed with an appropriate carrier; the unlabeled aglycone should be mixed with labeled carrier. Further purification and crystallization to constant specific activity (and to constant isotopic ratio when double-labeling is used) should confirm the structure assigned to the aglycone. Double conjugates should be submitted to alternative hydrolysis by β-D-glucuronidase or sulfatase, and subsequent acetylation of the hydroxyl groups. After solvolysis of the acetylated product, the derivatized aglycone is characterized and identified by standard methods [138]. Honma and Nambara [156] reported the structure of the double conjugate of 2-hydroxyestradiol. In the identification procedure, enzymic hydrolysis was omitted. The NMR data indicated that the glucuronic acid moiety was attached to position 17. The position of the sulfate group was determined after methylation of the conjugate, followed by acid hydrolysis and identification of the aglycone.

Numerous metabolites of estrone, estradiol, estriol, and epiestriol have been extensively studied, and include the characterization of estriol-3 glucosiduronic acid [210], several metabolites of 17-estradiol glucosiduronic acid [111], 17β-estradiol [80], and various conjugated metabolites of 16-epiestriol [138]. Identification of the latter metabolites was obtained by methylation, hydrolysis, and crystallization of the aglycone with a carrier steroid to constant specific activity and, in some cases, to constant isotopic ratio, followed by acetylation and crystallization. 16-Epiestriol-16 glucuronide from human urine was identified by converting it into its methyl ester with diazomethane and into the acetyl derivative with labeled acetic anhydride and pyridine [160]. Reverse isotope-dilution with a synthetic sample was employed to confirm the structure assignment. Honma and Nambara [156] deduced the structure of biliary estrone metabolites from physicochemical data and direct comparison with authentic specimens. Glucuronic acid conjugates were converted into methyl esters, and these were acetylated. The derivatives were compared with synthetic samples or hydrolyzed with acid under mild conditions, and the identity of the aglycone confirmed.

Alkaloid molecules such as morphine and related compounds may contain two hydroxyl groups and can give various conjugates with glucuronic acid. The hydroxyl group at C-3 in the morphine molecule is of the phenolic type, and the whole molecule exhibits absorption in the UV region. This property is the basis for determining whether the conjugate is a mono- or a di-glucuronide, and whether the glucosyluronic acid moiety is attached to O-3. The free phenolic hydroxy group at 3-position in morphine-like molecules [161] exhibits reversible pH dependence in UV spectra. The addition of a base causes a bathochromic shift to higher wavelengths, and the addition of acid brings back the original UV spectral pattern. The presence of a free phenolic group is given by a positive test with ferricyanide [162]. Phenols give a color reaction and a precipitate. Kaul et al. [103] examined the metabolites of apomorphine. The monoglucuronide structure was assigned to two glucuronic acid conjugates isolated from rabbits on the basis of UV analysis. Further distinction between the metabolites conjugated on O-3 and O-4 was made, based on the assumption that the 3-position is less hindered and thus more susceptible to conjugation. Fujimoto and Way [163] isolated a morphine conjugate from human urine. Its UV characteristics indicated that no free phenol group was present in the molecule, thus leading to the conclusion that the metabolite was morphine-3 glucuronide. Codeine [162], morphine-3 and -6 glucuronide [47, 162] were isolated and characterized by comparison of their UV spectra and optical rotation with those of synthetic samples. Dihydromorphine and hydromorphone glucuronides were isolated and characterized after the administration of hydromorphone [91]. In both conjugates, the glucuronic acid moiety was shown to be attached at the 3-position of the aglycone since no bathochromic shift was observed upon addition of alkali.

In the N-glucuronide series, several types of conjugates can be formed. Sulfonamide drugs may have multiple nitrogen atoms at different positions in the molecule, including an aromatic amino group (N^4), sulfonamido group (N^1), and an imido group in the heterocyclic ring. Conjugates linked to glucuronic acid through the aromatic amino group can be readily distinguished from the other types by its lability in acid and by the fact that β-D-glucuronidase does not act upon this type of N-glucuronide. UV and IR spectral data form the basis for further distinction between possible derivatives. Tautomeric imido forms, which have a substituent on the ring-nitrogen atom, exhibit an absorption band in their IR spectra due to SO_2 symmetrical stretching frequencies at lower values: 940 cm^{-1} [73]; 1120 to 1145 cm^{-1} [19], and amido forms in the range of 1145 to 1170 cm^{-1} The glucosyluronic group on sulfathiazole was further characterized as the N^1-substituent by only one maximum in its UV spectra [73]. Heterocyclic N-substituents (imido forms) usually have two absorption maxima in their UV spectra.

I. Quantitative Determination of Glucuronic Acid in Conjugates

Qualitative and quantitative assays of glucuronic acid in glucuronic acid conjugates can be performed directly on biological material or on purified metabolites, with naphthoresorcinol or carbazole as the reagent. Both

reagents give a color reaction with the products of acid degradation of carbohydrates. Strong acid degradation products of glucuronic acid give an
organic soluble blue pigment. The colored product can be extracted from
the aqueous phase with ethyl acetate, ether, or 1-butanol, and estimated
colorimetrically at 560 to 570 nm.

Various procedures proposed for the Tollens test [25] for glucuronic
acid in conjugates differ in the composition of naphthoresorcinol reagent,
the mode of performing the assay, the sensitivity, and the solvent used for
the extraction. Mead et al. [64, 65] reported the application of the procedure as modified by Paul [164] where urine was treated with naphthoresorcinol, sulfuric acid, and chloramin T. After the mixture was boiled for
2 h, the colored product was extracted into ethyl acetate. Glucuronic acid
was estimated [165] after prehydrolysis of conjugated material in urine
with HCl by heating a mixture of the hydrolysate with aqueous naphthoresorcinol at 100°C. Mazzuchin et al. [31] elaborated a modification with
phosphoric acid in the reagent solution. HCl and naphthoresorcinol were
added to the reaction mixture, which was heated to 100°C and cooled. The
colored product was extracted into 1-butanol or ethyl acetate. Glucurono-
lactone standards were recommended, parallel with the samples since the
reagent was unstable. The accuracy was affected by variations in the stability of the reagent and the possible interference of other sugars, since
the reaction was not entirely specific for glucuronic acid. Glucuronic acid
assays were determined from 5 to 100 μg, but the best results were obtained with 5 to 50 μg, with an average error of 5%.

Dische [27] reacted hexuronic acid with carbazole for the selective assay of glucuronic acid where other sugars did not interfere. A glucuronic
acid solution was heated at 100°C with concentrated sulfuric acid. After
cooling, an alcoholic solution of carbazole was added and the mixture heated
again at 100°C. No extraction was necessary. The optical absorbance was
determined directly at 530 nm. The color was unstable and sensitive to
overheating and aqueous dilution. Color development was partially affected
by salts and impurities. Modifications have been reported [166]. Color
yield was increased by the addition of borate ions [167]. A procedure for
the degradation of glucuronic acid with sulfuric acid was elaborated in order
to obviate overheating; the stability of the color was increased, and greater
reproducibility achieved. The assay was reproducible for concentrations
above 4 μg/ml. The optical absorbance is a linear function of the concentration in the range of 4 to 40 μg of glucuronic acid per ml.

V. HYDROLYSIS WITH β-D-GLUCURONIDASE

Hydrolysis of presumptive glucuronic acid conjugates with β-D-glucuron-
idase (β-D-glucosiduronidase) has become an indispensable tool. The

properties, distribution, and assay of β-glucuronidase have been reviewed by several authors [21, 22, 168, 169].

The course of the hydrolysis is monitored by the assay of the liberated glucuronic acid or aglycone. Further processing of the incubation mixture after complete hydrolysis depends upon the choice of method for characterization of the hydrolysis products. Colorimetric estimation of glucuronic acid and chromogenic aglycones is conducted directly on aliquots of the incubation mixture. Direct chromatography can also be employed, especially if the experiment is performed with labeled material. If the major emphasis is on identification of the aglycone, extraction with organic solvents is performed first, followed by further separation and characterization of the metabolites.

In many papers, the only evidence given for the structure of conjugates was obtained by hydrolysis experiments with β-glucuronidase. Parallel experiments with D-glucaro-1, 4-lactone could provide additional evidence for the assignment of glucuronide structure.

There are numerous variations in the hydrolysis procedures and in the assays of the hydrolysis products, thus no general procedure exists. The choice of enzyme concentration depends on the nature of the substrate, the possible contaminants and inhibitors, and the origin and purity of the enzyme preparation. A survey of the papers published on glucuronides reveals that in too many instances inaccurate data on enzyme hydrolysis was presented; the quantitiy of substrate was either not mentioned or had not been determined. The concentration of enzyme sufficient to hydrolyze purified metabolite may not be adequate for hydrolysis of impure biological material which can contain endogenous inhibitors. Hydrolysis depends on pH and there are different optimal pH values with different enzyme preparations.

A. Conditions for Incubation with β-Glucuronidase

Enzyme preparations used for the hydrolysis of glucuronic acid conjugates differ in origin, purity, and activity. Although the commercial preparations of β-glucuronidase are usually not highly purified, repeated incubations can be conducted accurately. The bacterial and mammalian liver enzymes most frequently used are considered to contain no sulfatases. Preparations from invertebrates, Patella vulgata and Helix pomatia, contain sulfatases. Sulfatase-containing preparations will cause parallel hydrolysis of the sulfuric acid conjugates. The optimal pH for hydrolysis with mammalian enzyme and sulfatase-containing preparations lies between 4 and 5.5. The pH of the incubation mixture should be adjusted to 6 to 7 for optimal results with bacterial glucuronidase.

One Fishman unit (FU) of β-glucuronidase activity liberates 1 μg of phenolphthalein from phenolphthalein glucuronide in 1 h at 37°C. One international unit (IU) of enzyme hydrolyzes 1 μmol of phenolphthalein glucuronide in 1 min at 37°C. 1 FU is equivalent to 5.2×10^{-5} IU. Phenolphthalein glucuronide has been used as the standard for the determination of activity due to the chromogenic property of its aglycone. In alkaline media, the liberated aglycone produces a purple-pink color, and is subsequently quantified spectrophotometrically. A serious disadvantage of this substrate is the possible inhibition of the enzyme by the aglycone released. p-Nitrophenyl glucuronide was used since it produces a yellow color in alkaline media and does not inhibit the enzyme.

Unfortunately, numerous articles do not specify the units of activity of β-D-glucuronidase, nor do they give the experimental conditions of the incubations in sufficient detail. A brief survey of recent papers is given herewith with regard to the origin of the enzyme used and the quantities of enzyme required for hydrolysis of biological material and purified conjugates which differ considerably.

1. Hydrolysis with Mammalian Preparations

Hydrolysis with mammalian glucuronidase, mostly from bovine liver, is usually performed at pH 4.5 to 5.0 in acetate buffer at 37°C. The time of incubation may be as great as 72 h. Data for incubations of biological material have been reported for metabolites of phenacetin [141], various conjugates of steroids [170], metabolites of edrophonium chloride [ethyl(3-hydroxyphenyl)dimethylammonium chloride] [171], metabolites of 2-(p-aminobenzoyloxy)benzoic acid [172], and metabolites of lorazepam [46].

Data for the incubation of some partially or completely purified glucuronic acid conjugates is available on conjugates of $C_{19}O_2$ and $C_{21}O_2$ steroids in bile [126], metabolites of estrone and estradiol [79], metabolites of 2-pyridinethiol 1-oxide [100], metabolites of 3-hydroxyanthranilic acid [113, 114], metabolites of thyroxine [44], metabolites of niflumic acid {2-[3-(trifluoromethyl)anilino nicotinic] acid} [173], metabolites of estradiol [112], metabolites of estrone [156], metabolites of testosterone [86], metabolites of cortisol [83], and metabolites of norgestrel [85].

2. Hydrolysis with Bacterial Preparations

Commercial bacterial preparations used for the hydrolysis of glucuronic acid conjugates are usually obtained from Escherichia coli. Hydrolysis is usually performed at pH 6 to 7 in phosphate buffer at 37°C. The assay can be completed in minutes, but occasionally is conducted for several hours.

Data on incubations of biological material have been reported for metabolites of thyroxine [42], metabolites of cyproheptadine [174], metabolites of cis-5-fluoro-2-methyl-1-p-(methylsulfinyl)benzylidenyl)indene-3-

acetic acid [175], metabolites of tolamolol [48], and metabolites of morphine [176].

Data for incubations of purified metabolites were reported for double conjugates of estriol [137], conjugates of retinol and retinoic acid [50], conjugates of estrone and estradiol [79, 80, 111], conjugates of 3-(trifluoromethyl)-4-nitrophenol [94], conjugates of N-hydroxy-4-aminophenyl [101], metabolites of viloxazine [2-(2-ethoxyphenoxymethyl)2, 3, 5, 6-tetrahydro-1, 4-oxazine] [96].

3. Hydrolysis with β-Glucuronidase Preparations Containing Sulfatase

Conjugate hydrolyses with mixed-enzyme preparations are not specific for either sulfates and glucuronides. Although sulfatase activity can be inhibited by KH_2PO_4, mammalian or bacterial enzymes are best for specific hydrolysis. Incubations are usually performed at pH 4.5 to 5.5 at 37°C for several hours.

Data on the hydrolysis of biological material with mixed enzymes were reported for metabolites of mycophenolic acid [177], metabolites of imipramine and demethylimipramine [178], metabolites of vanillin and isovanillin [179], and metabolites of lofepramine [180].

Data on the hydrolysis of purified metabolites were reported for conjugates of sulfadimethoxine [19], double conjugate of estriol [137], 4-[3-(dimethylamino)propyl]-3, 4-dihydro-2-(1-hydroxyethyl)-3-phenyl-2H-1, 4-benzothiazine [54], conjugates of 16-epiestriol [110], and metabolites of 3-methylcholantrene [181].

B. Separation and Characterization of Aglycones

Related unconjugated metabolites and the parent drug may interfere with the characterization and identification of the aglycone produced by β-glucuronidase. Repeated extraction with organic solvents at neutral pH is often a convenient method for the removal of unconjugated, nonpolar components that could interfere with the assay of the liberated aglycone and is very often applied for pretreating biological fluids.

The incubation mixture obtained from the hydrolysis with β-glucuronidase can be processed by (1) paper chromatography, (2) gel chromatography, ion-exchange, or counter-current distribution, and (3) extraction of the aglycone with an organic solvent and subsequent characterization by various physicochemical methods.

1. Parallel chromatography of untreated and enzyme-treated material should be performed. If the enzyme has hydrolyzed the presumed glu-

curonic acid conjugate, the reaction will result in altered chromatographic behavior. For comparison purposes, cochromatography of appropriate standards is recommended. Low concentrations of aglycones in incubation mixtures and the presence of salts make it difficult to achieve very good chromatographic separation. The use of labeled parent drugs facilitates the quantification of specific compounds. Redistribution of activity before and after hydrolysis is a reliable indication that glucuronic acid conjugates are affected by the action of β-glucuronidase.

Paper or thin-layer chromatography for the estimation of hydrolysis products in incubation mixtures was reported for indomethacin metabolites [51], conjugates or sulfadimethoxine [19], metabolites of edrophonium chloride [171], conjugates of thyroxine and 3, 5, 3'-triiodothyronine [42], conjugates of thyroxine [45], and conjugates of isoetharine [1-(3,4-dihydroxyphenyl)-2-isopropylamino-1-butanol] [182].

2. Aglycones released in reaction with β-glucuronidase can be isolated from incubation mixtures by processing on ion-exchange resins, as with metabolites of phenacetin [141] and dopamine [104]. The chromatographic patterns of enzyme-treated and untreated urines were compared for checking phenacetin by UV absorption of eluted material, and dopamine products were monitored after elution by TLC.

Radioactive steroid aglycones were separated from incubation mixtures on Sephadex G-25 [129] and DEAE-Sephadex separated the hydrolysis products of safrole metabolites [110]. Counter-current distribution was used to separate steroid aglycones after the hydrolysis of double steroid conjugates [137].

3. The method most frequently used is the extraction of the aglycone with subsequent separation and characterization.

In general, paper or thin-layer chromatography of concentrated extracts give better results than the chromatography of the unconcentrated incubation mixtures, and are frequently employed. Products of the hydrolysis of numerous metabolites have been estimated in this manner for metabolites of retinol and retinoic acid [50], conjugate of N-hydroxy-ar-phenylacetanilide (N-hydroxy-4-acetamidobiphenyl) [183], conjugate of 4-nitro-3-(trifluoromethyl)phenol [94], metabolites of 18-homoestriol [184], metabolites of thioureidobenzene fungicides [185], metabolites of testosterone [86, 139], conjugates of p-hydroxyphenobarbital [186], metabolites of lofepramine [180], and metabolites of cyproheptadine [174].

Characterization of the aglycones by means of UV spectra were reported for metabolites of chloropromazine [49], conjugate of N-acetyl-N-phenylhydroxylamine [187], various 1-thioglucosiduronic acids [188, 189], metabolites of pyridinethione [100], and conjugate of N-hydroxy-4-acetamidobiphenyl [183].

Characterizations of aglycones according to their fluorogenic properties were reported for metabolites of mycophenolic acid [177] and 4-hydroxy-anthranilic acid, liberated from its glucuronic acid conjugate [113, 114].

Gas chromatography for the separation and characterization of aglycones is frequently used, especially for steroid aglycones, and profiles the steroid content of biological fluids. Gas-chromatographic quantitations were reported for corticosteroids [170, 190], probenecid metabolites [52], N-hydroxy-4-biphenylamine [101], metabolites of the alkaloid naltrexone [191], and the separation of the aglycones from conjugated compounds in cow's milk [92]. Partition column chromatography was used for the separation of steroid aglycones [80, 111, 126]. Isolation, followed by acetylation and thin-layer chromatography were also effected [192, 193].

Estrogens released in an enzymic hydrolysis can be estimated by use of the Kober reagent. The colored Kober chromogen is formed by the addition of hydroquinone and sulfuric acid to the extracted aglycones and is estimated spectrophotometrically. This method was applied to the assay of steroids in urine [194-196]. Total amounts of estrogen steroids are obtained, but individual metabolites are not distinguished. The method can also be applied to previously separated and purified steroids.

If appropriated labeled standards are available and steroid yields after hydrolysis are high, crystallization to constant specific activity can be applied [112, 120].

C. Comparative Action of β-Glucuronidase from Various
   Sources on Glucuronic Acid Conjugates

Detailed and quantitative studies are available to compare the activity of β-glucuronidase from various sources.

Comparative hydrolyses of steroid conjugates were reported [193, 196-199]. Several enzyme preparations were evaluated by examining the hydrolysis of two glucuronic acid conjugates of 3-methoxy-4-hydroxyphenyl glycol in urine [200]. Other pertinent studies were on the enzyme hydrolysis of the conjugate of N-acetyl-N-phenylhydroxylamine with both mammalian and bacterial preparations [187], the efficiency of β-glucuronidase from various sources in the hydrolysis of morphine glucuronide [201], and the kinetics of the hydrolysis of several synthetic glucosiduronic acids and 1-O-acylglucuronic acids with bacterial and bovine liver β-glucuronidase [202].

Bacterial β-glucuronidase was shown to be the more effective agent to hydrolyze glucuronic acid conjugates with respect to the quantity of the enzyme required and the length of the incubation time necessary for complete hydrolysis.

D. Quantitative Assay of Liberated Glucuronic Acid and Aglycones

Rates of hydrolysis with β-glucuronidase can be determined by monitoring
the hydrolysis products with time. If the aglycones have chromogenic properties, direct colorimetric estimation of the aglycones released is feasible.
The liberated glucuronic acid can be assayed with naphthoresorcinol, carbazole, or benzidine. Successful quantitative estimation of the hydrolysis
products can be accomplished only with conjugates purified from biological
materials.

1. Determination of Glucuronic Acid with Naphthoresorcinol and Carbazole

The method of Fishman and Green [26] for the direct assay of glucuronic
acid conjugates described in Section II.A can be applied for the determination of enzymically released glucuronic acid. The hydrolysis of steroid
enol glucosiduronic acids was studied by using this method [198].

Wagner [203] reported a modified procedure with naphthoresorcinol
reagent. Liberated glucuronic acid was determined in the presence of unhydrolyzed glucosiduronic acid when the conjugate did not decompose under
the experimental conditions used. The method was applicable to conjugates
of the phenol ether type. The reaction mixture with naphthoresorcinol was
heated at 70°C, and phosphoric acid was added to the naphthoresorcinol instead of sulfuric acid. Ball and Double [204] applied this method to the
enzymic hydrolysis of the conjugate of the potently cytotoxic compound
N,N-bis(2-chloroethyl)-4-aminophenol ("p-hydroxyaniline mustard").

Yuki and Fishman [28] proposed use of the carbazole method for differential analysis of glucuronic and glucosiduronic acids. Free glucuronic
acid was first oxidized by iodine, and the glucuronic acid equivalent in the
conjugate was determined with carbazole. The total glucuronic acid was
also obtained by the carbazole reaction. The glucuronic acid liberated by
enzymic hydrolysis was calculated from the difference between the experimentally determined amounts of total and conjugated glucuronic acid. All three
methods can be applied only to stable, ether-type glucuronic acid conjugates.

2. Determination of Glucuronic Acid with Benzidine

Jones and Pridham [205, 206] reported a colorimetric method for the determination of glucuronic acid with benzidine that was modified by Tomašić
and Keglević [207] to assay glucuronic acid in the presence of labile glucuronic acid conjugates. The reaction of glucuronic acid with benzidine
in acetic acid was conducted on aliquots of incubation mixtures. In a
series of experiments with labile 1-O-acyl-β- and -α-D-glucuronic acids
[202], unhydrolyzed substances were not affected by the benzidine reagent.
The results obtained for glucuronic acid only reflected the enzymically liberated glucuronic acid.

Unfortunately, the benzidine reagent is carcinogenic and must be handled carefully. The possibility of aglycone reaction with benzidine should be checked beforehand, since benzidine is not an exclusively specific reagent for carbohydrates.

E. Inhibition of Hydrolysis with D-Glucaro-1,4-Lactone

The fact of hydrolysis with β-glucuronidase is considered as evidence for a glucuronide structure of metabolites. However, β-glucuronidase may not be specific and may be contaminated by sulfatases. Labile conjugates could have been chemically cleaved during the incubation and assay procedures. Thus, parallel experiments with the specific inhibitor D-glucaro-1,4-lactone (originally called saccharo-1,4-lactone) should be conducted to verify the assignment of glucuronide structure to the metabolites.

A general procedure for effective inhibition by D-glucaro-1,4-lactone cannot readily be deduced from the literature since the quantities of inhibitor and substrate are frequently omitted. In general, proper degrees of inhibition may have to be experimentally determined by modifying the quantities in a particular experiment.

Inhibition studies conducted on biological material were for: edrophonium metabolites [171], thyroxine and 3,5,3'-triiodo-L-thyronine metabolites [42], metabolites of tetrahydrocortisone [55], metabolites of 1- and 2-naphthol [35], and lorazepam metabolites [46].

Applications to the hydrolysis of purified conjugates were for: indomethacin metabolites [51], conjugate of N-acetyl-N-phenylhydroxylamine [187], morphine conjugates [47], various estrogen conjugates [80,112, 212], thyroxine metabolites [44,45], conjugate of p-nitrobenzenethiol [189], conjugate of 4-nitro-3-(trifluoromethyl)phenol [94], conjugates of 18-homoestriol [184], and metabolites of 16-epiestriol [138].

VI. CONCLUSIONS

The various methods applicable to the analysis of glucuronic acid conjugates have been surveyed. No one general method or combination of techniques can be applied to any conjugate disregarding its structure and stability. The choice of the analytical method must consider the properties of the presumed glucuronic acid conjugate and its purity. The choice of the method for isolation depends on the biological material or mixture containing the metabolite.

In most cases glucuronic acid conjugates of steroids are fairly stable compounds, except for enol glucosiduronic acids. Extraction with organic solvents can separate steroid glucuronides from their lipophilic aglycone in biological fluids. Concentration on XAD resins is also an effective separation procedure. The multiple structurally related glucosiduronic acids that result with one steroid demands suitable separation methods such as

separation on DEAE-Sephadex in a gradient of sodium chloride, counter-
current distribution, and high-voltage paper electrophoresis. Purified
conjugates are most accurately characterized by comparison with synthetic
samples. Gas chromatography and mass spectrometry are not always
applicable to steroid metabolites, due to the difficult preparation of sufficiently volatile derivatives. Paper and thin-layer chromatography are not
often used for the analysis of intact glucuronides, since their mobilities
are very low in standard chromatographic systems. If a particular synthetic steroid conjugate is not available, the steroid aglycone can be characterized after hydrolysis of the conjugate with acid or with β-glucuron-
idase. The most reliable results are obtained with labeled compounds.
Radioactively labeled aglycone can be mixed with an appropriate carrier,
and recrystallized to constant specific activity or, if a double label was
used, to a constant isotopic ratio.

The assay of a steroid aglycone after hydrolysis can be performed by
the Kober reaction with hydroquinone, which yields colored products with
steroids. In addition to glucuronic acid conjugates of steroids, glucuronides of an aryl or alkyl aglycone and other stable "ether" glucuronides
have been extensively studied and can be readily isolated. Appropriate
derivatives can be prepared from ether glucosiduronic acids to enable
characterization by comparison with synthetic samples or by GC and MS
analysis. This group of glucuronic acid conjugates is the only one to give
satisfactory results by GC and MS analysis. Most of these conjugates
usually have well-defined R_f values in paper and thin-layer chromatography.
Enzymic hydrolysis can be monitored by direct assay of the free glucuronic
acid in aliquots of incubation mixtures by use of naphthoresorcinol or carbazole reagents.

The group of alkaloid glucuronic acid conjugates is represented by
morphine glucuronide and the conjugates of morphine-like compounds.
The heterocyclic aglycone permits the successful isolation by adsorption
on charcoal or the isolation and separation by chromatography on ion-
exchange resins. Data obtained by paper and thin-layer chromatography
and UV and IR spectral data can characterize intact conjugates. TLC and
paper-chromatographic parameters are well elaborated for morphine and
morphine-like derivatives. Aglycones released by enzymic or acid hydrolysis can be subsequently identified by gas chromatography of appropriate derivatives or quantitated by fluorescence. Conjugates that differ
in the position of attachment of the glucosyluronic group to the aglycone
can be distinguished by their UV and IR spectral data or by comparison
with an authentic specimen.

Conjugates of N-hydroxy compounds, sensitive to alkali, require mild
conditions for isolation and very careful treatment. Isolation is accomplished by conversion into the lead salt, chromatography on DEAE-Sephadex
and Sephadex G-10, or a combination of these methods. Intact conjugates
can be characterized by R_f values and comparison with synthetic samples.

However, because of their instability, it is more accurate to characterize the aglycone after enzymic hydrolysis.

Mild conditions are also required to isolate the alkali-labile 1-O-acyl-glucuronic acids. The most frequent methods are: extraction with organic solvents, conversion into lead salts, countercurrent distribution, chromatography on DEAE-Sephadex, and preparative, paper, and thin-layer chromatography. Reports on isolation and characterization are scarce, and few attempts to characterize intact 1-O-acylglucuronic acids have been reported in the last few years. The conjugates are susceptible to enzymic hydrolysis, which can be monitored by the determination of the liberated glucuronic acid with benzidine. Evidence for the structure of these conjugates is mainly based on the qualitative and quantitative determination of glucuronic acid content, on R_f values, and on the physicochemical data obtained for the aglycone.

N-Glucuronides differ in their stability dependent on the aglycone. The method of analysis for a particular conjugate should consider this factor. Lead salt techniques and chromatography on ion-exchange resins are methods for isolation with characterization by UV and IR spectral data and R_f values available for intact glucuronides. Conjugates of aromatic amines and carbamoyl compounds are not hydrolyzed by β-glucuronidase, whereas the conjugates of drugs of the sulfonamide type are susceptible to enzymic hydrolysis.

S-Glucuronides are stable compounds and, theoretically, any of the discussed methods can be applied for analysis, but they have not yet been extensively studied. Preparative thin-layer or paper chromatography, extraction with organic solvents, and filtration on Sephadex G-10 were proposed. Intact conjugates are characterized according to R_f values. Normally, hydrolysis with an enzyme or an acid is performed, followed by characterization of the aglycone. Accurate characterization may depend on the preparation of sufficiently volatile derivatives for GC and MS analysis, which has not been extensively applied to S-glucuronides.

The isolation and characterization of conjugates are greatly facilitated by the use of labeled compounds independent of conjugate stability or linkage. Detection and identification of labeled metabolites not only is accurate, but the metabolites arising from an administered or parent compound may be more readily distinguished from naturally occurring constituents of biological material.

VII. APPENDIX

The following table presents paper and thin-layer chromatographic parameters of some glucuronic acid conjugates, including ether glucuronides, N-hydroxy compounds, 1-O-acylglucuronic acids, N-glucuronides, and S-glucuronides.

APPENDIX

Paper and Thin Layer Chromatographic Parameters of Glucuronic Acid Conjugates

Ether glucuronides

Conjugate of	Solvent system	R_f	Ref.
Phenol	1-Propanol – aq. NH_3 (sp. gr. 0.88), (7:3)	0.45^a	[38]
4-Hydroxyphenol(hydroquinone)	1-Propanol – aq. NH_3 (sp. gr. 0.88), (7:3)	0.20^a	[38]
1-Naphthol	1-Butanol – aq. NH_3 (sp. gr. 0.88) – H_2O, (4:1:5)	0.40^a	[35]
2-Naphthol	1-Butanol – aq. NH_3 (sp. gr. 0.88) – H_2O, (4:1:5)	0.33^a	[35]
m-Aminophenol	1-Butanol – AcOH – H_2O, (4:1:5)	0.14^a	[14]
Salicylic acid^d	1-Butanol – AcOH – H_2O, (4:1:5)	0.56^a	[14]
4-Aminosalicylic acid^d	1-Butanol – AcOH – H_2O, (4:1:5)	0.17^a	[14]
4-(Acetamido)phenol	Acetone – 1-butanol – H_2O, (5:4:1)	0.25^b	[41]
4-Nitro-3-(trifluoromethyl)phenol	$CHCl_3$ – MeOH – aq. NH_3, (8:4:1)	0.38^b	[94]
Phenolphthalein	1-Propanol – pyridine – H_2O, (1:1:1)	0.78^a	[35]
Retinol	Benzene – $CHCl_3$ – MeOH – AcOH, (5:5:5:1)	0.30^b	[50]
Thiamphenicol	1-Butanol – EtOH – aq. NH_3 (28%) – H_2O, (4:4:1:2)	0.44^b	[75]
Chloropromazine	Isopentyl alc. – H_2O – EtOH – HCOOH (88%), (2:2:3:2)	0.33^a	[49]

Edrophonium	2–Butanol – EtOH – H_2O – AcOH, (32:8:12:1)	0.14^a	[171]
Edrophonium	2–Butanol – EtOH – H_2O – AcOH, (32:8:12:1)	0.63^b	[171]
H–88[e]	Benzene – EtOAc – MeOH – HCOOH, (1:5:1:1)	0.46^b	[95]
PE[f]trinitrate	EtOAc – AcOH – MeOH – H_2O, (15:1:2:2)	0.50^b	[59]
PE[f] dinitrate	EtOAc – AcOH – MeOH – H_2O, (15:1:2:2)	0.33^b	[59]
PE[f] mononitrate	EtOAc – AcOH – MeOH – H_2O, (15:1:2:2)	0.12^b	[59]
3–Hydroxyindole(indoxyl)	2–Propanol – aq. NH_3 – H_2O, (8:1:1)	0.31^b	[132]
Morphine (3–yl)	1–Butanol – AcOH – H_2O, (4:1:5)	0.35^b	[47]
Morphine (6–yl)	1–Butanol – AcOH – H_2O, (4:1:5)	0.65^b	[47]
Hydromorphone	1–Butanol – AcOH – H_2O, (35:10:3)	0.27^b	[91]
Dihydromorphine	1–Butanol – AcOH – H_2O, (35:10:3)	0.36^b	[91]
Cortisol	1–Butanol – H_2O	0.41^a	[140]
11–Deoxycortisol	1–Butanol – H_2O	0.61^a	[140]
Corticosterone	1–Butanol – H_2O	0.49^a	[140]
11–Dehydrocorticosterone	1–Butanol – H_2O	0.40^a	[140]
THA[g] (3–yl)	0.10 M THAC[h] in $CHCl_3$ – EtOAc, (1:1), 0.20 M KCl in H_2O	0.24^a	[116, 117]
THA[g] (21–yl)	0.10 M THAC[h] in $CHCl_3$ – EtOAc, (1:1), 0.20 M KCl in H_2O	0.36^a	[116, 117]

APPENDIX (Continued)

Conjugate of	Solvent system	R_f	Ref.
Estrone	$CHCl_3$ – EtOH, (23:2)	0.63[b]	[56]
Estradiol	$CHCl_3$ – EtOH, (23:2)	0.59[b]	[56]
N–Hydroxy compounds			
N–Acetyl–N–2–fluorenyl hydroxyl–amine	Isopropyl alc. – H_2O – HCOOH, (40:9:1)	0.66[c]	[68]
N–Hydroxy–4'–phenylacetanilide	EtOH – 0.5 M ammonium acetate, pH 5.0, (6:1)	0.62[c]	[183]
N–Hydroxy–4–biphenylamine	1–Butanol – 1–propanol – H_2O, (2:1:1)	0.40[b]	[101]
1–O–Acylglucuronic acids			
Benzoyl	1–Butanol – AcOH – H_2O, (4:1:2)	0.67[a]	[37]
Salicyl	EtOAc – MeOH – H_2O – AcOH, (60:30:9:1)	0.38[b]	[208]
Salicyl	1–Butanol – AcOH – H_2O, (4:1:5)	0.69[a]	[14]
p–Aminosalicyl	1–Butanol – AcOH – H_2O, (4:1:5)	0.28[a]	[14]

3-Hydroxyanthraniloyl	1-Butanol – 1-propanol – EtOH – H_2O, (3:6:4:2)	0.20[c]	[114]
Retinoyl	Benzene – $CHCl_3$ – MeOH – AcOH, (5:5:5:1)	0.27[b]	[50]
Indomethacin-3-yl	MeOH – 1-butanol – benzene – H_2O, (2:1:1:1)	0.75[a]	[51]
5-Methoxy-2-methylindole-3-acetyl	MeOH – 1-butanol – benzene – H_2O, (2:1:1:1)	0.55[a]	[51]
1-(p-Chlorobenzoyl)-5-hydroxy-2-methylindole-3-acetyl	MeOH – 1-butanol – benzene – H_2O, (2:1:1:1)	0.69[a]	[51]
N-Glucuronides			
Sulfadiazine	Aq. EtOH (80%)	0.17[a]	[43]
Sulfadimethoxine (N^4 conjugate)	Aq. EtOH (80%)	0.25[a]	[19]
Sulfadimethoxine (N^1 conjugate)	Aq. EtOH (80%)	0.55[a]	[19]
Prontosil[1]	1-Butanol – aq. NH_3 (sp. gr. 0.88) – H_2O, (10:1:1)	0.27[a]	[40]
Meprobamate	1-Butanol – AcOH – H_2O, (4:1:5)	0.57[a]	[211]
7-Amino-5-nitro-1 H-indazole	Ether – isopropylamine, (19:1)	0.33[a]	[36]

APPENDIX (Continued)

Conjugate of	Solvent system	R_f	Ref.
S-Glucuronides			
Diethyldithiocarbamic acid	1-Butanol – AcOH – H_2O, (4:1:1)	0.60[a]	[20]
2-Pyridinethione	Methanol	0.62[b]	[100]

[a] Paper chromatography.

[b] Thin-layer chromatography on silica gel.

[c] Thin-layer chromatography on cellulose.

[d] Ether type conjugates.

[e] 3-(2-Hydroxyethyl)-1-[3-(trifluoromethyl)phenyl]2,4(1 H, 3 H)quinazolinedione.

[f] Pentaerythritol.

[g] 3α,21-Dihydroxy-5β-pregnane-11,20-dione.

[h] Tetraheptylammonium chloride.

[i] 4-(2',4'-Diaminophenylazo)benzenesulfonamide.

ACKNOWLEDGMENTS

I am grateful to the NIAMDD, National Institutes of Health, for their support while writing this chapter. I am indebted to Drs. Dina Keglević and S. R. Tipson for the critical reading of the manuscript and I wish to thank them for helpful discussion and suggestions.

REFERENCES

1. R. T. Williams, Detoxication Mechanisms, 2nd ed., Wiley, New York, 1959.
2. W. H. Fishman, Chemistry of Drug Metabolism, C. C. Thomas, Springfield, Illinois, 1961.
3. C. A. Marsh, in Glucuronic Acid, Free and Combined (G. J. Dutton, ed.), Academic Press, New York and London, 1966, pp. 4-136.
4. R. L. Smith and R. T. Williams, in Glucuronic Acid, Free and Combined (G. J. Dutton, ed.), Academic Press, New York and London, 1966, pp. 457-491.
5. G. J. Dutton, in Glucuronic Acid, Free and Combined (G. J. Dutton, ed.), Academic Press, New York and London, 1966, pp. 186-299.
6. J. Pryde and R. T. Williams, Biochem. J., 27, 1197 (1933).
7. M. Neeman and Y. Hashimoto, J. Amer. Chem. Soc., 84, 2972 (1962).
8. H. Tsukamoto, H. Yoshimura, and K. Tatsumi, Chem. Pharm. Bull. (Tokyo), 11, 1134 (1963).
9. M. F. Jayle and J. R. Pasqualini, in Glucuronic Acid, Free and Combined (G. J. Dutton, ed.), Academic Press, New York and London, 1966, pp. 507-543.
10. D. S. Layne, in Metabolic Conjugation and Metabolic Hydrolysis, Vol. 1 (W. H. Fishman, ed.), Academic Press, New York and London, 1970, pp. 40-43.
11. C. C. Irving, in Metabolic Conjugation and Metabolic Hydrolysis, Vol. 1 (W. H. Fishman, ed.), Academic Press, New York and London, 1970, pp. 66-87.
12. C. C. Irving, R. Wiseman, Jr., and J. T. Hill, Cancer Res., 27, 2309 (1967).
13. I. A. Kamil, J. N. Smith, and R. T. Williams, Biochem. J., 53, 137 (1953).
14. H. Tsukamoto, K. Kato, and K. Yoshida, Chem. Pharm. Bull. (Tokyo), 12, 731 (1964).
15. D. Keglević, N. Pravdić, and J. Tomašić, J. Chem. Soc., C, 511 (1968).
16. J. Tomašić and D. Keglević, Croat. Chem. Acta, 44, 493 (1972).

17. R. Bugianesi and T. Y. Shen, Carbohyd. Res., 19, 179 (1971).
18. R. T. Williams, Ann. N. Y. Acad. Sci., 179, 141 (1971).
19. J. W. Bridges, M. R. Kibby, and R. T. Williams, Biochem. J.,
     96, 829 (1965).
20. G. J. Dutton and H. P. Illing, Biochem. J., 129, 539 (1972).
21. G. A. Levvy and J. Conchie, in Glucuronic Acid, Free and Combined
     (G. J. Dutton, ed.), Academic Press, New York and London, 1966,
     pp. 301-364.
22. M. Wakabayashi, in Metabolic Conjugation and Metabolic Hydrolysis,
     Vol. 2 (W. H. Fishman, ed.), Academic Press, New York and
     London, 1970, pp. 519-602.
23. P. Millburn, in Metabolic Conjugation and Metabolic Hydrolysis,
     Vol. 2 (W. H. Fishman, ed.), Academic Press, New York and
     London, 1970, pp. 1-74.
24. G. A. Sandberg, W. R. Slaunwhite, Jr., and R. Y. Kirdani, in
     Metabolic Conjugation and Metabolic Hydrolysis, Vol. 2 (W. H.
     Fishman, ed.), Academic Press, New York and London, 1970,
     pp. 123-152.
25. B. Tollens, Ber., 41, 1788 (1908).
26. W. H. Fishman and S. Green, J. Biol. Chem., 215, 527 (1955).
27. Z. Dische, J. Biol. Chem., 167, 189 (1947).
28. H. Yuki and W. H. Fishman, Biochim. Biophys. Acta, 69, 576
     (1963).
29. S. Green, C. Anstiss, and W. H. Fishman, Biochim. Biophys. Acta,
     62, 574 (1962).
30. R. Rava, G. Della Pietra, M. Carteni, and F. Cedrangolo, Ann.
     Inst. Super. Sanita, 7, 478 (1974).
31. A. Mazzuchin, R. J. Walton, and R. J. Thibert, Biochem. Med.,
     5, 135 (1971).
32. D. Schachter, J. Clin. Invest., 36, 297 (1957).
33. D. Schachter and J. G. Manis, J. Clin. Invest., 37, 800 (1958).
34. J. M. Perel, A. B. Gutman, T. F. Yu, and P. G. Dayton, Clin.
     Res., 18, 342 (1970).
35. I. D. Capel, P. Millburn, and R. T. Williams, Xenobiotica, 4,
     601 (1974).
36. N. M. Woolhouse, B. Kaye, and A. M. Monro, Xenobiotica, 3,
     511 (1973).
37. J. W. Bridges, M. R. French, R. L. Smith, and R. T. Williams,
     Biochem. J., 118, 47 (1970).
38. I. D. Capel, M. R. French, P. Millburn, R. L. Smith, and R. T.
     Williams, Xenobiotica, 2, 25 (1972).
39. D. H. Hutson, E. C. Hoadley, and B. A. Pickering, Xenobiotica,
     1, 593 (1971).
40. R. Gingell, J. W. Bridges, and R. T. Williams, Xenobiotica, 1,
     143 (1971).

41. R. L. Smith and J. A. Timbrell, Xenobiotica, 4, 489 (1974).
42. D. A. R. Sinclair and J. G. Eales, Gen. Comp. Endocrinol., 19, 552 (1972).
43. M. Atef and P. Nilsen, Xenobiotica, 5, 167 (1975).
44. C. H. Bastomsky, P. W. Horton, and J. Shimmins, J. Nucl. Med., 14, 34 (1973).
45. C. H. Bastomsky, Endocrinology, 92, 35 (1973).
46. R. T. Schillings, S. F. Sisenwine, M. H. Schwartz, and H. W. Ruelius, Drug Metab. Disp., 3, 85 (1975).
47. H. Yoshimura, K. Oguri, and H. Tsukamoto, Biochem. Pharmacol., 18, 279 (1969).
48. B. A. Wood, D. A. Stopher, and A. M. Monro, Xenobiotica, 5, 183 (1975).
49. A. H. Beckett, M. A. Beaven, and A. E. Robinson, Biochem. Pharmacol., 12, 779 (1963).
50. K. Lippel and J. A. Olson, J. Lipid Res., 9, 168 (1968).
51. R. E. Harman, M. A. P. Meisinger, G. E. Davis, and F. A. Kuehl, Jr., J. Pharmacol. Exp. Ther., 143, 215 (1964).
52. A. M. Guarino, W. D. Conway, and H. M. Fales, Eur. J. Pharmacol., 8, 244 (1969).
53. P. G. Dayton, J. M. Perel, R. F. Cunningham, Z. H. Israili, and I. M. Weiner, Drug Metab. Disp., 1, 742 (1973).
54. S. J. Lan, T. J. Chando, A. I. Cohen, I. Weliky, and E. C. Schreiber, Drug Metab. Disp., 1, 619 (1973).
55. K. W. Miller, E. C. Heath, K. H. Easton, and J. V. Dingell, Biochem. Pharmacol., 22, 2319 (1973).
56. E. C. Heath and J. V. Dingell, Drug Metab. Disp., 2, 556 (1974).
57. M. D. Melgar, F. J. Leinweber, M. C. Crew, and F. J. Di Carlo, Drug Metab. Disp., 2, 46 (1974).
58. F. J. Leinweber, M. D. Melgar, M. C. Crew, and F. J. Di Carlo, Drug Metab. Disp., 2, 40 (1974).
59. M. C. Crew, M. D. Melgar, and F. J. Di Carlo, J. Pharmacol. Exp. Ther., 192, 218 (1975).
60. I. A. Kamil, J. N. Smith, and R. T. Williams, Biochem. J., 50, 235 (1951).
61. I. A. Kamil, J. N. Smith, and R. T. Williams, Biochem. J., 53, 129 (1953).
62. D. Robinson and R. T. Williams, Biochem. J., 59, 159 (1955).
63. D. Robinson and R. T. Williams, Biochem. J., 62, 23P (1956).
64. J. A. R. Mead, J. N. Smith, and R. T. Williams, Biochem. J., 68, 61 (1958).
65. J. A. R. Mead, J. N. Smith, and R. T. Williams, Biochem. J., 68, 67 (1958).
66. A. Yamamoto, H. Yoshimura, and H. Tsukamoto, Chem. Pharm. Bull. (Tokyo), 10, 522 (1962).

67. H. Tsukamoto, H. Yoshimura, and K. Tatsumi, Life Sci., 2, 382 (1963).
68. J. T. Hill and C. C. Irving, Biochemistry, 6, 3816 (1967).
69. K. Kato, H. Ide, I. Hirohata, and W. H. Fishman, Biochem. J., 103, 647 (1967).
70. P. R. Rao, T. R. Seshadri, and P. Sharma, Curr. Sci., 42, 811 (1973).
71. T. Uesugi, M. Ikeda, R. Hori, K. Katayama, and T. Arita, Chem. Pharm. Bull. (Tokyo), 22, 2714 (1974).
72. M. Arcos and S. Lieberman, J. Clin. Endocrinol. Metab., 25, 808 (1965).
73. T. Uno and M. Ueda, Chem. Pharm. Bull. (Tokyo), 11, 709 (1963).
74. S. Y. Yeh, H. I. Chernov, and L. A. Woods, J. Pharm. Sci., 60, 469 (1971).
75. T. Uesugi, M. Ikeda, Y. Kanei, R. Hori, and T. Arita, Biochem. Pharmacol., 23, 2315 (1974).
76. F. Marcucci, R. Bianchi, L. Airoldi, M. Salmona, R. Fanelli, C. Chiabrando, A. Frigerio, E. Mussini, and S. Garattini, J. Chromatogr., 107, 285 (1975).
77. R. L. Gustafson, R. L. Albright, J. Heisler, J. A. Lirio, and O. T. Reid, Jr., Ind. Eng. Chem. Prod. Res. Develop., 7, 107 (1968).
78. H. L. Bradlow, Steroids, 11, 265 (1968).
79. R. Hobkirk and M. Nilsen, Steroids, 15, 649 (1970).
80. R. Hobkirk and M. Nilsen, J. Clin. Endocrin. Metab., 32, 779 (1971).
81. K. Takeda, M. Noto, and M. Murakami, Clin. Chim. Acta, 36, 163 (1972).
82. A. R. Robinson, G. O. Henneberry, and R. H. Common, Biochem. Biophys. Acta, 326, 93 (1973).
83. S. Miyabo and L. Kornel, J. Steroid. Biochem., 5, 233 (1974).
84. J. H. Grose, W. Nowaczynski, O. Kuchel, and J. Genest, J. Steroid Biochem., 4, 551 (1973).
85. S. F. Sisenwine, H. B. Kimmel, A. L. Liu, and H. W. Ruelius, Acta Endocrinol. (Copenhagen), 73, 91 (1973).
86. M. Matsui, Y. Kinuyama, and M. Hakozaki, Steroids, 24, 557 (1974).
87. C. Gwilliam, A. Paquet, D. G. Williamson, and D. S. Layne, Can. J. Biochem., 52, 452 (1974).
88. J. M. Fujimoto and R. I. H. Wang, Toxicol. Appl. Pharmacol., 16, 186 (1970).
89. N. Weissman, M. L. Lowe, J. M. Beattie, and J. A. Demetriou, Clin. Chem., 17, 875 (1971).
90. S. Y. Yeh and L. A. Woods, J. Pharm. Exp. Ther., 173, 21 (1970).

91. S. Roerig, J. M. Fujimoto, and R. I. H. Wang, Proc. Soc. Exp. Biol. Med., 143, 230 (1973).
92. C. R. Brewington, O. W. Parks, and D. P. Schwartz, J. Agr. Food. Chem., 21, 38 (1973).
93. T. T. L. Chang, C. H. F. Kuhlman, R. T. Schillings, S. F. Sisenwine, C. O. Tio, and H. W. Ruelius, Experentia, 29, 653 (1973).
94. J. J. Lech, Toxicol. Appl. Pharmacol., 24, 114 (1973).
95. R. Kodama, T. Yano, K. Furukawa, K. Noda, and H. Ide, Xenobiotica, 5, 39 (1975).
96. D. E. Case and P. R. Reeves, Xenobiotica, 5, 113 (1975).
97. C. G. Beling, Acta Endocrinol. (Copenhagen), Supp., 43, 79 (1963).
98. E. R. Smith and A. E. Kellie, Biochem. J., 104, 83 (1967).
99. S. L. Cohen and E. Oran, Steroids, 17, 155 (1971).
100. B. L. Kabacoff, C. M. Fairchild, and C. Burnett, Food Cosmet. Toxicol., 9, 519 (1971).
101. J. L. Radomski, A. A. Rey, and E. Brill, Cancer Res., 33, 1284 (1973).
102. D. A. Blake, R. S. Rosman, H. F. Cascorbi, and J. C. Krantz, Biochem. Pharmacol., 16, 1237 (1967).
103. P. N. Kaul, E. Brochmann-Hanssen, and E. L. Way, J. Pharm. Sci., 50, 840 (1961).
104. I. Merits, D. J. Anderson, and R. C. Sonders, Drug Metab. Disp., 1, 691 (1973).
105. H. Yoshimura, S. Ida, K. Oguri, and H. Tsukamoto, Biochem. Pharmacol., 22, 1423 (1973).
106. J. B. Knaak, J. M. Eldridge, and L. J. Sullivan, J. Agr. Food Chem., 15, 605 (1967).
107. L. J. Sullivan, J. M. Eldridge, J. B. Knaak, and M. J. Tallant, J. Agr. Food Chem., 20, 980 (1972).
108. A. S. Kenneth, K. R. Hallmark, M. E. Carroll, and J. G. Wagner, Res. Comm. Chem. Pathol. Pharmacol., 6, 845 (1973).
109. P. I. Jaakonmaki, K. L. Knox, E. C. Horning, and M. G. Horning, Eur. J. Pharmacol., 1, 63 (1967).
110. W. G. Stillwell, M. J. Carman, L. Bell, and M. G. Horning, Drug Metab. Disp., 2, 489 (1974).
111. R. Hobkirk and M. Nilsen, Steroids, 14, 533 (1969).
112. R. Hobkirk and M. Nilsen, J. Steroid. Biochem., 5, 15 (1974).
113. M. Watanabe, K. Ohkubo, and Z. Tamura, Biochem. Pharmacol., 21, 1337 (1972).
114. M. Watanabe, K. Minegishi, and Y. Tsutsui, Cancer Res., 32, 2049 (1972).
115. A. F. Hofman, J. Lipid Res., 8, 55 (1967).
116. V. R. Mattox, J. E. Goodrich, and R. D. Litwiller, J. Chromatogr., 66, 337 (1972).

117. V. R. Mattox, R. D. Litwiller, and J. E. Goodrich, Biochem. J., 126, 533 (1972).

118. V. R. Mattox, R. D. Litwiller, and J. E. Goodrich, Biochem. J., 126, 545 (1972).

119. R. Hobkirk, P. Musey, and M. Nilsen, Steroids, 14, 191 (1969).

120. R. Y. Kirdani, W. R. Slaunwhite, Jr., and A. A. Sandberg, J. Steroid Biochem., 1, 265 (1970).

121. G. R. Goertz, O. C. Crepy, O. E. Judas, J. E. Longchampt, and M. F. Jayle, Clin. Chim. Acta, 51, 277 (1974).

122. H. Jirku and M. Levitz, J. Clin. Endocrinol. Metab., 29, 615 (1969).

123. E. Sandberg, E. Gurpide, and S. Lieberman, Biochemistry, 3, 1256 (1964).

124. P. K. Siiteri, Steroids, 2, 687 (1963).

125. J. Sjövall, K. Sjövall, and R. Vihko, Steroids, 11, 703 (1968).

126. T. Laatikainen and R. Vihko, Eur. J. Biochem., 10, 165 (1969).

127. I. Huhtaniemi, J. Endocrinol., 59, 503 (1973).

128. O. Jänne, Clin. Chim. Acta, 29, 529 (1970).

129. M. J. Tikkanen and H. Adlercreutz, Acta Chem. Scand., 24, 3755 (1970).

130. H. Adlercreutz, B. Soltmann, and M. J. Tikkanen, J. Steroid Biochem., 5, 163 (1974).

131. L. Kornel, J. Clin. Endocrinol. Metab., 24, 956 (1964).

132. O. B. Martinez and D. A. Roe, J. Nutr., 102, 365 (1972).

133. W. Wortmann, D. Y. Cooper, and J. C. Touchstone, Steroids, 20, 321 (1972).

134. V. R. Mattox, J. E. Goodrich, and R. D. Litwiller, J. Chromatogr., 108, 23 (1975).

135. R. Y. Kirdani and R. L. Priore, Anal. Biochem., 24, 377 (1968).

136. R. L. Priore and R. Y. Kirdani, Anal. Biochem., 24, 360 (1968).

137. U. Goebelsmann, N. Wiqvist, and E. Diczfalusy, Acta Endocrinol. (Copenhagen), 59, 595 (1968).

138. B. De la Torre, N. Wiqvist, and E. Diczfalusy, Acta Endocrinol. (Copenhagen), 75, 159 (1974).

139. R. K. Rhamy and H. E. Hadd, Steroids, 22, 719 (1973).

140. V. R. Mattox, J. E. Goodrich, and W. D. Vrieze, Steroids, 18, 147 (1971).

141. C. A. Burtis, W. C. Butts, and W. T. Rainey, Jr., Amer. J. Clin. Pathol., 53, 769 (1970).

142. J. E. Mrochek, W. C. Butts, W. T. Rainey, Jr., and C. A. Burtis, Clin. Chem., 17, 72 (1971).

143. W. C. Butts, J. E. Mrochek, and D. S. Young, Clin. Chem., 17, 956 (1971).

144. J. E. Mrochek and W. T. Rainey, Jr., Anal. Biochem., 57, 173 (1974).

145.   G. D. Paulson, R. G. Zaylskie, and M. M. Dockter, Anal. Chem.,
       45, 21 (1973).
146.   T. Imanari and Z. Tamura, Chem. Pharm. Bull. (Tokyo), 15,
       1677 (1967).
147.   R. M. Thompson and D. M. Desiderio, Biochem. Biophys. Res.
       Commun., 48, 1303 (1972).
148.   R. M. Thompson, N. Gerber, R. A. Seibert, and D. M. Desiderio,
       Res. Commun. Chem. Pathol. Pharmacol., 4, 543 (1972).
149.   R. M. Thompson, N. Gerber, R. A. Seibert, and D. M. Desiderio,
       Drug Metab. Disp., 1, 489 (1973).
150.   R. M. Thompson, N. Gerber, and R. A. Seibert, Xenobiotica,
       5, 145 (1975).
151.   N. Gerber, R. A. Seibert, and R. M. Thompson, Res. Commun.
       Chem. Pathol. Pharmacol., 6, 499 (1973).
152.   W. J. A. VandenHeuvel, W. L. Gardiner, and E. C. Horning,
       Anal. Chem., 36, 1550 (1964).
153.   M. G. Horning, C. Stratton, J. Nowlin, D. J. Harvey, and
       R. M. Hill, Drug Metab. Disp., 1, 569 (1973).
154.   B. Jelus, B. Munson, and C. Fenselau, Anal. Chem., 46, 729
       (1974).
155.   S. Billets, P. S. Lietman, and C. Fenselau, J. Med. Chem.,
       16, 30 (1973).
156.   S. Honma and T. Nambara, Chem. Pharm. Bull. (Tokyo), 22,
       687 (1974).
157.   D. E. Case, Xenobiotica, 3, 451 (1973).
158.   J. B. Brown, Biochem. J., 60, 185 (1955).
159.   Y. A. Sa'at and W. R. Slaunwhite, Jr., Steroids, 13, 545 (1969).
160.   T. Nambara, Y. Matsuki, J. Igarashi, Y. Kawarada, and
       M. Kurata, Chem. Pharm. Bull. (Tokyo), 22, 2242 (1974).
161.   J. M. Fujimoto, W. E. Leong, and C. H. Hine, J. Lab. Clin.
       Med., 44, 627 (1954).
162.   S. Y. Yeh and L. A. Woods, J. Pharm. Exp. Ther., 175, 69
       (1970).
163.   J. M. Fujimoto and E. L. Way, J. Pharmacol. Exp. Ther., 121,
       340 (1957).
164.   J. Paul, Ph.D. Thesis, University of Glasgow, 1951.
165.   P. Cornillot, Clin. Chim. Acta, 7, 42 (1962).
166.   T. Bitter and H. M. Muir, Anal. Biochem., 4, 330 (1962).
167.   J. D. Gregory, Arch. Biochem. Biophys., 89, 157 (1960).
168.   R. E. Dohrman, β-Glucuronidase, Springer Verlag, Berlin, 1969.
169.   W. H. Fishman, in Methods in Biochemical Analysis, Vol. 15
       (D. Glick, ed.), Wiley (Interscience), New York, 1967, pp. 77–145.
170.   R. N. Beale, D. Croft, and R. F. Taylor, Steroids, 18, 621
       (1971).
171.   D. J. Back and T. N. Calvey, Brit. J. Pharmacol., 44, 534
       (1972).

172. R. D. Smyth, A. Polk, J. Diamond, B. J. Burns, and T. Herczeg, Xenobiotica, 4, 383 (1974).
173. S. J. Lan, T. J. Chando, I. Weliky, and E. C. Schreiber, J. Pharmacol. Exp. Ther., 186, 323 (1973).
174. K. L. Hintze, J. S. Wold, and L. J. Fischer, Drug Metab. Disp., 3, 1 (1975).
175. H. B. Hucker, S. C. Stauffer, S. D. White, R. E. Rhodes, B. H. Arison, E. R. Umbenhauer, R. J. Bower, and F. G. McMahon, Drug Metab. Disp., 1, 721 (1973).
176. S. Y. Yeh, J. Pharm. Exp. Ther., 192, 201 (1975).
177. R. J. Bopp, R. E. Schirmer, and D. B. Meyers, J. Pharm. Sci., 61, 1750 (1972).
178. M. H. Bickel, R. Minder, and C. Di Francesco, Experientia, 29, 960 (1973).
179. L. P. Strand and R. R. Scheline, Xenobiotica, 5, 49 (1975).
180. G. P. Forshell, Xenobiotica, 5, 73 (1975).
181. G. Takahashi and K. Yasuhira, Cancer Res., 35, 613 (1975).
182. F. M. Williams, R. H. Briant, C. T. Dollery, and D. S. Davies, Xenobiotica, 4, 345 (1974).
183. C. C. Irving, L. T. Russell, and E. Kriek, Chem. Biol. Interact., 5, 37 (1972).
184. S. F. Sisenwine, H. B. Kimmel, A. L. Liu, A. Segaloff, and W. H. Ruelius, Drug Metab. Disp., 1, 537 (1973).
185. P. G. C. Douch, Xenobiotica, 4, 457 (1974).
186. J. Alvin, T. McHorse, A. Hoyumpa, M. T. Bush, and S. Schenker, J. Pharmacol. Exp. Ther., 192, 224 (1975).
187. H. Ide, S. Green, K. Kato, and W. H. Fishman, Biochem. J., 106, 431 (1968).
188. C. Hétu and R. Gianetto, Can. J. Biochem., 48, 799 (1970).
189. H. P. A. Illing and G. J. Dutton, Biochem. J., 131, 139 (1973).
190. J. F. Van de Calseyde, R. J. H. Scholtis, N. A. Schmidt, and C. J. J. A. Leijten, Clin. Chim. Acta, 38, 103 (1972).
191. E. J. Cone, C. W. Gorodetzky, and S. Y. Yeh, Drug Metab. Disp., 2, 506 (1974).
192. J. C. Legrand, S. Legrand, F. Zogbi, and S. Guillemant, Ann. Biol. Clin., 25, 1199 (1967).
193. J. Dray, F. Tillier, F. Dray, and A. Ullmann, Ann. Inst. Pasteur, 123, 853 (1972).
194. R. E. Oakey, L. R. A. Bradshaw, S. S. Eccles, S. R. Stitch, and R. F. Heys, Clin. Chim. Acta, 15, 35 (1967).
195. M. R. Crowley, K. J. T. Garbien, and A. Rosser, Clin. Chim. Acta, 38, 91 (1972).
196. M. R. Crowley and A. Rosser, Clin. Chim. Acta, 49, 115 (1973).
197. K. D. Voigt, M. Lemmer, and J. Tamm, Biochem. Z., 332, 550 (1960).

198. M. Wakabayashi, H. H. Wotiz, and W. H. Fishman, Biochim. Biophys. Acta, 48, 198 (1961).
199. J. F. Becker, Biochim. Biophys. Acta, 100, 582 (1965).
200. P. A. Bond and D. R. Howlett, Biochem. Med., 10, 219 (1974).
201. F. Fish and T. S. Hayes, J. Forensic Sci., 19, 676 (1974).
202. J. Tomašić and D. Keglević, Biochem. J., 133, 789 (1973).
203. W. Wagner, Anal. Chim Acta, 29, 227 (1963).
204. C. R. Ball and J. A. Double, Biochem. Pharmacol., 23, 3173 (1974).
205. J. K. M. Jones and J. B. Pridham, Nature, 172, 161 (1953).
206. J. K. M. Jones and J. B. Pridham, Biochem. J., 58, 289 (1954).
207. J. Tomašić and D. Keglević, Anal. Biochem., 45, 164 (1972).
208. A. Robertson, J. P. Glynn, and A. K. Watson, Xenobiotica, 2, 339 (1972).
209. D. Robinson, J. N. Smith, and R. T. Williams, Biochem. J., 59, 153 (1955).
210. U. Goebelsmann, K. Sjöberg, N. Wiqvist, and E. Diczfalusy, Acta Endocrinol. (Copenhagen), 50, 261 (1965).
211. H. Tsukamoto, H. Yoshimura, and K. Tatsumi, Chem. Pharm. Bull. (Tokyo), 11, 421 (1963).
212. R. Hobkirk, R. N. Green, M. Nilsen, and B. A. Jennings, Can. J. Biochem., 52, 9 (1974).
213. H. R. Schulten and D. E. Games, Biomed. Mass Spectrom., 1, 120 (1974).

Numbers in brackets are reference numbers and indicate that an author's work is referred to although his name is not cited in the text. Underlined numbers give the page on which the complete reference is listed.

A

Acenocoumarol, polarography, 27, 28
4-Acetamidophenol glucuronides,
    chromatography, 322
Acetanilide glucuronides, separa-
    tion, 299
Acetophenone oxime metabolites,
    discrimination of enantiomers,
    165
N-Acetyl-p-aminophenol glucuron-
    ide, isolation, 291
N-Acetyl-N-phenyl-hydroxylamine
    glucuronides, hydrolysis, 316,
    317, 319
Acetylsalicylic acid, fluorometric
    assay, 240
Actinomycin D, fluorometric assay,
    239
Aldosterone glucuronides, isola-
    tion, 293, 297
5-Alkyl-2-thiohydantoin, fluoro-
    metric assay, 240
Alloxan, fluorometric assay, 240
Allylmorphine, fluorometric assay,
    236
Allylnormorphine, fluorometric
    assay, 240
Alprenolol:
    GLC, 51, 125
    metabolites, GLC, 125

p-Aminobenzoic acid:
    fluorometric assay, 236, 240
    glucuronide, chromatography,
        300
2-(p-Aminobenzoyloxy)benzoic
    acid glucuronides, hydrolysis,
    314
7-Aminoclonazepam, fluoro-
    metric assay, 240
7-Amino-3-hydroxy-clonazepam,
    fluorometric assay, 240
7-Amino-5-nitro-1H-indazole
    glucuronides, chromatography,
    325
m-Aminophenol glucuronides,
    chromatography, 322
Aminopterin, fluorometric assay,
    236
p-Aminosalicylic acid:
    fluorometric assay, 236, 240
    glucuronides:
        chromatography, 322, 324
        isolation, 291
Amitryptiline, GLC, 51, 84, 86,
    102, 131
Amobarbital, fluorometric assay,
    236
Amphetamine:
    enantiomers:
        separation, 187
        urinary excretion, 150